GRANT'S DISSECTOR

7th edition

GRANT'S DISSECTOR

7th edition

Eberhardt K. Sauerland, M.D.

Professor of Anatomy

University of Texas Medical Branch

Galveston, Texas

The Williams
& Wilkins Company
Baltimore

THE WILLIAMS & WILKINS COMPANY
428 E. Preston Street
Baltimore, Md. 21202, U.S.A.

Made in the United States of America

By J. C. B. GRANT AND H. A. CATES
First Edition, April 1940
  Reprinted February 1942

Second Edition, July 1945

Third Edition, May 1948
  Reprinted August 1951

Fourth Edition, June 1953
  Reprinted September 1956
  Reprinted August 1957

By J. C. B. GRANT
Fifth Edition, August 1959
  Reprinted June 1961
  Reprinted January 1965

Sixth Edition, September 1967
  Reprinted April 1968
  Reprinted August 1970

**Library of Congress Cataloging
in Publication Data**

Grant, John Charles Boileau, 1886–1973.
Grant's dissector.

First-5th ed. published under title: A handbook for dissectors.
1. Human dissection. I. Sauerland, Eberhardt. II. Title. [DNLM: 1. Dissection. QS130 G762h 1974] QM34.G75 1974 611′.0028 73-18162 ISBN 0-683-07555-1

Composed and printed at the
WAVERLY PRESS, INC.
Mt. Royal and Guilford Aves.
Baltimore, Md. 21202, U.S.A.

Preface to the sixth edition

This handbook is a guide to the orderly and consecutive display of the structures of the human body, region by region. An effort has been made to discriminate between the more important structures for which **bold type** is used and the less important which appear in *italics*. If the student will follow the instructions given within, he should be able to proceed successfully alone at such times as the help of an instructor is not available.

On account of the dimishing number of hours made available to the student for the study of Practical Anatomy, the changes made in this edition have largely been directed towards saving time and speeding dissection by various means, such as: shortening the text, increasing the number of headings and subheadings, moving structures from bold type to italics, and supplying an illustration where it can adequately replace the printed word or where the pace of progress is unduly slow.

Moreover, since some cadavers can be dissected with relative ease and others only with difficulty and more time, the less fortunate dissector might profitably seek advice regarding omissions he might judiciously be permitted; these will in part depend upon the dissected material and the specimens available to him for study.

Many parts of the text have been modified or re-written, including the female pelvis and perineum, the cranial nerves, and the middle ear. Alternative procedures and sequences are suggested. Instructions for the dissection of the fetus and of the bull's eye have been added.

Although this handbook is well illustrated, many students seek additional visual aid. Of those who have used the author's Atlas in conjunction with the Dissector, some remark that they would have been saved a great deal of time and trouble if appropriate references to plates in the Atlas were noted in the margins of the pages of the Dissector. To fit this need, unobtrusive references are made throughout the text, thus: (*Atlas, 123*).

To Professor J. S. Thompson of the University of Toronto and Professor C. H. Sawyer of the University of California at Los Angeles I am indebted for their courtesy and kindness in allowing me free access to the anatomical material in their respective schools.

To those who have provided me with ideas and suggestions for the improvement of this handbook I am indeed most grateful, and particularly to Professors R. V. Gregg, R. D. Laurenson, G. F. Lewis, R. G. MacKenzie and E. K. Sauerland, and Mr. D. W. Schwartz. Their contributions are incorporated in this edition.

To Mrs. Dorothy Chubb, who made the new illustrations and many of the earlier ones, I express my thanks for the thought and skill she devoted to them. And, here I repeat to Miss Nancy Joy, Head of Department of Art as Applied to Medicine in the University of Toronto, my thanks for the artistic help given in previous editions, and also to Dr. Brock Brown.

I would also thank Mr. Francis E. Old Jr., who, representing the Publishers, has taken a personal and active interest in the preparation of this book and has with his customary courtesy met all my tedious requests.

J. C. Boileau Grant
Toronto
May, 1967

Preface to the seventh edition

In January 1972, Professor J. C. Boileau Grant asked me to prepare the 7th edition of his DISSECTOR and to adapt this handbook to the everchanging needs of our medical school curricula. In my efforts to make the necessary changes I was not alone. Dr. Grant advised me frequently and made, as usual, brilliant suggestions. This great man and teacher is now dead at the age of 87. Only days before his death on August 14, 1973, Dr. Grant read the last pages of the manuscript. As an indication of his approval, he concluded his final communication with his old school motto '*laus finem*'. I am immensely grateful to Dr. Grant for his trust, advice, and his friendship.

Since new medical curricula have reduced the number of hours available for gross anatomical studies, it was our objective to save time whenever possible. Consequently: – (1) The text is concise. (2) Numerous illustrations replace the printed word. (3) The text contains hundreds of references to appropriate illustrations in *Grant's Atlas of Anatomy* (6th ed.). These references ensure the most efficient use of the Atlas during dissection or review. (4) Since rapid and competent dissection often depends on thorough knowledge of pertinent bony reference points, a brief discussion of important bony landmarks is included for each anatomical region. (5) Several new procedures allow efficient dissection without sacrificing clarity or detail (e.g., *en bloc* removal and study of the G.I. tract and its associated glands; facilitated approach to intrapelvic and perineal structures by partial disarticulation of right hip bone; rapid exposure of brain stem and cranial nerves by removal of wedge of occipital bone; etc.).

Courses in physical examination (with emphasis on thoracic and abdominal structures) are being offered by many medical and dental schools during the freshman year. To accomodate the needs of students taking these courses, we have covered thorax and abdomen in the initial chapters. Pelvis, extremities, and head and neck follow in logical sequence. However, the dissections may be carried out in any sequence desirable. A detailed dissection of the brain was deleted from this edition since, in most cases, anatomical studies concerning the brain are incorporated in special neuroanatomy courses. If time permits, special projects may be desirable (dissection of bull's eye; fetus; lumbar approach to kidney; certain joints). Appropriate procedures for these projects are described in the *Appendix*.

The clinical significance of gross anatomical structures was stressed whenever possible. Such clinically relevant comments (in fine print) are intended to demonstrate the practical importance of gross anatomy and to arouse the student's interest.

In addition to Professor Grant, I am indebted to Professor David S. Maxwell (U.C.L.A.) for critically reading the manuscript and making most valuable suggestions. Furthermore, I am most grateful to my colleagues in the Anatomy Department at the University of Texas Medical Branch, particularly to Professor Donald Duncan, for providing me with ideas and suggestions for the improvement of this edition. My wife deserves special thanks for her understanding, patience, and contributions.

Finally, I thank the editors and staff of the Williams and Wilkins Company, and particularly Miss Sara A. Finnegan, for their interest and efforts in preparing this book.

E. K. Sauerland
September 1973

Contents

Chapter 4. PELVIS AND PERINEUM

Chapter 5. LOWER EXTREMITY

Chapter 6. BACK

Chapter 7. UPPER EXTREMITY

APPENDIX

CHAPTER 1

INTRODUCTION TO DISSECTION

When the student is assigned to a cadaver or subject, he assumes responsibility for its proper care. He will find the subject already preserved or embalmed, the arteries occasionally injected with a (red) coloring matter, the veins sometimes full of clotted blood, and sometimes empty. The whole body has been kept moist by adequate wrappings or by submersion into suitable preservative fluid. It is the duty of the dissector to uncover only the parts on which he is engaged, to inspect every part periodically, and to renew and moisten wrappings as occasion demands. No part must ever be left exposed to the air needlessly. Special attention must be given to the face, hands, feet, and external genitalia. Once a part is allowed to become dry and hard, it can never be fully restored, and its proper dissection is impossible. Plastic bags are particularly useful to prevent drying.

Instruments

The dissector should procure the following instruments (fig. 1-1):

1. **Two pairs of forceps** about 12 to 15 cm long, with handles transversely ridged to prevent slipping, ends blunt and rounded, and gripping surfaces corrugated. The second pair is needed for distracting the tissue.
2. **A seeker or probe** consisting of a rigid steel probe with blunt bent tip. Pointed needle-like seekers, as well as abruptly hooked ones, should be banned from the dissecting room.
3. **A scalpel,** preferrably with detachable knife blades. The blade should be about 3.5 to 4 cm long. The cutting edge must possess some convexity near the point since in ordinary dissecting the movement is a circular one. The blade must be kept sharp at all times, particularly in the vicinity of the tip, for this is the part constantly used (fig. 1-3). No one can do good work with a blunt knife. The rounded end of the handle can be conveniently used to separate soft tissues.
4. **Two pairs of scissors:** A larger, heavy dissecting scissors with two sharp points (sharp-sharp type), about 15 cm in length. A fine pair of scissors with two sharp points for the dissection of delicate structures.

Dissection

Light and Working Conditions. Be sure that the light falls on the part under investigation. Adequate light is essential for efficient dissection. Work in a position that is comfortable and not tiring. Make use of wooden blocks to stabilize parts of the cadaver and to maintain its most suitable posture. Protect your clothing by wearing a long white coat or an apron.

Purpose of Dissection. There is no substitute for a three-dimensional approach to the structures of the body. Observe and palpate the topographic relations of various structures to each other. Feel the texture of blood vessels, nerves, and various tissues. Test the rigidity of bones and the strength of ligaments. Add to your theoretical knowledge the three-dimensional concept which is so necessary for an intelligent approach to surgery and physical examination.

Efficiency. Time is immensely valuable. Learn as much as possible in the shortest possible time. The following suggestions will help you to increase your efficiency:

1. Acquire a *theoretical concept* of the area under investigation *before* you attempt to dissect it. You don't dig around and happen to find 'something interesting.' You must deliberately search for certain structures.
2. Make full use of a good *atlas*.
3. Always palpate *bony landmarks* since they are keys in your search for related soft structures. It is mandatory to have a skull on hand when dissecting the head.

4. *Use your time wisely.* To spend an hour tracing the terminal twigs of a cutaneous nerve, when the general skin area supplied by the nerve is obvious, is spending an hour for little gain. To spend 3 minutes to define the exact fiber direction of a ligament, is to spend 3 minutes for great gain since a knowledge of the movements restrained or prevented by that ligament is the reward.

5. Demonstrate the *essential features* of a given anatomical region with *clarity*. Remove fat, connective tissue, and smaller veins. If a clear-cut display of the arteries is obtained, the general arrangement of the companion veins will be obvious.

Dissecting Techniques. Keep in mind that a variable amount of subcutaneous fat lies immediately deep to the skin. In that fat course superficial nerves and vessels, particularly veins. Therefore, in removing skin, all fat should be left behind. In those subjects nearly devoid of fat, one needs to exercise special care in order not to go too deep. If, during removal of skin, you see brownish muscular fibers shining through the filmy deep fascia, you are too deep. Always remember to put *traction on the skin* as it is being removed, to keep the *sharp knife* directed against it, and to leave the fat in place (unless specified otherwise). In this manner, you will work faster and encounter fewer difficulties (figs. 1-2 and 1-3).

The unnecessary destruction of many soft structures can be avoided and a great deal of time can be saved by utilizing the following safe and efficient technique: As illustrated in figure 1-4, use a pair of scissors of the sharp-sharp type and gently force the blades apart in a direction parallel to the structures of interest. Use the same technique with a fine pair of scissors to prepare delicate blood vessels and fine nerve filaments.

Terminology

Anatomical Position (fig. 1-5). Anatomists have agreed to relate everything they describe to a universally approved and accepted position of the body. It is that position in which the body stands erect with the feet together, arms by the side, and the palms facing forward. That the dissector is, on most occasions, working with the subject lying on its back makes not the slightest difference. When he says this or that structure is *inferior* to this or that muscle, he is understood by all anatomists to mean it is nearer the feet.

Figure 1-6 illustrates such essential terms as *superior* (*cranial*), *inferior* (*caudal*), *anterior* (*ventral*), and *posterior* (*dorsal*). The terms *coronal*, *sagittal*, and *transverse* (*horizontal*) are explained in figure 1-7.

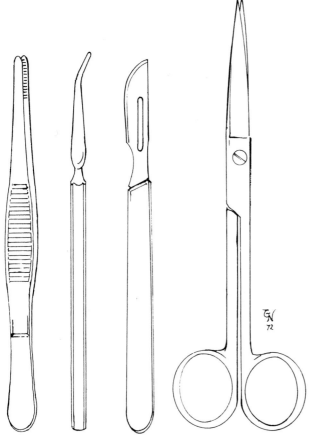

FIG. 1-1. Dissecting instruments.

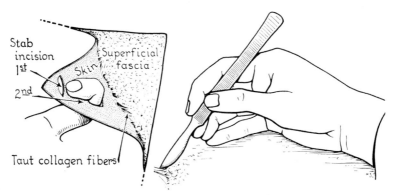

FIG. 1-2. When removing skin, apply traction.

FIG. 1-3. When dissecting, rest the hand. Eliminate unsteady movements.

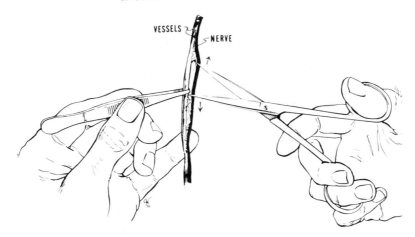

FIG. 1-4. Scissor technique: Separating delicate structures.

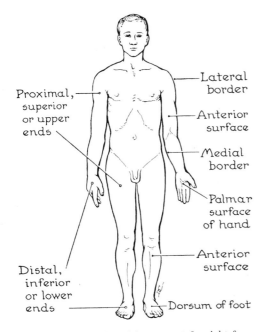

FIG. 1-5. Anatomical position, except for right forearm.

Descriptions

Anatomical structures can be precisely described. Learn and practice to give an *accurate account* of each important structure in an *orderly* and *logical fashion*. Always project yourself into a future professional situation: Remember, you must give orderly and logical accounts when reporting on radiological findings, on performed surgery or autopsies, etc. Your ability to recall facts will be greatly enhanced if you adopt the following schemes or similar ones:

Muscle:
1. Shape, size, and position.
2. Attachments (origin and insertion):
   a. Fleshy
   b. Fibrous (tendinous or aponeurotic).
3. Actions and uses

4. Nerve supply (spinal nerve; cranial nerve)
5. Immediate relations (anterior; posterior; etc.).

Bone:
1. Type or class (long; short; flat; irregular; sesamoid).
2. Situation (where in the body).
3. Shape, size, and appearance.
4. Parts (e.g. body, borders, processes, foramina; articulate surfaces).
5. Attachments of muscles, ligaments, and septa.
6. Ossification and epiphyses.

Joint:
1. Type or class (suture or synchondrosis; symphysis or syndesmosis; synovial joint of the plane, uniaxial, biaxial, or multiaxial variety).
2. 'Proximal' bone concerned.
3. 'Distal' bone concerned.
4. Articular capsule (fibrous capsule; synovial membrane).
5. Ligaments.
6. Bursae.
7. Movements.

Blood Vessel or Nerve:
1. Size, source, and situation.
2. Course and terminal branches.
3. Structures supplied.
4. Immediate relations and accompanying structures.
5. Variations and anomalies.

Variations

No cadaver will conform in all details of its anatomical construction to the patterns outlined in the pages of this Dissector. This manual describes the most usual patterns encountered in the adult. Minor and even major variants frequently occur: Arteries may arise from other sources than those indicated or may pursue different courses. Muscles may have extra heads of origin or be absent entirely. Organs may vary

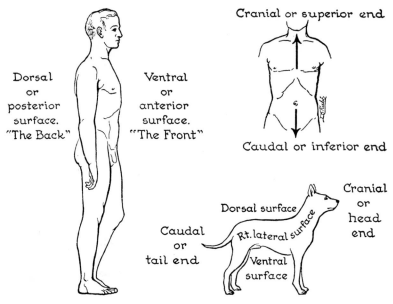

FIG. 1-6. Essential terms.

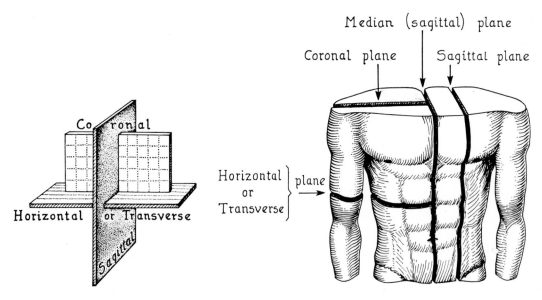

FIG. 1-7. Fundamental planes in the body: sagittal, coronal, transverse. (From *Grant's Method of Anatomy*.)

from their accepted shape and (or) be found in other than 'normal' positions. The usual anatomical relations may be distorted by disease processes.

Regard the cadaver you are working on as a 'typical example.' By all means, examine as many different subjects as possible. Only in this manner will you be able to familiarize yourself with the accepted 'normal' and with variations and anomalies.

Illustrations

The line drawings and schemes shown in this book are intended to orient the dissector and to facilitate his approach to a given anatomical region. They are designed to offer explanations, increase comprehension, and attract attention to a useful point of reference. The additional use of a good atlas is highly desirable.

Students who are using *Grant's Atlas of Anatomy* will find throughout the text of this Dissector references to appropriate plate numbers in the 6th edition of the Atlas. For example: (*Atlas, 213*).

CHAPTER 2

THORAX

Thoracic Wall

Bony Landmarks

Refer to individual bones or to an articulated skeleton. Study the following:

Vertebra (*Atlas, 357, 358*). It consists of a weight-bearing **body** and a protective vertebral arch which is made up of two rounded pedicles (roots) and two flat plates or **laminae.** At the junction of pedicle and lamina, a **transverse process** projects laterally, and **articular processes** project superiorly and inferiorly. At the junction of the two laminae, a **spinous process** projects posteriorly in the median plane. The bodies and transverse processes of the thoracic vertebrae have facets for the ribs (fig. 2-1; *Atlas, 366*).

Place your index finger into the **vertebral foramen** of a vertebra (fig. 2-2 or *Atlas, 369*). Observe that the size of the vertebral foramina differs from vertebra to vertebra (*Atlas, 366, 370, 371*). In the articulated vertebral column, the vertebral foramina collectively form a bony tube, the **vertebral canal**. This canal encloses and protects the important spinal cord. Understand that access to the contents of the spinal canal is possible by surgical removal of the laminae (laminectomy).

Rib (fig. 2-3; *Atlas, 398, 399*). Identify **head, neck, tubercle,** and **body.** On the external surface, observe the **angle** where the body takes a bend and also a twist; therefore, a rib will not lie flat on a table. The lower border of a typical rib is sharp and flange-like to shelter a costal groove for the intercostal nerve and vessels (figs. 2-10, 2-11). Note the distinctly different shape of the first rib. It is a superlative in being the highest, shortest, broadest, and most curved.

Sternum (*Atlas, 393–397*). Identify the wide upper segment, the **manubrium.** The **body** is made up of four distinguishable segments or **sternebrae.** The pointed lower extremity of the sternum is the **xiphoid process** [Gk., xiphos = sword]. It is cartilaginous in youth, but ossified in the middleaged and older person.

Refer to an articulated skeleton and understand the following:

1. Two adjacent vertebral bodies are united by a fibrocartilaginous **intervertebral disc.** This is a joint of the symphysis variety (fig. 2-4; *Atlas, 384–387*).

2. Two adjacent vertebral arches are united by their articular processes (fig. 2-4).

3. An **intervertebral foramen** is completed between the pedicles of two adjacent vertebrae. It transmits the spinal nerve of the corresponding segment (fig. 2-4).

4. The head of a rib articulates typically with two vertebral bodies and the intervening disc. The tubercle of a rib articulates with the transverse process of the vertebra with the same segmental number. Example (fig. 2-4). The head of rib 5 articulates with vertebral bodies T_4 and T_5. The tubercle of rib 5 articulates with the transverse process of T_5.

5. The anterior extremity of each rib is connected to the sternum by means of a bar of hyaline cartilage. These costal cartilages become progressively longer from 1st to 7th rib (*Atlas, 391*). Costal cartilages 8, 9, and 10 reach only as far as the cartilage next above.

6. Ribs 11 and 12 have free pointed ends; therefore, they are also known as 'floating ribs.'

In addition, identify the following bony structures or landmarks related to the dissection of the thoracic wall (fig. 2-5 or *Atlas, 11, 11.1*):

1. **Jugular notch** (suprasternal notch)
2. **Sternal angle** marking the junction of manubrium with body of sternum. At this level, the 2nd rib can be palpated.
3. Medial end of **clavicle** marking the sternoclavicular joint.
4. Lateral end of clavicle marking the acromioclavicular joint.
5. **Acromion** of scapula forming the point of the shoulder.
6. **Coracoid process** of scapula.

As a useful practical exercise for the students's future activities in **physical diagnosis,** the following study is recommended (fig. 2-6): With a grease pencil mark the subject's sternum, clavicle, and ribs 2 through 6. Identify and number the intercostal spaces (I.C.S.). The 2nd I.C.S. is located between ribs 2 and 3. The mammary papilla (nipple) lies at the level of I.C.S. 4 in the male, more inferiorly in the female. Outline the **borders of a normal heart:** The apex lies in I.C.S. 5 and about 8 to 10 cm to the left of the midsternal line. Mark the right border by a vertical line 2.5 cm (1″) lateral to the right sternal margin. The inferior border crosses the junction between xiphoid process and body of sternum. The left

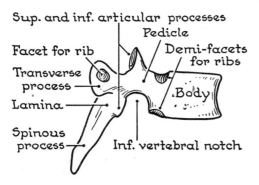

FIG. 2-1. Typical thoracic vertebra (side view). (From *Grant's Method of Anatomy.*)

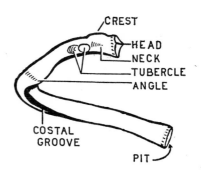

FIG. 2-3. Typical left rib, from behind. (From *Grant's Method of Anatomy.*)

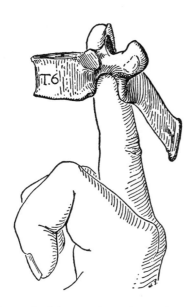

FIG. 2-2. A vertebral foramen is not larger than a finger ring. (From *Grant's Method of Anatomy.*)

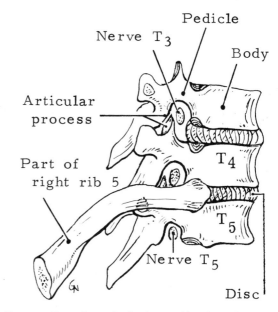

FIG. 2-4. Part of vertebral column, thoracic region: intervertebral disc, intervertebral foramen with spinal nerve, rib attachment.

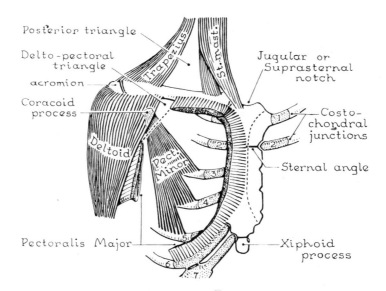

FIG. 2-5. Landmarks of thoracic region.

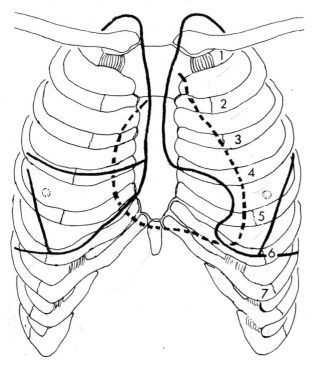

FIG. 2-6. Projections of heart (*broken line*) and lungs (*heavy solid lines*) on anterior chest wall.

border curves upward from the apex to I.C.S. 2, about 2.5 cm from the left sternal margin. Part of the aortic arch projects on I.C.S. 1, just to the left of the manubrium. In the living person in erect posture these borders will shift. Outline the **borders of the lungs:** The apex of each lung extends up into the neck for about 2.5 cm (cupula). The anterior borders of both lungs approach the midsternal line. The left lung deviates laterally at the level of ribs 4 and 5 to form the cardiac notch. Mark the approximate position of the horizontal fissure which begins near the right midaxillary line and extends forward along the right 4th intercostal cartilage. The oblique fissures of both lungs extend downward and end near the 6th costochondral junction.

Plan for Dissection

Prior to dissection of muscles, due consideration must be given to the superficially positioned mammary gland. The thoracic wall is covered anteriorly by muscles which belong to the upper extremity. These muscles (pectoralis major and minor; subclavius) must be dissected and reflected before the intercostal spaces and their contents can be approached. Subsequently, the anterior thoracic wall will be removed to provide access to the thoracic cavity.

Skin Incisions

Make the following skin incisions (fig. 2-7):
1. From jugular notch A along the clavicle and across the acromion B to point E, about 10 cm distal to the acromion.
2. From A to the xiphisternal junction C.

3. From C horizontally lateralward until stopped by the table D.
4. From C upward and along the anterior axillary fold to point E. Avoid the nipple. From E halfway around the medial side of the arm to point F.

Reflect the outlined flaps and discard them.

Dissection

Mammary Gland (*Atlas, 12, 12.1*). Since it is a modified skin gland, it lies in the superficial fascia. The rounded contour of the female breast is due to the superficial fat lying in compartments bounded by areolar septa, the **suspensory ligaments of Cooper.** These septa pass from the deep fascia to the deep layer of the skin. With the rounded handle of the knife, scoop collections of fat out of their compartments. Subsequently, trace some of the lactiferous ducts which converge on the tip of the **nipple.** Note that the nipple rises from the center of the pigmented **areola.**

If time permits, try to identify an orifice of one of the 15 to 20 lactiferous ducts. Attempt to pass a bristle or fine wire into the duct, and trace it to the corresponding lobe of glandular tissue. Finally, remove the gland and observe that it can be easily separated from the fascia of the underlying pectoralis major muscle.

In advanced carcinoma of the breast, the tumor may invade the pectoralis muscle and its fascia. Understand that this condition leads to a fixation of the breast lesion to the chest wall.

Cancer of the breast (and its accompanying fibrosis) also has a tendency to shorten Cooper's ligaments. Understand that the resulting traction of Cooper's ligaments on the skin leads to a characteristic dimpling of the skin.

Platysma (*Atlas, 13, 526*). Look for its brownish-red muscle fibers as they cross the clavicle. The platysma is no thicker than a sheet of paper. Turn the platysma upward. Observe one or more of the **supraclavicular nerves.** These nerves cling to the deep

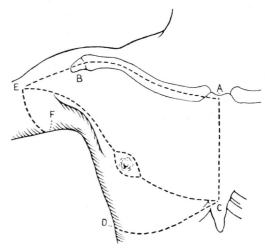

FIG. 2-7. Skin incisions for dissection of thoracic wall.

surface of the platysma and send twigs through it to
the skin. They are cutaneous nerves from C$_{3, 4}$ (*Atlas,
472*). The supraclavicular nerves do *not* supply the
platysma. The muscle fibers of the platysma are
innervated by a branch of the 7th cranial nerve.

Cutaneous Branches of Spinal Nerves (*Atlas, 13*).
The dissection of these branches can be intelligently
performed only if the student is familiar with the
disposition of a typical spinal nerve (fig. 2-8 or *Atlas,
13.1*). **Anterior cutaneous twigs** emerge from the
intercostal spaces just lateral to the sternal margin.
Be familiar with the area of their distribution, but do
not dissect these very small nerves. The **lateral
cutaneous branches** are substantially larger, and one
representative (segments 4, 5, or 6) should be dissected: Make a vertical cut through the superficial fascia
just lateral to the sternum. Make a horizontal cut
corresponding to the lower horizontal skin incision.
Reflect the flap of superficial fascia lateralward.
Identify an intercostal space by fingertip palpation
between two ribs. Search for the lateral cutaneous
branch where it leaves its intercostal space and passes
between the digitations of the serratus anterior (fig.
2-9; *Atlas, 13*). Free the nerve. Trace its anterior and
posterior branch for a short distance.

Pectoralis Major (*Atlas, 13*). Clean its whole
anterior surface. Identify the **clavicular part** and the
sternocostal part (on rare occasions absent; *Atlas, 27
A*). Trace the tendon of the muscle to its insertion in
the humerus. Observe that: (1) the anterior lamina of
the tendon belongs to the clavicular head; (2) the
posterior lamina is folded on itself and belongs to the
sternal head. Superior to the clavicular head, and
between it and the adjacent deltoid muscle, lies the
deltopectoral triangle. It transmits the **cephalic
vein,** which is a superficial vein of the upper limb
(*Atlas, 4*). Realize that the pectoralis major constitutes the most important part of the anterior wall of
the axilla (*Atlas, 15.1*). Palpate your own anterior
axillary fold, and activate its muscular components.

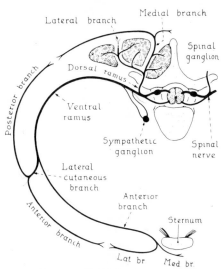

FIG. 2-8. Typical spinal nerve.

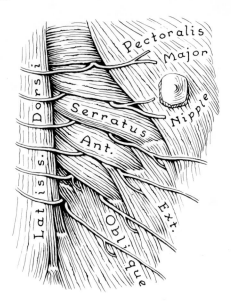

FIG. 2-9. Anterior and posterior branches of lateral cutaneous
nerves.

Pass a finger upward behind the *clavicular head* of
the pectoralis major. Palpate its nerve supply, the
lateral pectoral nerve, entering the deep surface of
the muscle. Detach the clavicular head close to the
clavicle, and reflect it toward the arm. Cut nerve and
blood vessels close to the muscle.

Relax the *sternal head* of the pectoralis major by
flexing and adducting the arm of the cadaver. Gently
insinuate your fingers behind the sternal head. Your
fingers are now in the space between the posterior
surface of the pectoralis major and the **clavipectoral
fascia,** which envelopes the pectoralis minor (*Atlas,
14.1*). Palpate the vessels and nerves entering the
pectoralis major. Detach the sternal head from its
sternal and costal origins (fig. 2-5), and reflect it
toward the arm. Note that the **medial pectoral nerve**
pierces the **pectoralis minor** before it enters the
sternal head of the pectoralis major (*Atlas, 16, 16.1*).
Leave arterial branches and nerves attached to the
muscle for subsequent identification.

Pectoralis Minor and Subclavius. After reflection
of the pectoralis major, the **clavipectoral fascia** is
exposed. It encloses the subclavius (a slender muscle
immediately inferior to the clavicle) and the pectoralis minor (*Atlas, 14.1*). Trace the cephalic vein as it
crosses the pectoralis minor tendon anteriorly and
pierces the clavipectoral fascia (*Atlas, 14*). Piercing
the clavipectoral fascia with the vein are the thoracoacromial artery and the lateral pectoral nerve. Detach
the pectoralis minor from its costal origin and reflect
it upward. Leave the muscle attached to its insertion
in the coracoid process of the scapula. Remove the
remains of the clavipectoral fascia and any fat that
might exist between the pectoralis minor and the rib
cage. Now, the **thoracoacromial artery** can be conveniently traced to its origin from the axillary artery
(*Atlas, 3 anterior view, 16*). Lateral to the pectoralis

minor identify the **lateral thoracic artery.** To obtain a clearer picture of this vessel, free it from the surrounding fat. Remove small veins. Trace the cephalic vein to the axillary vein. Do *not* disturb or destroy the contents of the axilla.

Intercostal Muscles (*Atlas, 406*). Define the **external intercostal muscles** which run obliquely downward and forward between the adjacent borders of two ribs. Note that the muscles do not extend forward beyond the ends of the bony ribs. More anteriorly, the muscles are replaced by the **external intercostal membrane.** Incise this membrane at the 4th intercostal space (ICS 4). Insert the flat handle of the knife or forceps deep to the membrane. Push the handle along ICS 4 into the aerolar tissue deep to the external intercostal muscle. With the handle as a guide, cut the muscle from the rib above and turn it down (fig. 2-10). Follow the external intercostal laterally until you reach the digitations of the serratus anterior. Observe the external intercostal becoming progressively thicker posteriorly.

The fibers of the **internal intercostal muscles** run at right angles to the external intercostal fibers (*Atlas, 406*). The internal intercostals extend from the most anterior portion of the intercostal space laterally as far as the angles of the ribs. In I.C.S. 4, carefully detach the internal intercostal from rib 5 below, and reflect it upward. Now, with the aid of a probe, locate the 4th intercostal nerve just below rib 4 (fig. 2-10). Subsequently, identify the intercostal vessels. (The innermost intercostal muscles are posteriorly located and do not reach as far anterior as the external intercostals; fig. 2-12. They will be seen later, p. 12).

Without waste of time, remove additionally the intercostal muscles from I.C.S. 2, 3, and 5. Resect the muscles as far laterally as the digitations of the serratus anterior. Be careful not to damage the subjacent costal pleura.

About 1 cm from the margin of the sternum, notice the **internal thoracic** (internal mammary) **vessels** (*Atlas, 406*). Realize that these vessels are attached to the anterior thoracic wall by numerous fine arterial branches, venous tributaries, and by muscle slips of the **transversus thoracis** (fig. 2-12; *Atlas, 407*). The next objective is to remove the anterior thoracic wall,

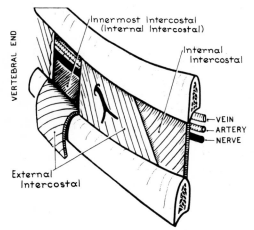

FIG. 2-10. An intercostal space.

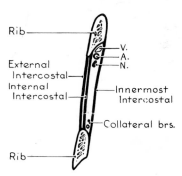

FIG. 2-11. Intercostal space on coronal section: intercostal muscles, intercostal nerve and vessels. (From *Grant's Method of Anatomy*.)

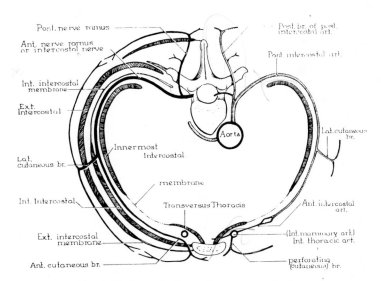

FIG. 2-12. Intercostal muscles, nerve, and artery.

but to leave the anterior thoracic vessels behind and intact. Proceed as follows: With your fingers, free ribs 2 to 5 from the subjacent pleura. The pleura must be moist. If it is not, moisten it. Gently tear the transversus thoracis from the internal surface of the ribs so that the internal thoracic vessels may be freed. Next, with a rib cutting tool, transect ribs 2 to 5 close to the digitations of the serratus anterior. Cut through the sternum at I.C.S. 5. With a saw, carefully (not too deep!) cut across the manubrium sterni at I.C.S. 1. Now, gently elevate the inferior part of the sternum together with the attached portions of severed ribs. Reflect the anterior chest wall upward and remove it.

In the removed and isolated anterior thoracic wall, examine one of the **sternocostal joints** (*Atlas, 404*). Cut through fine ligaments and the joint capsule, and open the synovial cavity. Understand that slight gliding movements occur in the sternocostal joints during (respiratory) movements of the ribs.

Clean the **internal thoracic artery** (*Atlas, 406, 407*). Follow the vessels toward the diaphragm. To facilitate dissection, remove the costal cartilage of rib 6. Observe that the internal thoracic artery ends in I.C.S. 6 by dividing into the **superior epigastric artery** (medially located) and the **musculophrenic artery.** Later (p. 27) the superior epigastric artery will be dissected in the sheath of the rectus abdominis where it anastomoses with the inferior epigastric artery (*Atlas, 106*). The musculophrenic artery supplies the lower intercostal muscles and the adjacent part of the diaphragm. Note: The origin of the internal thoracic artery from the subclavian artery will be displayed after removal of the lungs (p. 12).

Pleural Cavity

General Remarks and Definitions

The thoracic cavity contains two **pleural sacs** and the **mediastinum.** The mediastinum [L., quod per medium stat = which stands in the middle] is the thick median partition between the two pleural cavities. It contains the heart and many other important structures, such as the aorta, trachea, and esophagus. The two pleural cavities occupy the lateral parts of the thoracic cavity. During development, the lungs invaginate the pleural cavities (fig. 2-13 or *Atlas, 412.1*). Each **lung** is completely covered with a smooth glistening membrane, the **pulmonary or visceral pleura.** Each lung is attached to the mediastinum by an isthmus through which the airways and blood vessels enter or leave the organ. This area of attachment to the mediastinum is known as the root of the lung. Here, the visceral pleura is continuous with the parietal pleura which lines the walls of the pleural cavity.

Parietal Pleura (fig. 2-13 or *Atlas, 412.1*). The parietal pleura can be subdivided into the following

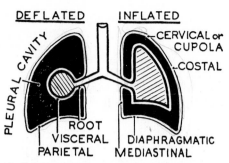

FIG. 2-13. Scheme of pleurae and pleural cavity. (From *Grant's Method of Anatomy*.)

portions: **costal** pleura (lining the rib cage); **mediastinal** pleura (lining the mediastinum); **diaphragmatic** pleura (lining the diaphragm); and **cupola** (cervical pleura, extending into the neck).

The lines along which costal pleura becomes diaphragmatic and mediastinal are known as **pleural reflections.** At *three sites* these reflections are so acute that the two portions of the parietal pleura are not only continuous but also *in actual contact with one another* by their inner or serous surfaces. No lung tissue with its visceral pleura intervenes between the apposing pleural layers. These sites of reflections of parietal pleura are known as **pleural recesses** (fig. 2-14). The **right and left costodiaphragmatic recesses** are found at the most inferior limits of the parietal pleura. Here the diaphragm lies so close to the costal wall as to bring costal and diaphragmatic surfaces of the parietal pleura into apposition. During ordinary inspiration, the thin inferior margin of the lung does not extend into the costodiaphragmatic recess. The **costomediastinal recess** is defined as the parietal pleural reflection from the anterior portion of the thoracic wall to the mediastinum.

Understand that the two pleural cavities are two separate and closed *potential spaces*. Normally, there is only a small amount of serous lubricating fluid in the pleural cavity. This substance reduces friction between parietal and visceral pleura during respiratory movements.

Under pathological conditions, the *potential space* of the pleural cavity may become a *real* one. If air is allowed to enter the pleural cavity (pneumothorax), the lung collapses due to its elasticity (compare fig. 2-13). If blood is accumulated in the pleural cavity, we speak of 'hemothorax.'

Pleurisy is an inflammation of the pleurae. It usually leads to the formation of pleural adhesions between parietal and visceral pleura. You may encounter such adhesions in the cadaver. These adhesions must be broken down before the lung can be completely mobilized.

Plan for Dissection

The right and left pleural cavities must be explored. This should be done both before and after removal of the lungs. Subsequently, the right and left side of the mediastinum will be examined, and nerves and vessels related to the posterior thoracic wall will be dissected.

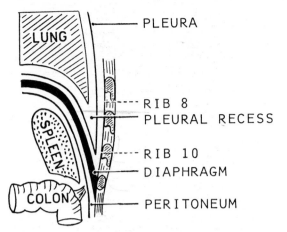

FIG. 2-14. The left costodiaphragmatic pleural recess.

Dissection

Incise both pleural sacs (if not already damaged), and place your hand into the **pleural cavity.** Palpate the root of the lung. Verify that it is attached to the mediastinum. All other portions of the lung are free within the pleural cavity; (however, you may encounter pleural adhesions in various places as a result of old pleurisy. Sever these adhesions with your fingers). Explore with your hand the various parts of the **parietal pleura: costal, diaphragmatic, mediastinal,** and **cupola.** Place your fingers into the **costomediastinal recess.** Find it on the left side in the region where the heart lies close to the anterior thoracic wall. Palpate the extensive and deep right and left **costodiaphragmatic recesses.** In addition, study the three recesses on cross section (*Atlas, 431*).

Root of Lung. The mediastinal pleura becomes visceral pleura at the root of the lung. Verify this fact by palpation. The connecting portion between parietal and visceral pleurae is a tube or sleeve of pleura (fig. 2-15, *A* and *B*). In its upper half lie all the structures that pass from and to the lung (fig. 2-15*C*). This is the actual **root** of the lung. The lower half of the sleeve is empty (except for a few lymph vessels). It is collapsed and known as the **pulmonary ligament** (fig. 2-15*C*). This ligament reaches caudally nearly to the diaphragm. Palpate the pulmonary ligament by passing your finger below its sharp free lower border.

Removal of Lung. Place your hand into the pleural cavity between lung and mediastinum. With one hand push the lung laterally, thereby stretching and exposing the root of the lung. With a scalpel in the other hand, carefully transect the root in the middle between lung and mediastinum. Take care *not* to cut into the mediastinum. Remove both lungs and store them in a plastic bag for future study.

Exposure. To facilitate exploration and dissection, enlarge the thoracic opening in the following manner: Reflect the digitations of the serratus anterior from ribs 2 through 5 back to the midaxillary line. Subsequently, cut these ribs at the midaxillary line.

Pleural Cavity and Reflections. Explore again the extent of the **costodiaphragmatic recess.** Push your fingers deep into it. If available, use white gauze or absorbent cotton to stuff one of the recesses. In the midaxillary line, identify I.C.S. 9 (about two finger's breadth above the costal margin). Pass a probe or needle horizontally through the thoracic wall at I.C.S. 9. The probe should appear in the costodiaphragmatic recess, close to the line of reflection between costal and diaphragmatic pleura (compare fig. 2-14).

Pleural Tap. The aspiration of pathological material (serous fluid; fluid mixed with tumor cells; blood; pus; etc.) from the pleural cavity is of important diagnostic value. The pleural tap is performed in the midaxillary line or slightly posterior to it. Usually, I.C.S. 6, 7, or 8 are selected for the needle puncture.

Refer to figures 2-10 and 2-11 and determine where the needle should pierce the I.C.S. in reference to the upper and lower rib. The needle should be passed close to the superior border of the lower rib to avoid injury to the intercostal nerve and vessels.

If the puncture needle is passed through I.C.S. 8 or 9 and pushed too deep, it will penetrate the diaphragm. After penetration of the diaphragm, the needle would reach the spleen on the left side (fig. 2-14), or the liver on the right side (*Atlas, 124, 125*).

Follow the right and left layers of the **mediastinal pleura** dorsally. Behind the pericardial sac, they pass to the sides of the esophagus. Posterior to the esophagus the two layers come together (fig. 2-16) to form a 'mesoesophagus.' This meso passes to the descending aorta where the two layers separate to reach the sides of the vertebral bodies. Subsequently, each layer becomes costal pleura. Verify these facts. Place one hand in each pleural cavity and bring the fingertips together posterior to the lower portion of the esophagus (fig. 2-16).

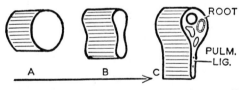

FIG. 2-15. Diagram of root of lung and of pulmonary ligament. (From *Grant's Method of Anatomy.*)

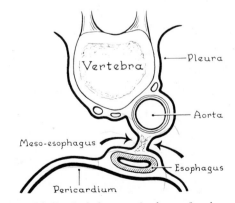

FIG. 2-16. Mediastinal layers of pleura forming a 'mesoesophagus.'

Note that certain structures are conspicuous through the mediastinal pleura. With the pleura intact, briefly identify on the *right side* (*Atlas, 428*): Superior vena cava; azygos vein and tributaries; phrenic nerve running anterior to root of lung; sympathetic trunk; and intercostal nerves and vessels. The esophagus is subpleural from end to end, except where it is crossed by the arch of the azygos vein. Superior to this venous arch, palpate the elastic trachea. It lies anterior to the esophagus. On the *left side* identify (*Atlas, 429*): Large bulge of heart; phrenic nerve; aortic arch; descending aorta; sympathetic trunk; and intercostal nerves and vessels. The esophagus is subpleural at both ends: (1) above the aortic arch; and (2) just before it pierces the diaphragm.

Removal of Costal and Mediastinal Pleura. Peel off the parietal pleura from the rib cage, starting at the level of the cut ribs 2 to 5. Next, gently remove it where it covers the vertebral column, aorta, esophagus, and pericardium (fig. 2-16). Be careful *not* to injure the **phrenic nerve.** This nerve is positioned between mediastinal pleura and pericardium, about 1.5 cm anterior to the root of the lung (*Atlas, 428, 429*).

With the pleura removed, demonstrate the following structures (*Atlas, 428, 429*): The **phrenic nerve** which is immediately subpleural throughout its course in the thorax. Above the cupola, identify the **subclavian artery,** and trace the **internal thoracic artery** to it. Observe a long and slender branch of the internal thoracic artery, the **pericardiacophrenic artery.** This artery accompanies the phrenic nerve toward the diaphragm. Clean one intercostal nerve, artery, and vein.

Sympathetic Trunk (fig. 2-17; *Atlas, 428, 429, 429.1*). It is bilateral. Find it on the neck of rib 1. Follow it inferiorly. It crosses successively the heads of ribs 2 to 9. Subsequently, it lies on the sides of the lower thoracic vertebrae. Note that the sympathetic trunk has a series of swellings, the **sympathetic ganglia,** one for each segment. Find the following branches:

1. **Rami communicantes.** At each segment, a **white ramus communicans** (preganglionic) passes from intercostal (spinal) nerve to sympathetic ganglion. A **gray ramus communicans** (postganglionic) passes from sympathetic ganglion to intercostal nerve. You may not be able to distinguish white from gray rami. However, demonstrate the fact that *two rami communicate* with each intercostal nerve and its corresponding sympathetic ganglion. Understand the functional significance of these rami (*left half* of fig. 2-18).

2. **Splanchnic nerves.** Identify the largest of the three splanchnic nerves, the **greater splanchnic nerve.** Demonstrate that it receives contributions from several sympathetic ganglia (fig. 2-17). The nerve carries preganglionic sympathetic fibers to the abdomen. Understand the functional significance of the splanchnic nerve (*right half* of fig. 2-18).

Explore the inner aspect of ICS 4. Note that the **innermost intercostal muscles** are posteriorly located and do not reach as far anterior as the external intercostals (*Atlas, 405*). Observe that the intercostal nerve and vessels are positioned between the planes of intercostal muscles (fig. 2-19).

Lungs

Refer to the two isolated lungs (*Atlas, 414–416*). Identify the surfaces and borders. The **surfaces** are **costal, medial** (having a mediastinal and vertebral part), and **basal** or **diaphragmatic.** The borders are anterior and inferior. They are thin and sharp. The

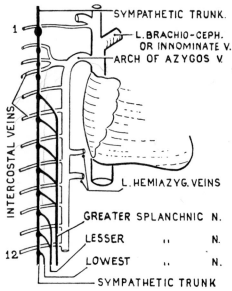

FIG. 2-17. Sympathetic trunk and splanchnic nerves.

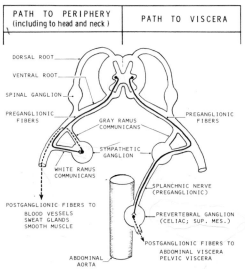

FIG. 2-18. General plan of sympathetic nerve distribution.

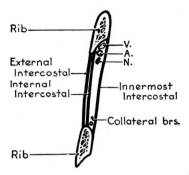

FIG. 2-19. Position of intercostal nerve and vessels between intercostal muscles. (From *Grant's Method of Anatomy*.)

apex of the lung rises as high as the neck of the first rib, but not higher. The right lung is shorter but more voluminous than the left. Each lung is divided into an **upper** and a **lower lobe** by an **oblique fissure.** Identify these lobes and observe that: most of the lower lobe lies at the back of the thoracic cavity; most of the upper lobe lies at the front. The upper lobe of the right lung is further subdivided by a **horizontal fissure,** thereby producing in front a small **middle lobe.** This lobe reaches lateralward only as far as the midaxillary line.

In the well embalmed and hardened lung, **contact impressions** from topographically related structures can be observed. On the mediastinal surface of the *right lung (Atlas, 415),* identify the **cardiac impression** and the **groove for the esophagus.** On the mediastinal surface of the *left lung (Atlas, 416),* identify the **cardiac impression** and the continuous **groove for aortic arch and descending aorta.**

Examine the **hilus** of both lungs. Observe the relative positions of **bronchus, pulmonary artery,** and **pulmonary veins** *(Atlas, 415, 416).* Generally, the bronchus lies posterior, the artery superior, and the veins inferior. The **right upper bronchus** has a special location. It is higher than any other bronchus, and even higher than the pulmonary artery (fig. 2-20 or *Atlas, 416.1*). Therefore, this bronchus has also been named 'eparterial bronchus.'

There are additional structures at the hilus: Bronchial arteries which are nutrient vessels for the lung tissue. Lymph nodes and vessels. Autonomic nerve fibers. Be aware of these structures, but do not make a special effort to dissect them.

Dissection. The fat-free lung tissue is readily forced apart with the blunt ends of two pairs of forceps. Use this technique. Identify the **main bronchus.** If the root of the lung was cut close to the lung tissue, the main bronchus was left behind in the mediastinum. In this case, only the subsidiary bronchi can be seen at the hilus. In the *left lung,* identify the **superior (upper) and inferior (lower) lobar bronchi.** In the *right lung,* identify the **upper, middle, and lower bronchi** (fig. 2-20 or *Atlas, 416.1*).

Next, identify the **segmental bronchi** (*Atlas,*

424–427). Verify by palpation that they contain pieces of cartilage. Pass a probe into each segmental bronchus. Follow each structure for 2 to 3 cm into the lung tissue. Remove intervening (black) lymph nodes. Cut away some lung tissue near the hilus. Identify:

Right Lung (*Atlas, 417):*
Superior lobe
1. apical
2. posterior
3. anterior
Middle lobe
4. lateral
5. medial
Inferior lobe
6. superior
7. medial basal
8. anterior basal
9. lateral basal
10. posterior basal
Left Lung (*Atlas, 420):*
Superior lobe
1. + 2. apical-posterior
3. anterior
4. superior lingular
5. inferior lingular
Inferior lobe
6. superior
7. medial basal
8. anterior basal
9. lateral basal
10. posterior basal

Select one segmental bronchus. Open it with a pair of scissors, and follow it and its ramifications far into the lung tissue. Sufficient knowledge of the segmental bronchial distribution is a necessary prerequisite for pulmonary radiology and surgery.

Identify the **pulmonary artery** and its branches

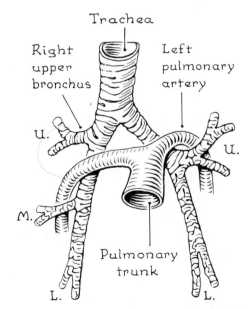

FIG. 2-20. Relationship of pulmonary arteries to bronchi.

which carry deoxygenated blood (*Atlas, 419, 422*). These vessels are distributed together with the bronchial tree.

Mediastinum

Definitions and Subdivisions

The thick median region between the two pleural sacs is the mediastinum (*Atlas, 412*). It extends from the superior aperture of the thorax to the diaphragm, and from the sternum to the bodies of the 12 thoracic vertebrae. Purely for descriptive purposes, this extensive region is arbitrarily subdivided into subsidiary parts (fig. 2-21).

A horizontal plane at the level of the sternal angle cuts the intervertebral disc between thoracic vertebrae 4 and 5. Above this imaginary plane lies the **superior mediastinum** (*S* in fig. 2-21). This plane is especially convenient since it indicates the level of the upper border of the fibrous pericardium and the level of the bifurcation of the trachea, i.e. the upper border of the root of the lung.

The remaining portion of the mediastinum (inferior to the superior mediastinum) is divided into three parts: (1) **anterior mediastinum** (*A* in fig. 2-21), the small and unimportant portion between sternum and pericardium; (2) **middle mediastinum** (*M* in fig. 2-21), containing the pericardium with the enclosed heart and the roots of the great vessels; (3) **posterior mediastinum** (*P* in fig. 2-21), the portion behind the pericardium and in front of the bodies of the lower 8 thoracic vertebrae. Certain structures traversing the length of the mediastinum (e.g. esophagus, vagus, phrenic nerve, thoracic duct) lie, of course, in more than one mediastinal subdivision.

It must be stressed that, in the living person, the mediastinum is a highly mobile region. Observe the loose fat and areolar tissue of the mediastinum. Recognize that it is perfectly suited to accommo-date movements and volume changes in the thoracic cavity (e.g. movements of trachea during respiration; pulsations of great vessels; volume changes of esophagus).

Middle Mediastinum

The **middle mediastinum** contains the pericardium (with adjacent phrenic nerves), the **heart,** and the roots of the great vessels passing to and from the heart. The **pericardium** or pericardial sac (*Atlas, 412.2*) is a double-walled sac enclosing the heart and pierced by the roots of the 8 vessels (2 arteries, 2 caval veins, 4 pulmonary veins). Its outer surface, now fully exposed, is fibrous and appears dull. This fibrous layer gradually thins out on the surfaces of the eight vessels that pierce it. The fibrous layer is lined inside with the serous pericardium. At the roots of the great vessels, the serous pericardium is reflected on to the surface of the heart as the **visceral layer of the serous pericardium,** also called the **epicardium** (fig. 2-22). Observe that the pericardium adheres firmly to the central tendon of the diaphragm. Thus, the pericardial sac is influenced by the movements of the diaphragm.

Plan for Dissection

The pericardial sac must be opened to provide access to the heart. After manual exploration of the pericardial cavity and its two sinuses, the heart should be skillfully detached from its 8 great vessels. Subsequently, the isolated heart can be dissected.

Inspection and Manual Exploration

With a pair of forceps, pinch up a fold of parietal pericardium near its upper end. With the scissors nick the fold, and enter the pericardial cavity. Produce a U-shaped flap of parietal pericardium by cutting along its right, lower, and left borders. Turn up the U-shaped flap. Sponge the interior of the pericardial sac with soap and water.

Notice the contrast between the inner lining of smooth, glistening serous pericardium and the outer rough and dull fibrous pericardium. Observe that the visceral layer of serous pericardium intimately invests the heart. Push a probe upward in front of the ascending aorta to the superior limit of the cavity.

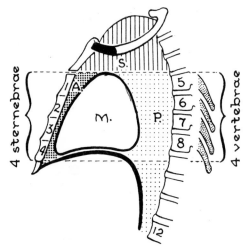

FIG. 2-21. Four subdivisions of mediastinum.

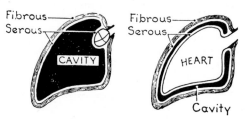

FIG. 2-22. Layers of pericardium. (From *Grant's Method of Anatomy.*)

Establish that the superior limit corresponds approximately to the level of the sternal angle (*Atlas, 432, 433*).

With your fingers explore the lines of reflections from the visceral to the parietal (serous) pericardium (*Atlas, 441* illustrates these lines of reflections). With the heart still in the pericardial cavity, insinuate your *left* index finger between the superior vena cava and ascending aorta. Then, push the finger behind the pulmonary artery. Now, your finger lies in a serous-lined tunnel known as **transverse pericardial sinus.** Leave your finger in the sinus. Next, with your *right* hand, lift up the apex of the heart and push two fingers behind the heart into the **oblique pericardial sinus** (*Atlas, 441*). It is a serous-lined cul-de-sac bounded on the right by (1) the inferior vena cava; and (2) the right lower and upper pulmonary veins. On the left, the sinus is bounded by (1) the lower pulmonary vein; and (2) the upper pulmonary vein. Palpate and observe that your right and left fingers are separated by (two layers of) serous pericardium.

Review the projection of the heart on the anterior chest wall (p. 7 and fig. 2-6). Study the surfaces of the heart *in situ* (*Atlas, 433*): The **right border** consists of the **right atrium.** The **left border** is formed by the **left ventricle** which is responsible for the **apex** of the heart. At the upper end of the left border the **auricle of the left atrium** can be seen. The **lower border** belongs to the **right ventricle,** except for a small portion on the extreme left, which belongs to the left ventricle.

Removal of Heart

Removal of the Heart. The 8 great vessels must be severed, but the posterior wall of the pericardial sac should be left intact (*Atlas, 441*). Again identify the transverse pericardial sinus. Mark it by placing a pencil or probe through it. Then cut across the stems of the **aorta** and the **pulmonary trunk.** Next, cut the **inferior vena cava** as low as possible within the pericardial sac. Then transect the **superior vena cava** about 1 cm above its junction with the right atrium. Lift the heart forward and upward by its apex. Then, cut across the **four pulmonary veins** where they bound the oblique sinus. Do not injure the left atrium. Now, the heart is held in place merely by the two layers of pericardium that separate the oblique from the transverse sinus. Incise these two layers and remove the heart. Your field of dissection should compare with *Atlas figure 441.*

Note: The heart can be conveniently replaced into the pericardial sac. This should be done whenever clarification of orientation is required (e.g. *anterior* or *posterior* papillary muscle; *plane* of base of heart, or *plane* of interventricular septum). Hold the isolated heart in your hand. Hold it in its anatomical position in reference to your own chest. Use the roots of the pulmonary veins and of the venae cavae as reference structures. Pass two pencils or probes through the openings of the pulmonary veins in the left atrium, as indicated

in figure 2-23. Pass one probe from the superior vena cava through the right atrium into the inferior vena cava (fig. 2-23). In the anatomical position, the probes through the venae cavae are in a vertical position, whereas the probes through the pulmonary veins are horizontally oriented.

Heart

Identify the **coronary sulcus** (*Atlas, 434, 435*), a groove that runs obliquely around the heart, separating atria from ventricles. At the right angles to the coronary sulcus are the **anterior and posterior interventricular grooves or sulci.** These sulci separate the ventricles from one another and, therefore, denote the position of the interventricular septum (fig. 2-28). The sulci contain blood vessels.

Cardiac Vessels. When dissecting the vessels, it will be necessary to remove piecemeal the epicardium and fat. Using blunt forceps, begin with the two **coronary arteries** which originate from the **ascending aorta.** On leaving the aorta, the two coronary arteries pass forward, one on each side of the root of the pulmonary trunk (fig. 2-24 or *Atlas, 437*).

Follow the **left coronary artery** (fig. 2-24 or *Atlas, 437*). Between the left auricle and the pulmonary trunk, it divides into an **anterior interventricular branch** and a **circumflex branch.** The anterior interventricular branch follows the interventricular

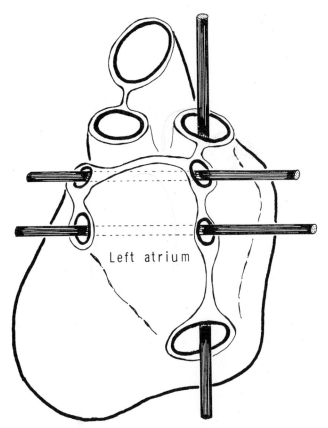

Left atrium

FIG. 2-23. Posterior aspect of heart in anatomical position. *Horizontal rods* pass through left atrium. *Vertical rod* passes through right atrium.

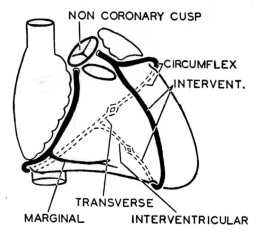

FIG. 2-24. Coronary arteries. (From *Grant's Method of Anatomy*.)

sulcus to or beyond the apex. The circumflex branch follows the coronary sulcus around the left border to the posterior surface of the heart.

Now, trace the **right coronary artery.** It follows the coronary sulcus to the right border and then onto the diaphragmatic surface of the heart. Usually, it reaches the posterior interventricular sulcus in which it descends toward the apex as the **posterior interventricular branch.** Note a branch which arises close to the origin of the right coronary artery, ascends along the anteromedial wall of the right atrium, and passes toward the superior vena cava. This is the **superior vena caval branch** (nodal artery) which supplies the important sinuatrial node of the specialized conduction system.

Expect to find variations of the arteries and their branching patterns. These are extremely common (*Atlas, 439*). In about two-thirds of the cases, the right coronary artery is *dominant*, i.e. it crosses to the left side to supply the left ventricular wall and ventricular septum. The left coronary artery, in addition to supplying all of the left ventricle and ventricular septum, may send branches to the right ventricular wall (left coronary artery *dominance*; about 15%). In about one-fifth of the cases, the coronary arterial pattern is *balanced*.

Cardiac Veins (fig. 2-25 or *Atlas, 438*). Most veins of the heart are tributaries of the **coronary sinus.** The coronary sinus is a sizable venous channel which lies in the posterior part of the coronary sulcus. The coronary sinus is about 2 to 2.5 cm in length. It empties into the right atrium. There are numerous tributaries of the coronary sinus. Identify the following two important **tributaries:**

1. **Great cardiac vein.** It begins at the apex and ascends in the anterior interventricular sulcus. In the coronary sulcus, it turns to the left and is continuous with the coronary sinus.
2. **Middle cardiac vein.** It ascends in the posterior interventricular sulcus and ends in the coronary sinus.

One or two **anterior cardiac veins** run from the

anterior aspect of the right ventricle across the coronary sulcus to open directly into the right atrium.

Right Atrium. Open the right atrium in the following manner (fig. 2-26 or *Atlas, 444.1*): Make a short cut through the tip of the right auricle. Next, cut with scissors through the atrial wall from the initial incision toward the inferior vena cava. Then, cut horizontally above the inferior vena cava, almost to the coronary sulcus. Turn the flap of atrial wall, and open the right atrium widely. Remove blood clots, and wash area thoroughly with cold water. Observe the following features (fig. 2-27; *Atlas, 443*):

1. A smooth posterior atrial wall (Note: 'posterior' in reference to the anatomical position of the heart).
2. A rough anterior atrial wall. It has comb-like parallel ridges, the **pectinate muscles.**
3. Posterior and anterior walls are separated by a vertical ridge, the **crista terminalis.**
4. The smooth posterior part receives the following veins: **superior vena cava, inferior vena cava, and coronary sinus.**
5. **Valve of inferior vena cava.**
6. **Valve of coronary sinus.** It guards the opening of the coronary sinus, which empties into the right atrium between the opening of the inferior

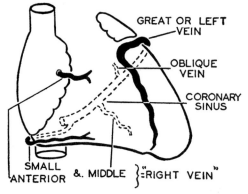

FIG. 2-25. Cardiac veins. (From *Grant's Method of Anatomy*.)

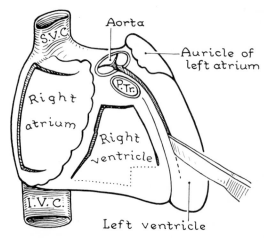

FIG. 2-26. Incisions for opening right atrium and both ventricles. (From *Grant's Atlas of Anatomy*.)

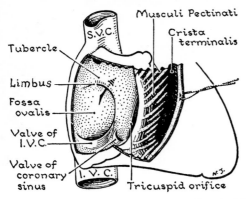

FIG. 2-27. Interior of right atrium. (From *Grant's Method of Anatomy*.)

vena cava and the atrioventricular orifice.

7. The large **atrioventricular or tricuspid orifice,** leading forward to the right ventricle.

8. **Fossa ovalis,** an oval depression of the interatrial wall. It is the remnant of the fetal foramen ovale.

Parts of the important specialized **conduction system** of the heart are topographically related to the right atrium. These structures are too small to be visible in gross dissection. However, in view of their functional importance, familiarize yourself with their approximate locations. Point a probe to the vicinity of two important parts of the conduction system (*Atlas*, *445.1*):

1. **Sinuatrial node** (S-A node). It lies in the crista terminalis, at the junction between right atrium and superior vena cava. It is supplied by the nodal artery (p. 16).

2. **Atrioventricular node** (A-V node). It lies in the lower part of the interatrial septum, near the coronary sinus opening.

Right Ventricle. Open the right ventricle in the following manner (fig. 2-26 or *Atlas*, *444.1*): Pass a blunt instrument or your little finger down the pulmonary trunk (artery). Determine the level of the pulmonary valves. Make a short transverse incision into the right ventricular wall below the level of the pulmonary valves. Insert your finger through the opening, and guide the scissors for the following cuts: 1 cm away from and parallel to the coronal sulcus toward the inferior border of the heart. Next, cautiously from the left end of the initial transverse incision, about 2 cm from and parallel to the anterior interventricular sulcus, toward the inferior border of the heart. Turn the flap of right ventricular wall, and open the chamber widely. Remove blood clots, and wash area thoroughly with cold water. Observe the following features (*Atlas*, 444):

1. The right ventricle is crescentic in cross section (fig. 2-28). The interventricular septum is convex toward this chamber since the pressure is higher on the arterial than on the venous side.

2. The **atrioventricular orifice,** situated dorsally,

is large enough to admit the tips of three (average sized) fingers.

3. The atrioventricular orifice is guarded by **three cusps,** hence the name **tricuspid valve.** The cusps are continuous with one another at their bases. Toward the edges, they are disposed as *anterior, septal,* and *posterior.* Small secondary cusps may be present and may obscure the general arrangement.

4. The **chordae tendineae,** tendinous strands which pass from the margins and ventricular surfaces of the cusps into the apices of papillary muscles (the strands are arranged like the cords of a parachute).

5. **Papillary muscles.** The *anterior* papillary muscle is the largest and most prominent. Its chordae tendineae are attached to the anterior and posterior cusps. The other papillary muscles are much smaller and irregular in disposition. They are designated: *posterior* and *septal.* The septal papillary muscles are very small and multiple.

6. The interior wall of the right ventricle is roughened by muscular ridges and bridges. These are known as the *trabeculae carneae* [L., trabs = wooden beam; carneus = fleshy].

7. **Septomarginal trabeculae** (moderator band), stretching from the interventricular septum to the base of the anterior papillary muscle.

8. The **orifice of the pulmonary trunk** (pulmonary orifice) lies above and in front. The cone-shaped portion of the chamber below the orifice is the **conus arteriosus** or **infundibulum.** The blood, of necessity, takes a U-shaped course in passing from the orifice of entrance to the orifice of exit.

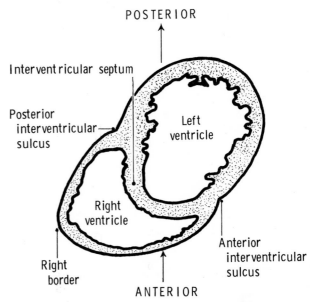

FIG. 2-28. Horizontal section through right and left ventricles. *Arrows* indicate sagittal plane.

9. The **valve of the pulmonary trunk** (pulmonary valve) consists of three semilunar valvules or cusps—an *anterior*, a *right*, and a *left* (fig. 2-29).

Left Atrium. Open this chamber by means of an inverted U-shaped incision through the posterior wall. Leave the openings of the pulmonary veins intact. Turn the flap downward. Remove blood clots, and wash thoroughly with cold water. Observe the following features:

1. The entrances of the **four pulmonary veins** into the right and left sides of the atrium (compare *Atlas*, 435).
2. The opening of the tubular left **auricle.**
3. The site of closure of the **foramen ovale,** situated anteriorly and to the right (anatomical position of heart!), and usually defined by a curved ridge.
4. The left **atrioventricular or mitral orifice** opening through the lower half of the anterior wall, into the left ventricle.
5. The atrial wall is smooth, except for small pectinate muscles in the left auricle.
6. Compare the thickness of the right and left atrial walls. The wall of the left atrium is distinctly thicker than that of the right atrium.

Left Ventricle. Open the left ventricle in the following manner (fig. 2-26 or *Atlas*, 444.1): Make a cut 1 cm to the left of, and parallel to, the anterior interventricular groove. The cut is through a wall about 1 to 1.5 cm in thickness. It should extend from the inferior border of the heart of the root of the aorta. Guide the cut with a finger passed through the left atrioventricular orifice into the left ventricle. Extend the incision along the entire length of the ascending aorta. Carefully cut exactly between the right and left coronary cusps of the aortic valve. During the prescribed cut, the circumflex artery and the great cardiac vein must be severed. Now, open the left ventricle and the length of the ascending aorta widely. Remove blood clots, and wash thoroughly with cold water. Observe the following features (*Atlas*, 445):

1. The ventricular cavity is cone-shaped in outline and circular on cross section (compare fig. 2-28).
2. The muscular wall is about 1 to 1.5 cm in thickness, but much thinner at the apex. In the

normal (not necessarily in the diseased) heart, the left ventricular wall is about three times as thick as the right one.

3. The **left atrioventricular or mitral orifice.**
4. The **left atrioventricular valve (bicuspid or mitral valve),** consisting of an *anterior* and a *posterior* cusp. The larger anterior cusp intervenes between the atrioventricular and aortic orifices.
5. **Chordae tendineae,** attached to two papillary muscles, *anterior* and *posterior*.
6. **Trabeculae carneae.**
7. **Aortic valve,** composed of three **semilunar cusps:** *right coronary, left coronary,* and *posterior or noncoronary* cusp. Observe the **nodule,** a small fibrous thickening at the middle of the free margin of each cusp (*Atlas*, 446.2). Study and probe the orifices of the two coronary arteries and their relation to the two coronary valvules (*Atlas*, 445).
8. The thick and extensive **muscular part of the interventricular septum.**
9. The **membranous part of the interventricular septum,** about the size of a fingernail. It is situated just below the attached margins of the right coronary and noncoronary cusps of the aortic valve. Palpate this thin membranous septum between your index fingers, one in each ventricle.

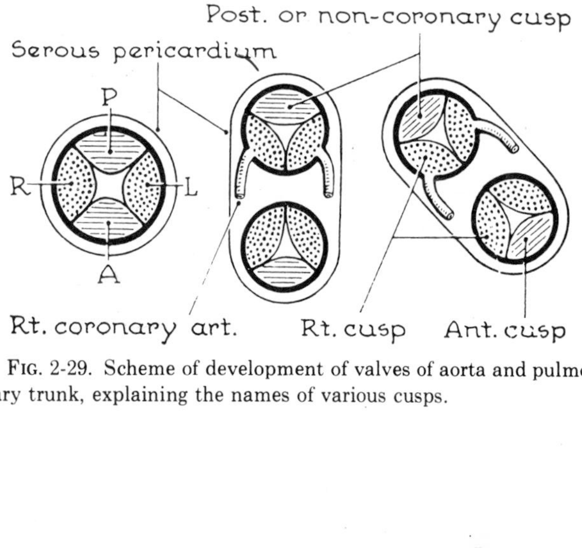

The thin membranous interventricular septum adjoins the atrial septum. During development, the membranous interventricular septum closes last. It may be the site of a congenital defect, the 'patent interventricular septum.'

Posterior Mediastinum

Posterior Mediastinum. Review the definition of the term 'posterior mediastinum' (p. 14; *P* in fig. 2-21 or *Atlas*, 413.1). Note that it is that portion of the mediastinum in front of the bodies of the lower 8 thoracic vertebrae and *behind* and also below the pericardium. Thus, it is logical to approach the structures in the posterior mediastinum through the already opened pericardial sac: Remove the posterior wall of the pericardial sac behind the oblique sinus (*Atlas*, 442). Now, the posterior relations of the heart can be examined. Most anteriorly and slightly to the right is the **esophagus.**

Temporarily, place the heart back into the opened pericardial sac. Examine its topographic relations to the esophagus. Understand why the posterior border of the heart can be best evaluated radiologically when the esophagus is filled with radioopaque material. The esophagus lies immediately posterior to the left atrium and part of the left ventricle. An enlargement of these chambers will indent the barium-filled esophagus and displace it posteriorly.

Certain heart murmurs in the left atrial area (regurgitant murmurs in mitral valve insufficiency) can be excellently recorded

FIG. 2-29. Scheme of development of valves of aorta and pulmonary trunk, explaining the names of various cusps.

with the aid of a small microphone channelled into the esophagus behind the heart.

In the region of the posterior mediastinum, study and clean the **esophagus,** a collapsed muscular tube (*Atlas, 442*). Give special attention to the two **vagal nerves** and their relations to the esophagus. Identify and clean the **right vagus** posterior to the root of the right lung (fig. 2-30; *Atlas, 428*). Follow the nerve to the esophagus. Similarly, identify the **left vagus** behind the root of the left lung, and follow it to the esophagus (*Atlas, 429*). Note that the vagal fibers separate and spread out on the esophagus as the **esophageal plexus** (fig. 2-30; *Atlas, 428*). Close to the diaphragm, the bundles of the esophageal plexus combine to form the two **vagal trunks,** and *anterior* and a *posterior* one. Due to the rotation of the gut during development, the bundles from the left vagus swing around to the anterior surface of the esophagus. The bundles from the right vagus come to lie dorsal to the esophagus (fig. 2-31). Identify the **vagal trunks** as they pass through the diaphragm together with the esophagus.

Pull the esophagus to the left and expose the azygos vein. From its arch, follow it caudally to the dipharagm (*Atlas, 428*). Study a diagram of the azygos system of veins (fig. 2-32 or *Atlas, 445, 455.1*). Note that the intercostal veins on the right side are tributaries to the azygos vein. Observe the cross channels (irregular) bringing blood from the left side via the hemiazygos veins.

Thoracic duct, (*Atlas, 453*). This is a thin-walled, pale, and easily torn structure found between the

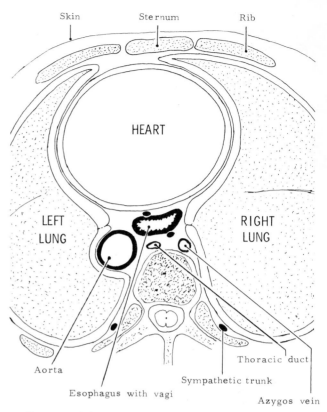

FIG. 2-31. Schematic cross section through thorax inferior to roots of lungs.

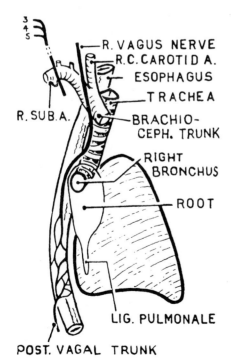

FIG. 2-30. The right vagus nerves applied to the trachea and esophagus.

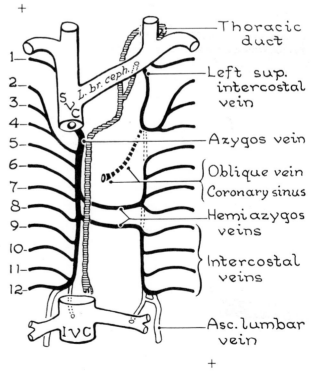

FIG. 2-32. Diagram of azygos system of veins. Axiom: In order to arrive in the right orvenous side of the heart, blood from the left side of the body must cross the median plane. (From *Grant's Atlas of Anatomy*.)

azygos vein and the descending aorta. Using the scissor technique, carefully free this fragile structure from the surrounding fatty areolar tissue. Commonly, the duct may be plexiform in the posterior mediastinum. Observe that the thoracic duct traverses the diaphragm together with the descending aorta (*Atlas, 452*).

Identify the **descending aorta.** Clean it from the surrounding fatty areolar tissue. Look for its small variable branches to the esophagus and trachea (*Atlas, 454*). Identify several of its paired posterior intercostal branches (*Atlas, 457.1*).

Note: The sympathetic trunks lie posterior to each lung and *not* between the mediastinal pleurae (fig. 2-31; *Atlas, 428, 429*). Therefore, the sympathetic trunks are *not* contained in any subdivision of the mediastinum. However, some of its branches, the **splanchnic nerves,** turn medially and forward and thus become part of the posterior mediastinum.

Superior Mediastinum

Review the **boundaries of the superior mediastinums** (p. 14; *S* in fig. 2-21 or *Atlas, 413.1*).
1. Superiorly: superior aperture of thorax (i.e. superior entrance into thorax bounded by manubrium, first thoracic vertebra and the two first ribs; *Atlas, 391*).
2. Posteriorly: thoracic vertebrae 1 through 4.
3. Anteriorly: manubrium of sternum.
4. Laterally: mediastinal pleurae of the two lungs.
5. Inferiorly: a plane from sternal angle to intervertebral disc T$_{4/5}$; this plane is just superior to the limit of the pericardium.

Identify the **thymus** (*Atlas, 448*). It is the fatty mass that lies immediately behind the manubrium in the anterior portion of the superior mediastinum. Observe that the arteries supplying the thymus are (in part) derived from the internal thoracic arteries. In the infant and child the thymus is a prominent organ of glandular texture. After puberty, the organ undergoes involution, and it may be scarcely recognizable in old age.

Remove the thymus but do not damage the left brachiocephalic vein which lies posterior to it (*Atlas, 448.1*). Now, clean the great veins (*Atlas, 449*). Halfway down the right margin of the manubrium, the two **brachiocephalic veins** (innominate veins) meet to form the **superior vena cava.** On the right side, identify again the **azygos vein.** It arches over the root of the lung to empty into the superior vena cava (*Atlas, 428, 455*). Cut the superior vena cava just superior to the entrance of the azygos vein. Reflect the great veins in order to expose the **arch of the aorta** and the great arteries arising from it (fig. 2-33 or *Atlas, 428.1*).

Clean the aortic arch and the three great arteries arising from it (fig. 2-34; *Atlas, 449, 452*):
1. **Brachiocephalic trunk** (innominate artery),

arising from the summit of the aortic arch.
2. **Left common carotid artery.**
3. **Left subclavian artery.** It lies immediately behind the left common carotid artery. Both arteries ascend almost vertically.

The **aortic arch,** by definition, begins and ends at the same level: this is the sternal angle anteriorly, and the intervertebral disc T$_{4/5}$ posteriorly. Observe that the aorta arches over the left bronchus (fig. 2-34) and then becomes the descending aorta. Further caudally, the esophagus is interposed between it and the pericardial sac (*Atlas, 442*). Verify that the aortic arch passes from front to back. Therefore, by necessity, the aortic arch is crossed by two nerves that descend vertically. These are: the **left phrenic nerve** and the **left vagus** (fig. 2-34; *Atlas, 449*).

Left Phrenic Nerve (fig. 2-33; *Atlas, 429, 449*). It descends from the neck, enters the thorax between the subclavian artery and subclavian vein, and reaches the aortic arch. After crossing the arch, it lies approximately 1 cm anterior to the root of the lung. Subsequently, it lies on the left side of the pericardial sac. Restore its position, and review the course of the nerve to the diaphragm.

Left Vagus (*Atlas, 429, 449–451*). It descends from the neck along the posterolateral side of the left common carotid artery. Find it in the angular interval between the left common carotid and subclavian arteries (fig. 2-34). Trace it across the left side of the aortic arch. Since it is on its way to the esophagus, it passes posterior to the root of the left lung; i.e. posterior to bronchus, pulmonary artery, and pulmonary veins (fig. 2-36). Use a probe and dissect bluntly the area where the vagus crosses the arch. Confirm that the concavity of the arch is connected to the left pulmonary artery by a stout, obliquely set cord. This is the **ligamentum arteriosum,** the remnant of the ductus arteriosus (fig. 2-35; *Atlas, 450*). Find and clean the **left recurrent laryngeal nerve.** It is an important branch of the left vagus. Locate it immediately posterior to the ligamentum arteriosum. Follow it for a short distance superiorly. Later (p. 153), the nerve will be followed to its termination in the larynx (*Atlas, 660*).

The aortic arch is also crossed by two slender cardiac nerves (*Atlas, 449*) which may now be difficult to find. They arise in the neck from the sympathetic trunk and from the vagus. They pass to the superficial cardiac plexus situated just to the right of the ligamentum arteriosum. Do not waste time searching for these fine fibers.

Identify the **right phrenic nerve.** Review the positions and relationships of the **right vagus** nerve (fig. 2-36; *Atlas, 428, 449, 450*). Note that this nerve takes a course along the right side of the trachea and toward the posterior aspect of the root of the lung. Some branches arise from the vagus and cross the trachea anteriorly (*Atlas, 450*); these are cardiac branches on their way to the deep cardiac plexus.

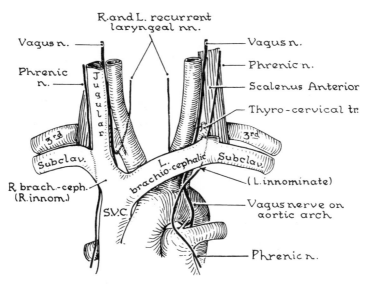

FIG. 2-33. Great veins and arteries, and related nerves.

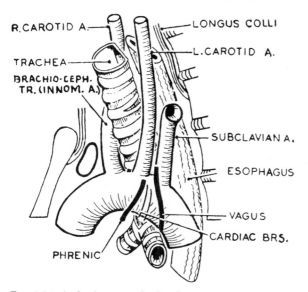

FIG. 2-34. Arch of aorta and related structures.

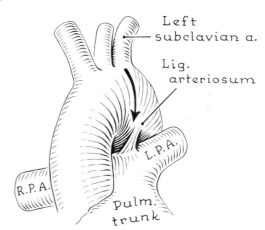

FIG. 2-35. Ligamentum arteriosum (obliterated ductus arteriosus).

The right recurrent laryngeal nerve, which cannot be demonstrated at this time, loops around the right subclavian artery (*Atlas*, 543.1). Since this vessel lies too high to be part of the superior mediastinum, the right recurrent laryngeal nerve is not part of it either. In contrast, the left recurrent laryngeal nerve with its close relation to the aortic arch traverses the superior mediastinum.

If not already done, detach the ascending portion of the aorta from the pericardial sac. Reflect the aortic arch to the left (let your partner hold it, or use a pin to hold it in the reflected position). Once again, identify the ligamentum arteriosum and the left recurrent laryngeal nerve. Observe and clean a number of fine branches from both vagi and sympathetic trunks as they course toward an area between the aortic arch and the bifurcation of the trachea (*Atlas*, 450). This is the site of the **deep cardiac plexus** which is much more extensive than the superficial cardiac plexus.

Observe the **tracheobronchial lymph nodes** on

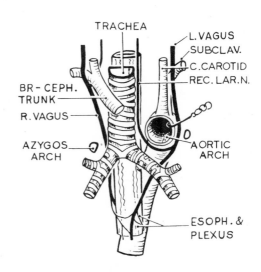

FIG. 2-36. Vagus and recurrent laryngeal nerve. Their relations to trachea and esophagus. (From *Grant's Method of Anatomy*.)

both sides of the trachea and in the vicinity of its bifurcation (*Atlas, 450, 452*). This mass of pigmented nodes fills the angle within the fork of the trachea and intervenes between the right pulmonary artery and esophagus. Be reasonably familiar with the passageways through which the nodes are drained (*Atlas, 453*).

Identify and study the **bifurcation of the trachea** (fig. 2-36; *Atlas, 450–452*). Palpate the anterior and posterior surface of the trachea near its bifurcation. Identify individual **tracheal rings.** Verify that these 'rings' are imperfect: Only the anterior two-thirds of the circumference consists of cartilage. Posteriorly, the tracheal tube is completed by a fibrous membrane. With sturdy scissors, incise the right main

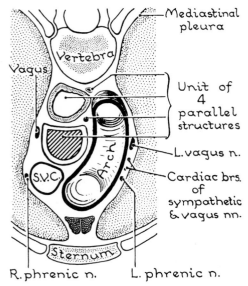

Fig. 2-37. Cross section through superior mediastinum at level of aortic arch.

bronchus. Carry the incision to the tracheal bifurcation. Identify the carina. It is a ridge on the inside of the tracheal bifurcation.

During bronchoscopy, the carina serves as an important landmark. It stands between the superior ends of the right and left main bronchi.

Foreign bodies (paper clips, small metal objects, etc.) are usually aspirated into the right main bronchus. Understand why: (1) the right main bronchus is more vertical, shorter, and wider than the left one (*Atlas, 451*); (2) the carina is usually positioned slightly to the left of the median plane.

Above the level of the aortic arch there are four parallel vertically running structures: **esophagus, trachea, left recurrent laryngeal nerve,** and **thoracic duct.** Study these relations in the cadaver and in a suitable cross section (fig. 2-37 or *Atlas, 448.1, 449.1*). Observe the **esophagus** in front of the vertebral column and projecting slightly to the left of the trachea. The **trachea** is immediately in front of the esophagus. In the angle between esophagus and trachea, the **left recurrent laryngeal nerve** ascends to the larynx. The thoracic duct is small, thin-walled, and easily torn. Make an attempt to find the thoracic duct above the level of the aortic arch. With a blunt probe, search in the area posterior to the left subclavian artery where it ascends subpleurally on the side of the esophagus (*Atlas, 448.1, 451*). Do not waste appreciable time. The structure will be examined again during dissection of the neck (p. 142; *Atlas, 453, 536 B*).

Realize that the superior mediastinum is only an arbitrary subdivision. Many vital structures on their way to or from the neck pass through this space. Therefore, this region should be reviewed again during dissection of the neck. Keep all dissected structures moist with preservative fluid to avoid deterioration.

CHAPTER 3

ABDOMEN

Anterior Abdominal Wall

General Remarks

The contents of the abdominal cavity are protected in front and on the flanks by a wall made up of several layers. These layers are (*Atlas, 113*):
1. Skin.
2. Superficial fascia:
   a. fatty layer (of Camper)
   b. membranous layer (of Scarpa).
3. External oblique. ⎫
4. Internal oblique. ⎬ **three flat muscles**
5. Transversus. ⎭
6. Fascia transversalis.
7. Extraperitoneal fatty areolar tissue.
8. Peritoneum.

On each side of the midline, extending down the length of the anterior abdominal wall, the three flat muscles are reinforced by a longitudinal strap-like muscle. This muscle, the **rectus abdominis,** is enclosed in a sheath produced by the aponeuroses of the three flat muscles (*Atlas, 105*).

The ventral rami of the lower six thoracic nerves enter and supply the abdominal wall (*Atlas, 107*). Note that T_{10} supplies the skin around the umbilicus (*Atlas, 664*). Three nerves (T_9, T_8, T_7) supply the region above the umbilicus; and three nerves (T_{11}, T_{12}, L_1) supply the region below the umbilicus. These segmental nerves run between the two innermost of the three flat muscles (fig. 3-1). (Similarly, the intercostal nerves run between the two innermost of the three intercostal muscles).

In the male, the **testes** are housed in a special outpouching of the anterior abdominal wall, the **scrotum.** The scrotum consists of skin and superficial fascia which is void of fat. Each testis is connected to intrapelvic structures via the **ductus deferens.** The duct and its associated vessels and nerves constitute the major components of the **spermatic cord.** This cord traverses the abdominal wall through an obliquely set canal, the **inguinal canal.** The inguinal canal is of great clinical importance, since loops of intestine may herniate through it. Therefore, this region of the anterior abdominal wall should be studied with particular attention.

In the female, the inguinal canal is relatively small. It contains the **round ligament of the uterus,** a tape-like structure corresponding in position to the spermatic cord of the male. Compare male with female cadavers. If you dissect a female cadaver, substitute in the text 'round ligament' for 'spermatic cord.'

Important Landmarks

Palpate the following (fig. 3-2 or *Atlas, 104.2 A*):
1. **Xiphisternal junction,** at the lower end of the body of the sternum.
2. **Costal margin,** consisting of the upturned ends of cartilages 7 to 10.
3. **Pubic symphysis,** marking the lowest limit of the anterior abdominal wall in the median plane.
4. **Pubic crest,** extending laterally from the symphysis.
5. **Pubic tubercle,** at the lateral end of the pubic crest.
6. **Inguinal ligament,** stretching from the pubic tubercle to the anterior superior iliac spine.
7. **Anterior superior iliac spine,** at the anterior end of the iliac crest.
8. **Tubercle of the crest,** at the most lateral point of the crest.

Plan for Dissection

The three flat muscles (external oblique, internal oblique, transversus) will be studied, particularly in the important inguinal region. The composition and contents of the rectus sheath will be explored. Finally, the anterior abdominal wall will be reflected so that:
1. Full access to the contents of the abdominopelvic cavity is insured.
2. Most components of the abdominal wall can be repositioned for future studies. These studies include a review of the inguinal canal and of the various layers of the abdominal wall.

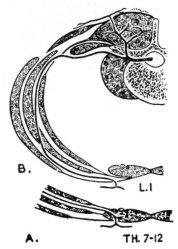

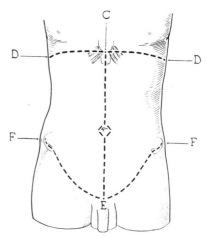

FIG. 3-3. Skin incisions.

FIG. 3-1. Course of a ventral nerve ramus in the abdominal wall. *A*, lower thoracic; *B*, 1st lumbar. (From *Grant's Method of Anatomy*.)

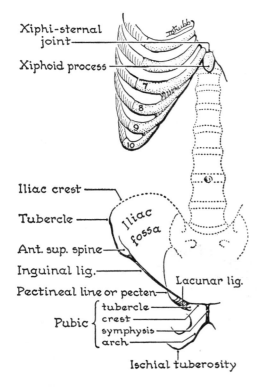

FIG. 3-2. Landmarks and boundaries of the anterior abdominal wall. (From *Grant's Method of Anatomy*.)

Skin Incisions

Place the cadaver into the supine position (face up). Put a block transversely beneath the lumbar region of the back. This procedure stretches the anterior abdominal wall. Make the following skin incisions according to fig. 3-3:

1. Make a midline skin incision from the xiphisternal junction to the symphysis pubis, encircling the umbilicus (C to E).
2. If not already done, make a transverse incision from the upper end of the vertical incision lateralward until stopped by the table (C to D).
3. From the lower end of the vertical incision cut along the pubic crest. Below the course of the inguinal ligament, extend the incision to the anterior superior iliac spine and along the iliac crest (E to F).
4. Reflect the skin of the abdomen laterally.

Dissection of Anterior Abdominal Wall and Inguinal Canal

The superficial fascia (Camper's fascia) may contain various amounts of fat. In this fascia observe the superficial epigastric vein. It passes downward from near the umbilicus toward the inguinal region (*Atlas, 105*).

The right and left superficial epigastric veins are of potential clinical importance: The veins and their anastomoses with the lateral thoracic veins constitute important collateral venous channels to the upper part of the body. These collateral channels are utilized and engorged in patients whose venous blood cannot freely return to the heart (obstruction of the inferior vena cava or portal vein). Under these pathological conditions, the superficial veins in the abdominal wall, especially around the umbilicus, become greatly dilated and tortuous. This phenomenon, known as *caput medusae*, is of important diagnostic value.

Scarpa's fascia (fig. 3-4) (the membranous, deep layer of the superficial fascia) lies immediately superficial to the aponeurosis of the external oblique. This fascia is best distinguished from the underlying aponeurosis at a point approximately 3 cm above the iliac crest and 5 cm behind the anterior superior iliac spine. At this point, incise Scarpa's fascia without cutting into the fleshy fibers of the external oblique. Make sure that the proper plane between Scarpa's fascia and muscular aponeurosis has been reached. Then, continue the incision medially to the midline, about 4 cm above the upper end of the pubic sym-

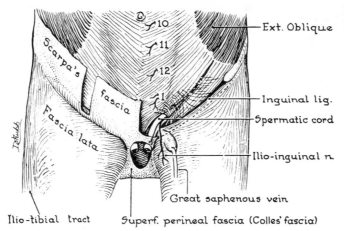

FIG. 3-4. Scarpa's and Colle's fasciae, external oblique, and superficial inguinal ring (penis and scrotum cut away).

physis. **Scarpa's fascia** ends by being attached to the **fascia lata** (i.e. deep fascia of the thigh) along a line 2 cm below the inguinal ligament. Infero-medially, Scarpa's fascia is attached along the pubic arch (where scrotum and skin of the thigh are continuous).

Insert your index finger between **Scarpa's fascia** and the **aponeurosis of the external oblique.** With gentle sweeping movements of the finger, demonstrate the verify that (fig. 3-4).

1. The finger is prevented from descending into the thigh.
2. The finger can be insinuated into the scrotum, but it cannot pass laterally into the thigh.
3. Above the symphysis pubis, the finger is prevented from crossing the median plane by a mass of fibroelastic tissue, the **fundiform ligament** of the penis or clitoris (*Atlas, 110*).

The clinician must be aware of the fascial arrangement of the external genitalia and of the lower abdominal wall. If the penile urethra is injured, urine may escape into the scrotum. From there it may readily spread upward into the lower abdominal wall between Scarpa's fascia and the aponeurosis of the external oblique (fig. 3-4).

Cutaneous Nerves (*Atlas, 105, 106*). Do not injure the underlying aponeurosis of the external oblique. Incise the superficial fascia 5 cm from the midline. Make this incision from the xiphoid process to the symphysis pubis. With the finger or the handle of a scalpel, detach the fascia medially for about 2.5 cm. Now, palpate the **anterior cutaneous nerves.** These nerves are in series with those in the thoracic region. The anterior cutaneous nerves of the abdomen are terminal twigs of the ventral rami (T_7 to L_1). About 4 cm above the pubic crest look for the **anterior cutaneous branch of the ilio-hypogastric nerve** (L_1), the lowest branch on the anterior abdominal wall (*Atlas, 106*). Review the distribution of a spinal nerve (*Atlas, 405*).

The fleshy fibers of the **external oblique** originate above the costal margin (*Atlas, 107*). Observe the fleshy digitations of the external oblique from each of the lower 8 ribs (the upper four interdigitate with serratus anterior, the lower four with the latissimus dorsi). Between the digitations observe the **lateral cutaneous nerves** (T_7 to T_{12}). Each nerve divides into a small posterior branch and a large anterior branch. The posterior branches turn backward over the latissimus dorsi. The anterior branches descend, in the superficial fascia, in line with the fibers of the external oblique (*Atlas, 107*). Trace at least one anterior branch forward to the abdominal wall.

Remove all remains of the superficial fascia. Clean the surface of the **external oblique.** Clearly distinguish between muscular and aponeurotic portion. Observe the curved line of union between these two portions (*Atlas, 105, 107*). Notice the **linea alba** (*Atlas, 106*). It is a whitish groove in the midline of the abdominal wall, formed by interlacing fibers from the right and left sides. About halfway between the xiphoid process and the pubic symphysis, the linea alba is interrupted by the umbilicus.

Carefully clean the aponeurosis of the external oblique in the **inguinal region.** Identify the following structures (*Atlas, 105, 108*).

1. **Superficial inguinal ring.** A triangular aperture in the aponeurosis for the passage of the spermatic cord in the male, or for the passage of the round ligament in the female. The base of the triangle is formed by the pubic crest; its sides are the medial and lateral crura.
2. **Lateral (inferior) crus.** It is formed by the portion of the inguinal ligament attached to the pubic tubercle. The spermatic cord rests on the lateral crus.
3. **Medial (superior) crus** (*Atlas, 108*).
4. **Intercrural fibers.** Lateral to the apex of the triangular gap. They prevent the crura from spreading apart (*Atlas, 108, 109*).
5. **Inguinal ligament** or Poupart's ligament (*Atlas, 109*). The free lower border of the aponeurosis of

the external oblique. Notice its attachment to the anterior superior iliac spine and to the pubic tubercle.

6. **External spermatic fascia.** A delicate, tubular prolongation of the fascia of the external oblique. It is carried down as the outermost covering of the spermatic cord (compare *Atlas, 113*, No. 3).

Identify but do not disturb the **spermatic cord** (round ligament) as it traverses the superficial inguinal ring (*Atlas, 105*). Note the **ilioinguinal nerve** which emerges from the ring lateral to the cord. This nerve sends sensory twigs to the external genitalia and the medial aspect of the thigh. Do not destroy the proximal portion of the nerve. It will be used as a guiding structure for finding the plane between the internal oblique and the transversus abdominis. Clean the space between the spermatic cord and the fundiform ligament of the penis. Remove fat and small external pudendal vessels contained in this space (*Atlas, 105*). Before proceeding, **review the external oblique,** particularly its aponeurosis in the **inguinal region.**

The next objective is to find the plane between the **external oblique** and the underlying **internal oblique.** Proceed as follows: With a pair of scissors, split the fleshy fibers of the external oblique for approximately 10 cm. Start the incision about 5 cm above the iliac crest and proceed in the direction of the muscle fibers. Insert two fingers into the incision, and separate the fibers of the external oblique from the fascia of the underlying internal oblique. Notice that the fibers of the internal oblique take a different direction (*Atlas, 106*). Enlarge the incision. Free the posterior (deep) surface of the external oblique as far as possible with your hand. Medially, the fingers cannot proceed beyond the rectus sheath which is partially formed by the aponeurosis of the external oblique. Extend the incision in the direction of the aponeurotic fibers of the external oblique. Cut as far as 2.5 cm above the superficial inguinal ring.

The next objective is to reflect the external oblique and **expose the internal oblique.** Proceed as follows:

1. Keep your hand as a guide in the plane between the two oblique muscles.
2. Cut the external oblique: From the iliac crest upward, curving medially about 5 cm in front of the digitations of the serratus anterior, to a point corresponding approximately to the 5th costal cartilage.
3. Reflect the lower part of the divided external oblique downward.
4. Reflect the larger upper part of the muscle medially until stopped by the rectus sheath. Now, the anterior surface of the internal oblique is exposed (*Atlas, 106*).

The next objective is to separate the **internal oblique** from the **transversus abdominis.** Clean the anterior surface of the internal oblique and demonstrate the course of its muscle fibers. Do not injure the

ilioinguinal nerve. Clean this nerve and follow it proximally to the point where it traverses the internal oblique (*Atlas, 106*). Now, use the nerve as a guiding structure to determine the plane between the internal oblique and the underlying transversus abdominis. Remember, the ilioinguinal nerve, a branch of L_1, runs in the space between the two innermost muscles (fig. 3–5). With a pair of scissors, split the internal oblique along its fiber course where it is traversed by the ilioinguinal nerve (about 2 to 3 cm above the lower border of the muscle). Insert your finger into the plane between the internal oblique and the transversus abdominis. Push the finger inferiorly and separate the lower borders of the two muscles. If difficulties are encountered, consider the possibility that the internal oblique and the transversus abdominis may be fused. Turn to the 'inguinal' portion of the internal oblique. Above the medial half of the inguinal ligament, it has a free, arched, lower border (fig. 3-6 or *Atlas, 111.1*). In the male subject, notice that some fibers of the internal oblique arise from the lateral portion the arched, lower border and descend as a covering for the spermatic cord and testis. This is the **cremaster muscle.**

The elicitation of the **cremasteric reflex** is part of every routine physical examination in the male patient. When the skin on the

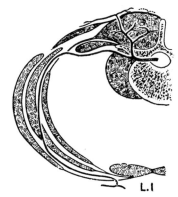

Fig. 3-5. Course of ventral nerve ramus L_1 in abdominal wall. (From *Grant's Method of Anatomy.*)

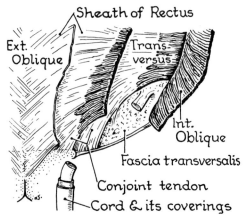

Fig. 3-6. Conjoined tendon and fascia transversalis.

inner side of the thigh is scratched, the testicle on the same side is drawn upward. The afferent fibers of this reflex are carried in the genital branch of the genitofemoral nerve (*Atlas, 248*). Sensory (afferent) fibers of this nerve supply the skin of the scrotum and the adjacent thigh. Motor fibers of this nerve supply the cremaster muscle (efferent reflex arc). Centrally in the spinal cord, the reflex involves segments L_1 and L_2.

Now, pick up the lower free, arched margin of the **transversus.** Notice that it takes a course very similar to that of the internal oblique. In fact, the two structures are often fused. Observe that aponeurotic fibers of both muscles 'join' as the **conjoined tendon (falx inguinalis).** The conjoined tendon is attached to the pubic tubercle and pecten pubis (fig. 3-6 or *Atlas, 111–112*). Hold the free lower margin of the transversus forward and upward. Sweep the handle of the scalpel between it and the underlying **fascia transversalis** (fig. 3-6; *Atlas, 113*, No. 6). This fascia is the internal investing layer which lines the entire abdominal wall. Notice that it is somewhat transparent. Through it you can see some yellowish **extraperitoneal fat** and areolar tissue. The next deeper layer is the **peritoneum** (*Atlas, 113*, No. 8). The peritoneum is the extensive serous membrane which lines the abdominopelvic cavity (this membrane cannot be seen at this time). Roll the spermatic cord laterally and observe the **inferior epigastric vessels** shining through the fascia transversalis (*Atlas, 111, 112*).

Great and prolonged increase in intraabdominal pressure could eventually produce an outward bulging of a sac whose walls are composed of peritoneum, extraperitoneal fat, and fascia transversalis. If this sac (hernial sac) protrudes *medial* to the inferior epigastric vessels, the condition of a **direct inguinal hernia** exist.

Rectus Abdominis (fig. 3-7; *Atlas, 105*). Reposition the cut halves of the external oblique. Outline the approximate location of the **rectus abdominis.** Note that the muscle is three times as wide cranially as it is caudally. The fleshy fibers of the rectus are inserted into the cartilages of ribs 5 to 7. The muscle arises from the symphysis and pecten pubis. Open the **rectus sheath** vertically to display its contents:
1. Below the umbilicus, keep the vertical incision about 12 mm from the midline.
2. Above the umbilicus, make the vertical incision about 25 mm from the midline.
3. Observe that the rectus sheath is firmly attached to the rectus muscle at the 3 **tendinous insertions.** Sever these connections with a scalpel.
4. Carefully mobilize the rectus muscle with your hands, but do *not* remove it. Note that the anterior branches of 6 spinal nerves (T_7 to T_{12}) pierce the rectus sheath laterally. These nerves enter and supply the muscle (fig. 3-8; *Atlas, 106*).
5. In the middle, divide the rectus muscle transversely. Carefully reflect the two halves upward and downward.
6. On the posterior (deep) surface of the inferior

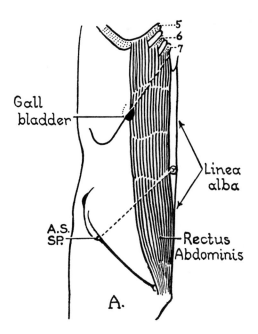

Fig. 3-7. Rectus Abdominis. (From *Grant's Method of Anatomy*.)

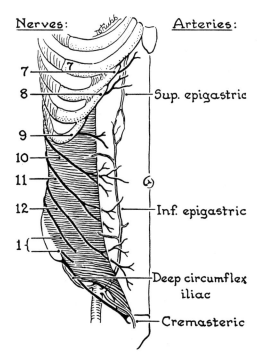

Fig. 3-8. Nerves and arteries within rectus sheath. (From *Grant's Method of Anatomy*.)

half, observe the large **inferior epigastric vessels.**
7. On the posterior (deep) surface of the superior half, note the smaller **superior epigastric vessels.**

The superior and inferior epigastric arteries and veins anastomose (fig. 3-8; *Atlas 106*). If the venous blood from the lower part of the body cannot return freely to the heart (obstruction of inferior vena cava or portal vein), the anastomosing inferior and superior epigastric veins provide an important collateral venous channel to the upper part of the body.

Study the **rectus sheath** (fig. 3-9). Examine the **posterior layer or wall** of the sheath. Identify the **arcuate line,** midway between the symphysis pubis and the umbilicus (*Atlas, 106*). At the level of the arcuate line, the inferior epigastric vessels enter the rectus sheath. Verify this.

The aponeuroses of the three flat abdominal muscles contribute to the formation of the **rectus sheath.** Below the arcuate line, all aponeurotic layers pass ventral to the rectus (fig. 3-9*a*); only the transversalis fascia remains dorsal to the muscle. Above the level of the arcuate line, the aponeurosis of the internal oblique splits: Together with the aponeurosis of the transversus it forms the posterior layer; together with the aponeurosis of the external oblique, it forms the anterior layer of the rectus sheath (fig. 3-9, *b* and *c*). At the level of the xiphoid process, only the aponeurosis of the external oblique contributes to the rectus sheath (fig. 3-9*d*).

Inferior to the arcuate line, remove the **transversalis fascia.** Remove the **extraperitoneal fat** and areolar tissue, and thus expose the **peritoneum.** Do *not* incise this membrane.

The **linea alba** is formed by decussating fibers of the aponeuroses of the right and left flat abdominal muscles (external oblique; internal oblique; transversus). Above the umbilicus the linea alba is a band,

about 2 cm wide (fig. 3-7 or *Atlas, 105.1*) Below the umbilicus it is a thin line since the two recti muscles come into contact with each other. The linea alba is a raphe or decussation, and therefore is extensile.

The next objective is to reflect the anterior abdominal wall in such a manner that:
1. Full access to the contents of the abdominopelvic cavity is ensured.
2. Most components of the abdominal wall can be repositioned for future studies.

Proceed in the following manner: Detach the fleshy fibers of the rectus from ribs 5 to 7, and sever the superior epigastric artery close to the muscle. Make a vertical incision through the linea alba, keeping on the left side about 1 cm from the midline (to preserve the obliterated umbilical vein). Make a 3 cm long vertical incision just left of the xiphoid process. Be careful not to injure the contents of the abdominal cavity. Place the index finger of one hand through the incision into the abdominal cavity. With your finger, pull the anterior abdominal wall forward, thereby creating a gap between abdominal wall and abdominal contents. Now, it is safe to extend the vertical incision inferiorly. Cut around the umbilicus on the left side so that it remains attached to the right side of the abdominal wall. Below the umbilicus, continue the incision on the left, about 5 mm from the midline and as close as possible to the left rectus sheath (to preserve the obliterated urachus). Continue the incision to the symphysis pubis.

Subsequently, place one hand into the left side of the abdominal cavity to separate abdominal wall from

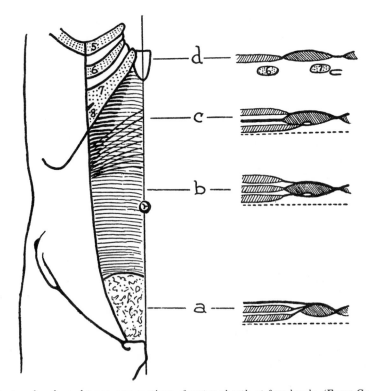

FIG. 3-9. Posterior wall of rectus sheath, and transverse sections of rectus sheath at four levels. (From *Grant's Method of Anatomy.*)

abdominal contents. With the scalpel in the other hand, detach the left abdominal wall from the rib cage. Starting at the xiphoid process, follow the inferior border of rib 10; then carry the cut to the left iliac crest. Reflect the left side of the anterior abdominal wall downward.

Before reflecting the right side of the abdominal wall, establish the following facts:

1. The **falciform ligament** spans the space between the anterior abdominal wall and liver (*Atlas, 125*).
2. Contained in the lower free margin of the falciform ligament is the **ligamentum teres.** This is the obliterated umbilical vein which, in the fetus, carried blood from the umbilical cord to the liver (Appendix, p. 167).

Make sure that your dissecting partners have seen these two structures. Now, detach the falciform ligament from the anterior abdominal wall and sever the ligamentum teres. Subsequently, reflect the right side of the anterior abdominal wall in the same manner as the left side.

Review the various layers of the **abdominal wall.** At the rib cage, observe the attachments of the three severed, flat abdominal muscles:

1. The origin of the **external oblique** from the *external* surface of the lower ribs.
2. The insertion of the **internal oblique** into the *inferior* surface of the lower ribs.
3. The origin of the **transversus abdominis** from the *inner* surfaces of the lower ribs.

Review the **inguinal canal** and its walls. Gently push a probe through the superficial inguinal ring parallel to the spermatic cord. Hold the probe in place while examining the inner aspect of the abdominal wall. Find the probe pushing against the **deep inguinal ring.** The length of the obliquely set inguinal canal is about 4 to 5 cm. Verify this. **Review the walls of the inguinal canal** (fig. 3-10).

1. *Ventral:* Mainly the **aponeurosis of the external oblique.**
2. *Caudal* (floor): **Inguinal ligament** and fibers of its medial end which are rolled under the spermatic cord. This is the **lacunar ligament** (*Atlas, 109*).
3. *Dorsal:* Reflex inguinal ligament (*Atlas, 109*), **conjoined tendon** (falx inguinalis), and fascia transversalis.
4. *Cranial* (roof): **Arches of internal oblique and transversus abdominis.**

The inguinal canal is like an arcade of three arches traversed by the spermatic cord (fig. 3-11). During standing, coughing, or vigorous straining, the abdominal muscles contract. The arched fleshy fibers of the internal oblique and transversus cause the roof of the canal to become lower and taut. The action is essentially that of a half-sphincter.

An enlarged or congenitally patent inguinal canal is a potential channel through which abdominal viscera may protrude. The protruding viscera are contained in a hernial sac, which is an

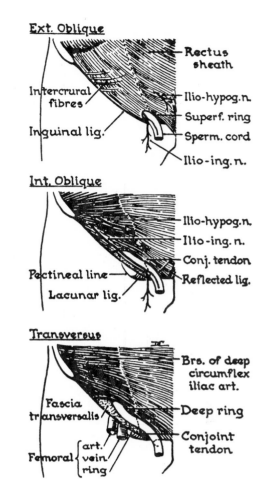

FIG. 3-10. Contribution of the three flat muscles to the inguinal canal. (From *Grant's Method of Anatomy.*)

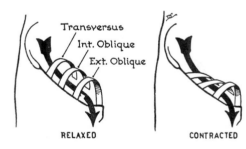

FIG. 3-11. The inguinal canal likened to an arcade of three arches traversed by the spermatic cord. (From *Grant's Method of Anatomy.*)

outpouching of the peritoneal membrane. Hernias through the inguinal canal are called **indirect hernias.** In contrast to the direct inguinal hernia, the indirect hernia is located *lateral* to the inferior epigastric vessels.

Briefly look at the peritoneal aspect of the umbilical region. The obliterated remains of four fetal structures radiate from it. These are:

1. The **ligamentum teres** of the liver (already seen).
2. The obliterated allantoid duct or **urachus,** as-

cending from the apex of the bladder (*Atlas, 205, 233*).

3. The **obliterated umbilical artery,** one on each side (*Atlas, 205, 233*).

Scrotum, Spermatic Cord, and Testis

Exposure of Spermatic Cord and Testis. Free the cord from the surrounding fat. Push your index finger into the scrotal sac so that the finger intervenes between testis medially and scrotal wall laterally. With the finger in this position, make an incision half way down the scrotum, through the skin, dartos, and superficial fascia. Free the testis and cord from the surrounding areolar tissue and shell it out of the scrotum. Snip the band of tissue which anchors the lower pole of the testis to the scrotum. This is the **gubernaculum testis.**

Observe that the **scrotal sac** is divided into two pouches by a median septum. Verify that the superficial fascia of the scrotum is void of fat. It contains a layer of involuntary muscle fibers, the **dartos,** which controls the surface area of the scrotum.

Coverings of the Cord (*Atlas, 113, 117*). Carefully incise the tubular coverings of the cord longitudinally:

1. **External spermatic fascia,** the thin outermost covering.
2. **Cremasteric fascia,** the middle covering. It is areolar and contains loops of cremaster muscle.
3. **Internal spermatic fascia,** the filmy innermost covering of the spermatic cord.

Constituents of the Cord. The **ductus (vas) deferens** is easily identified. It is located in the posterior portion of the cord, and is hard and cord-like in consistency. Using the sharp-sharp scissor technique, free it for 5 to 8 cm. Look for the small **deferent artery** that clings to it. Free a larger artery, the **testicular artery,** which runs with the **pampiniform plexus of veins.** Trace the ductus deferens up to the deep inguinal ring and note that it hooks around the lateral side of the inferior epigastric vessels. Be aware of, but do not search for other components of the cord: *Lymph vessels* which drain the testis (not the scrotum); *autonomic nerve fibers* running with the testicular artery and the ductus deferens.

Testis (*Atlas, 114–119*). Carefully remove any superficial areolar tissue that may adhere to the **tunica vaginalis testis.** The tunica vaginalis is a closed serous sac of peritoneal origin. During development, testis and epididymis invaginated into the posterior wall of this sac. Demonstrate the extent of the sac by injecting air or water into it (use syringe and fine needle). Observe that the (artificially distended) cavity covers the anterior, medial, and lateral surfaces of the testis.

Under pathological conditions, the potential space of the tunica vaginalis testis may be enlarged and distended by blood (hemato-

cele) or serous fluid (hydrocele). A hydrocele can eventually become as large as or larger than a fist. Taking into account the topographic relations of tunica vaginalis and testis, understand that in hydrocele the testis can *only* be palpated posterior to the swelling.

Incise the tunica vaginalis testis and inspect the interior of the serous sac. On the lateral side, identify the *sinus* of the epididymis which separates the testis from the **body of the epididymis** (*Atlas, 116*). The visceral layer of the sac covers the testis and the head of the epididymis. Carefully incise the sac at its reflection from the testis.

Trace the vas deferens to the tail of the **epididymis** (*Atlas, 118*). Here, the vas is thin-walled and easily torn. If time permits, unravel part of the epididymis. The epididymis consists of a single convoluted duct of considerable length. With a probe, free some of the 15 to 20 fine **efferent ductules** between superior pole of the testis and head of epididymis. From the cord, trace blood vessels to the testis (*Atlas, 119*).

Longitudinally, incise the front of the testis from upper to lower pole (*Atlas, 114*). Notice the thickness of its fibrous capsule, the **tunica albuginea.** Look for fibrous strands which divide the interior of the testis into numerous lobules. Tease some of these lobules apart, and note the fine thread-like **seminiferous tubules.**

Abdominopelvic Cavity

General Remarks

The **peritoneum** is a thin, translucent, serous membrane. To understand its complexities, certain fundamental facts must be appreciated:

1. It lines the walls of the abdominal cavity.
2. It forms a completely **closed sac** or cavity, except in the female where the mouths of the uterine tubes open into it.
3. Immediately outside of it is an extraperitoneal (subperitoneal) fatty layer. In this layer the organs and their vessels develop and lie.
4. 'Retroperitoneal' organs remain behind (retro) the sac and are merely covered in front with peritoneum. In general, this applies to the urinary system.
5. An organ which invaginates the sac is invested in peritoneum. The outer investment is the **serous coat** of the organ. In general, this applies to the gastrointestinal system.
6. The mobility of an organ depends to a great extent on its peritoneal covering.
7. Two layers of peritoneum are attached to each of the two curvatures of the stomach. They are the **omenta.** The **lesser omentum** is attached to the *lesser* curvature and the **greater omentum** is attached to the *greater* curvature.
8. **Mesenteries** are two layers of peritoneum

which 'sling' the intestine from the posterior abdominal wall. Vessels and nerves travel to and from the intestine between the two layers.

9. All other double layers and folds of peritoneum are called **peritoneal ligaments.**

10. **Folds or plicae** may be produced by blood vessels and ducts lifting the peritoneum off the body wall.

11. Everywhere within the peritoneal cavity, peritoneum is in contact with peritoneum. The cavity is merely a potential space containing a small amount of lubricating serous fluid. Thus, intra-abdominal organs can move upon each other without friction.

Under certain pathological conditions, the potential space of the peritoneal cavity may be distended into an actual space containing several liters of fluid. This accumulation of serous fluid in the peritoneal cavity is known as ascites. Also, other substances (e.g. blood from a ruptured spleen; bile from a ruptured bile duct; fecal matter from ruptured intestine) may accumulate in the abdominal cavity.

Inspection of Abdominal Cavity and Contents

Work will be much more pleasant if you clean the entire surface of the peritoneal cavity with a damp sponge. Always keep the cavity and its contents moist with mold-deterrent preservative fluid.

Inspect. Do not dissect at this time. Study the dispositions of various organs and of the peritoneum. You may encounter pathological conditions (e.g. cancer; enlarged liver or spleen; etc.). As a result of old inflammatory processes, *adhesions* (strands of fibrous tissue) may exist between the opposing surfaces of peritoneal membranes. These adhesions must be broken down with your fingers. **Identify**, merely identify the following structures (fig. 3-12; *Atlas, 124, 125*):

1. **Diaphragm,** forming the roof of the abdomen.
2. **Liver,** divided into a **right** and a **left lobe** by the **falciform ligament.** This ligament connects the liver to the diaphragm and to the anterior abdominal wall in the median plane. Place your opened hand into the potential space between diaphragm and right lobe of liver.
3. **Gall bladder.** It projects to the lateral margin of the right rectus abdominis (*Atlas, 105.1*). It is attached to visceral (inferior) surface of liver. Reaches beyond the sharp inferior border of the liver.
4. **Stomach or gaster** (*Atlas, 124–126*). It may be dilated and conspicuous or contracted and less evident. It is connected to the liver by the lesser omentum. From the caudal border of the greater curvature of the stomach hangs the fatty peritoneal apron, the **greater omentum** (fig. 3-12). Spread out this structure to appreciate its size and extent. It is draped over the transverse colon

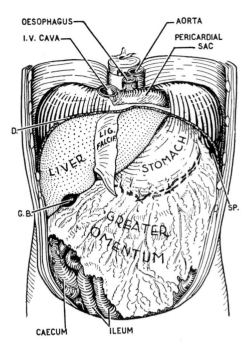

Fig. 3-12. Abdominal contents, undisturbed. *G.B.,* gall bladder; *SP,* Spleen; *D,* cut edge of diaphragm. (From *Grants' Method of Anatomy.*)

and portions of small intestine. If adhesions exist between small intestine and greater omentum, break them down with your fingers.

5. **Spleen of lien** (figs. 3–12, 3–13; *Atlas, 124*). It lies behind stomach in contact with the diaphragm. It is connected to the left part of the greater curvature of the stomach by two layers of peritoneum, the **gastrolienal (gastrosplenic) ligament** (*Atlas, 130.2*).

Now, reflect the greater omentum cranially over the costal margin and thereby uncover the following structures:

6. **Small intestine** (*Atlas, 124*). The mobile coils of the jejunum and ileum are visible (combined length approximately 6 meters). The small intestine terminates by emptying into the cecum, a large blind pouch of the large intestine (fig. 3-13).

7. **Large intestine** (fig. 3-13; *Atlas, 124*). The large intestine frames the small intestine on three sides:
   a. On the right side, the **ascending colon.**
   b. Superiorly, the **tranverse colon.**
   c. On the left side, the **descending colon** and the **sigmoid colon.**

In the abdomen, follow the **alimentary canal (G.I. tract)** from its beginning to its end. Realize that certain parts of the G.I. tract are not immediately accessible (e.g. duodenum; pancreas) and, therefore, cannot be demonstrated at this time. Study the names and general dispositions of the parts of the G.I. tract from proximal to distal ends (*Atlas, 124*):

Identify the **stomach.** The exit from the stomach is

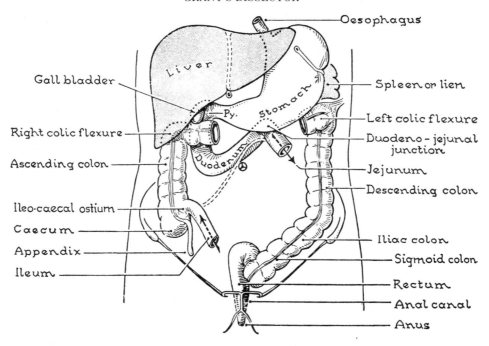

FIG. 3-13. Various parts of the digestive tract, and their dispositions. (From *Grant's Method of Anatomy*.)

the **pylorus.** Observe the right concave border of the stomach. This is the **lesser curvature.** The lesser curvature and the first 3 cm of the duodenum are the attachment sites for the **lesser omentum** which continues to the liver (*Atlas*, *126*, *130*). The lesser omentum is divisible into two parts: The **hepatogastric** and the **hepatoduodenal ligaments** (fig. 3-14). The left and inferior **greater curvature** of the stomach is long and convex. Attached to it is the **greater omentum.** The two important parts of the greater omentum are its **gastrocolic** (from gaster to colon) and **gastro-lienal** (from gaster to lien) **portions** (fig. 3-14).

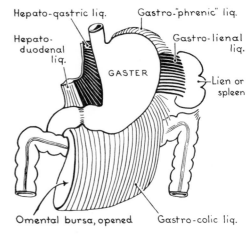

FIG. 3-14. Diagram of subdivisions of omenta.

The greater omentum varies remarkably from subject to subject. In the emaciated person, it may be as thin as a sheet of paper. In contrast, obese subjects usually have a greater omentum of considerable thickness and weight. In the living individual, the greater omentum is highly movable. It has a tendency to cover and seal off inflamed areas, thus preventing generalized infection of the peritoneal cavity (peritonitis). Occasionally, the greater omentum becomes part of the contents in a hernial sac.

Next, inspect the **small intestine.** It consists of three parts: **Duodenum, jejunum,** and **ileum:**

The **duodenum** (*Atlas*, *124*) immediately succeeds the pyloric portion of the stomach. Its first inch is mobile and was noted in association with the hepatoduodenal ligament (fig. 3-14). The remainder of the duodenum is inaccessible at the present time. Realize that it is C-shaped and molded around the head of the pancreas. The duodenum is attached to the structures ventral to the posterior abdominal wall. Find its termination, the **duodenojejunal junction:** Pull the mobile small intestine to the right side, then follow

the jejunum proximally as far as possible. Find the point where the immobile duodenum ends and the mobile jejunum begins. This is the duodenojejunal junction (*Atlas*, *163*; *163.1*).

Immediately succeeding the duodenum is the mobile part of the small intestine. It consists of **jejunum** (proximal ⅖) and **ileum** (distal ⅗). The ileum empties into the **cecum** at the **ileocecal orifice or junction.** Note that the distance between duodenojejunal junction and ileocecal junction is about 15 to 20 cm. Yet, the total length of small intestine accommodated between these two points is about 20 feet (or 6 meters). Find out how this is possible. Verify that the **root of the mesentery** of the mobile part of the small intestine stretches diagonally across the posterior wall from duodenojejunal to ileocecal junction (fig. 3-13; *Atlas*, *163*). This root is only 15 to 20 cm long. However, the **intestinal border of the mesentery** is elaborately ruffled to accommodate the substantial length of jejunum and ileum. The small intestine is so convoluted and mobile that you can pass many feet of it through your hands without knowing whether you are proceeding to its duodenal end or its cecal end. However, by placing a hand on each side of the mesentery and drawing the fingers forward (ventrally) from root to intestinal border, the convolutions are locally untwisted and the direction of the gut becomes obvious.

Next, turn your attention to the **large intestine** (*Atlas, 124*). It consists of **cecum** with attached **appendix, colon** (ascending; transverse; descending; sigmoid), **rectum,** and **anal canal.** Observe the following features:

1. **Cecum** [L., caecus = blind]. Extends caudalward beyond the ileo-cecal junction into the right iliac fossa. The length of its mesentery, i.e. the degree of its mobility varies considerably.

2. **Vermiform appendix** [L., vermis = worm; forma = shape; appendere = to hang on]. Opens into the cecum below the ileocecal orifice (fig. 3-13; *Atlas, 124; 170*). May occupy any position consistent with its length. Most commonly found retrocecal, i.e. behind the cecum (fig. 3-15). Its mesentery is a triangular fold of peritoneum, the mesoappendix (*Atlas, 169*).

3. **Ascending colon** [Gk., kolon = large intestine; hollow]. Has no mesentery; therefore, it is attached to the posterior abdominal wall. Ascends to the liver where it makes a right-angle bend. This is the **right colic flexure** or hepatic flexure (fig. 3-13).

4. **Transverse colon.** Extends transversely from **right colic flexure** to **left colic flexure** or splenic flexure. The left colic flexure is attached to the diaphragm by the **phrenicocolic ligament** which also forms a shelf to support the spleen. The left colic flexure is at a more superior level and a more posterior plane than the right colic flexure. Between the two flexures, the transverse colon is freely movable. Its mesentery, the **transverse mesocolon,** is con-

nected to the inferior border of the pancreas (fig. 3-16). Also adherent to the transverse colon is the **greater omentum** (fig. 3-16). The portion of the greater omentum between stomach and transverse colon is called the gastrocolic ligament (fig. 3-14).

5. **Descending colon.** Descends from the sharply curved left colic flexure to the pelvic brim. Is of considerably smaller caliber than the ascending colon. Its posterior surface is attached to the posterior abdominal wall.

6. **Sigmoid colon** [Gk., resembling old letter sigma]. Has long mesentery and, therefore, considerable freedom of movement. Identify the point where the mesentery, the **sigmoid mesocolon,** ends. Here, the sigmoid colon is continuous with the rectum (*Atlas, 202*).

7. **Rectum** [L., rectus = straight]. The rectum is only partially covered with peritoneum (*Atlas, 202, 203*). Its relation to other pelvic structures will be studied later (p. 51).

8. The outer longitudinal muscular coat of the large intestine is concentrated into three narrow bands, the **teniae coli.** The three teniae begin at the appendix (*Atlas, 165, 169*). The anterior tenia is easily visible in gross specimens (fig. 3-17).

9. Since the teniae are shorter than the other layers of the colon, they cause the formation of characteristic sacculations called **haustra** (fig. 3-17; *Atlas, 170*).

10. Appendices epiploicae are small bags of fat which hang from the colon throughout its length (fig. 3-17; *Atlas, 164*).

Now, return the greater omentum to its original position. Study the upper abdominal viscera and their disposition in the abdominal cavity:

Liver or Hepar [Gk., hepar = liver]. The largest organ in the body, weighing 1.2 to 1.6 kg. Note that its **right lobe** is about six times as large as the **left.**

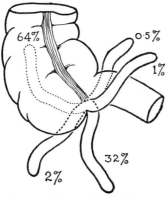

FIG. 3-15. Various positions of vermiform appendix. (From *Grant's Method of Anatomy.*)

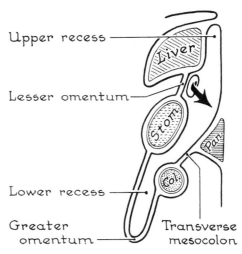

FIG. 3-16. Transverse colon (*col.*), its mesentery, and the greater omentum.

Observe the two surfaces of the liver, **diaphragmatic surface** and **visceral surface**:

1. **Diaphragmatic surface.** In contact with the diaphragm. Very extensive, convex, and smooth (*Atlas, 125*).

2. **Visceral surface.** In contact with viscera (stomach, duodenum, colon, right kidney). Concave and irregular, facing inferiorly, to the left and posteriorly. Pull the sharp lower margin of the liver forward, expose the visceral surface (fig. 3-18; *Atlas, 136, 136.1 C*), and observe two important structures:

   a. The **gallbladder.** Study its four contact relations: Liver, duodenum, colon, and anterior abdominal wall (fig. 3-19; *Atlas, 126.1*). These relations are of clinical importance: An inflamed gallbladder may become adherent to the intestinal tract. Subsequently, a cholecystoenteric fistula may develop through which gallstones and bile could enter the G.I. tract.

   b. The **porta hepatis** (*Atlas, 136*). The porta hepatis is the 'doorway' to the liver. Identify it by looking for a 5 cm transverse fissure through which vessels, ducts, and nerves enter and exit.

Once again identify the **lesser omentum** as it stretches from the lesser curvature of the stomach and from the initial portion of the duodenum to the visceral surface of the liver (fig. 3-18; *Atlas, 136*). Focus your attention on the right free margin of the lesser omentum, the **hepatoduodenal ligament.** Between the two peritoneal layers of this ligament are the structures that pass to the porta hepatis: **Hepatic**

artery, portal vein, bile passages, autonomic nerves and lymphatics. Stand on the right side of the cadaver. With the hand palm up, place your index finger behind (dorsal to) the hepatoduodenal ligament in the direction of the *arrow* shown in figure 3-18. Your finger will pass through the **epiploic foramen** (of Winslow) into the **omental bursa or lesser sac** (*Atlas, 126, 130.1*). In front of your finger is the hepatoduodenal ligament with its important contents.

Omental Bursa and Peritoneal Reflections

The **exploration of the omental bursa** (lesser sac) will be easier if its **anterior wall,** the **lesser omentum,** is partially removed: Break through the filmy membrane that stretches between lesser curvature of stomach and liver. Leave the hepatoduodenal ligament and its contents undisturbed. Place your hand into the widely opened lesser sac and study its extent:

1. Push your finger horizontally toward the far left. Here, the **peritoneal attachments of the spleen** are the boundaries of the lesser sac (fig. 3-20 or *Atlas, 130.2*).

2. Direct your fingers downward (figs. 3-20, 3-21; *Atlas, 130.1*). They will pass behind the stomach and, at the same time, in front of the pancreas

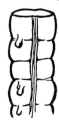

FIG. 3-17. Segment of colon showing appendices epiploicae, haustra, and one of the three teniae. (From *Grant's Method of Anatomy.*)

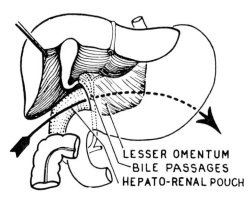

FIG. 3-18. Entrance into omental bursa through epiploic foramen.

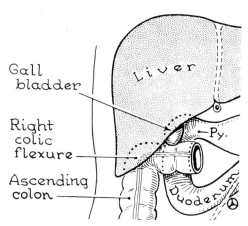

FIG. 3-19. Interrelation of gallbladder, duodenum, and colon.

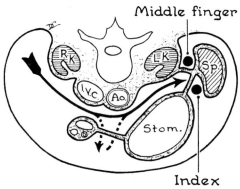

FIG. 3-20. Horizontal extent of omental bursa (lesser sac): To palpate 'pedicle' of spleen.

and transverse mesocolon. Then, the fingers will pass into the **lower recess** which lies between the two double layers of the gastrocolic ligament. Occasionally, the lower recess of the omental bursa is shut off from the main portion by adhesions. If these cannot be broken down, incise the anterior double layer of the gastrocolic ligament about 2.5 cm below the stomach and try to enter the lesser recess via that route.

3. Pass your middle finger upward in the median plane between liver and posterior aspect of diaphragm (fig. 3–21). Your finger is now in the **upper recess** of the omental bursa. Palpate the structures bordering this cul-de-sac (fig. 3–22): Posterior to your finger is the diaphragm; anteriorly the caudate lobe of the liver; to the left the abdominal portion of the esophagus; to the right the large inferior vena cava.

Next, examine the **peritoneal attachments of the spleen** (fig. 3–20 or *Atlas, 130.2*). Stand on the right side of the cadaver and push your right hand between diaphragm and spleen until the spleen lies scooped in

the palm. Pass your middle finger dorsal to the spleen until stopped by the **lienorenal ligament,** which stretches from spleen to kidney. Now, place your left fingers into the lesser sac and palpate the intervening lienorenal ligament. Next, leave your left hand in the omental bursa, place the right index finger between greater curvature of stomach and spleen, and palpate the intervening **gastrolienal ligament** (fig. 3–20 or *Atlas, 130.2*). Understand that these two ligaments, lienorenal and gastrolienal, suspend the spleen between kidney and stomach. They form a **pedicle** (stalk) which transmits blood vessels to and from the hilus of the spleen. From your observations and from the diagram in figure 3–20 it should be obvious that:

1. The lienorenal and gastrolienal ligaments are double layers of peritoneum.
2. Their inner layers are composed of peritoneum of the omental bursa (lesser sac).
3. Their outer layers are composed of peritoneum of the peritoneal cavity (greater sac).
4. Both ligaments form the left boundary of the omental bursa.
5. The spleen itself is covered with peritoneum of the greater sac.

Now, examine the **peritoneal attachments of the liver** (fig. 3–23; *Atlas, 130.3; 131*). Provide better access to the hepatic region by cutting the right costal cartilages 6 and 7 near the xiphisternal junction and by partially incising the diaphragm.

Once again identify the **falciform ligament of the liver** (*Atlas, 125*). Place your right hand between diaphragm and left lobe of liver; simultaneously, place your left hand between diaphragm and the larger right hepatic lobe. Verify that:

1. The hands cannot meet because of the intervening falciform ligament (compare fig. 3–24).
2. The hands can be pushed dorsally for a considerable distance between diaphragm and diaphragmatic surface of the liver *until* stopped by the

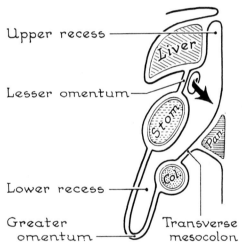

Fig. 3-21. Walls of omental bursa on median section (as seen from inside).

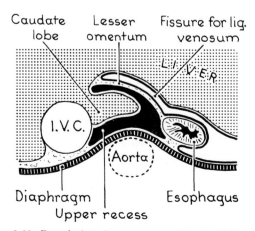

Fig. 3-22. Boundaries of upper recess of omental bursa (cross section viewed from below).

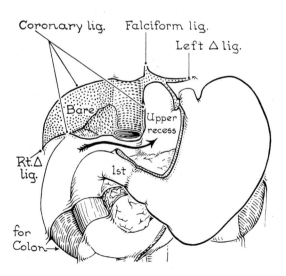

Fig. 3-23. Peritoneal attachments of the liver (liver removed).

reflections of peritoneum from liver onto the diaphragm (*Atlas, 130.3*).

These peritoneal reflections from liver onto diaphragm leave an irregular triangular area of the liver without peritoneal covering. Therefore, this uncovered area is called the **bare area** of the liver (*Atlas, 130.3; 136*). Figure 3–23 shows the area of the diaphragm which is in contact with the bare area of the liver. The peritoneal reflections around the bare area are called the **coronary ligament** (fig. 3–23; *Atlas, 130.3, 131*). The peritoneal fold attaching the left tip of the left hepatic lobe to the diaphragm is the **left triangular ligament.** Palpate it. The cranial reflection of the coronary ligament is continuous with the falciform ligament. The caudal part of the coronary ligament is reflected onto the diaphragm and the right kidney; therefore, it is alternatively called the **hepato-renal ligament** (*Atlas, 130.3*).

Below the hepatorenal ligament is a potential peritoneal space, the **hepatorenal pouch or recess** (of Morison). This pouch is bounded by liver, kidney, colon, and duodenum. It is surgically important. It lies at the lowest point of the peritoneal cavity when the subject is recumbent (fig. 3–25 or *Atlas, 130.4*).

Peritoneal Gutters (fig. 3–26). The mesentery of the mobile small intestine, the ascending colon, and the descending colon are attached to the posterior abdominal wall in a characteristic fashion. As a result, **four gutters** exist which can conveniently conduct materials (ascites; inflammatory material;

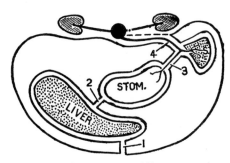

FIG. 3-24. Peritoneal investment of liver, stomach and spleen, and related peritoneal ligaments. *1*, falciform lig.; *2*, lesser omentum; *3*, gastrolienal lig.; *4*, lienorenal lig. (From *Grant's Method of Anatomy*.)

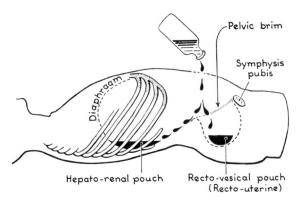

FIG. 3-25. Lowest parts of the peritoneal cavity.

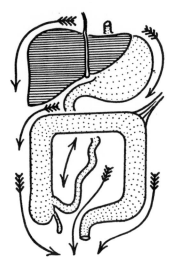

FIG. 3-26. Gutters in the peritoneal cavity. (From *Grant's Method of Anatomy*.)

blood; bile; etc.) from one point of the peritoneal cavity to another. Identify in the cadaver (fig. 3–26):

1. The **right lateral (paracolic) gutter,** to the right of the ascending colon. It may conduct fluid from the omental bursa *via* the hepatorenal pouch into the pelvis.
2. The **left lateral (paracolic) gutter** to the left of the descending colon. It is closed cranially by the phrenicocolic ligament.
3. The gutter to the right of the mesentery. It is closed cranially and caudally.
4. The gutter to the left of the mesentery. It opens widely into the pelvis.

Plan for Dissection

The vessels and ducts connecting the porta hepatis with other abdominal structures will be dissected. Next, the branches of the three unpaired abdominal arteries (celiac; superior and inferior mesenteric) will be followed to their fields of supply. On the other hand, the drainage of the G.I. tract into the portal venous system will be studied. Subsequently, the entire G.I. tract will be removed as a unit together with its 3 unpaired glands (liver, pancreas, and spleen). This *en bloc* extirpation offers several advantages:

1. No essential structures will be destroyed. The unity of the G.I. tract will be maintained.
2. By turning the removed viscera over, a posterior (dorsal) approach to organs, vessels, and ducts is possible.
3. The student will be able to study the G. I. tract repeatedly and in detail.
4. The organs can be replaced into the abdominal cavity, and topographical relations can be reestablished.

Bile Passages, Celiac Trunk, and Portal Vein

The following dissection requires time, patience, and adequate preparation on your part. Insert your finger into the epiploic foramen. Anterior to your finger lies the remaining free edge of the lesser omentum, the hepatoduodenal ligament, with its contents: Bile passages, hepatic artery, portal vein, autonomic nerves, and lymphatics. Replace the finger with a roll of white paper. Then, remove the peritoneum from the right free edge of the lesser omentum until the common **bile duct** is exposed (fig. 3–27; *Atlas, 147, 148*). The bile duct has the caliber of a pencil. It is thin-walled and usually empty and collapsed. By careful dissection, establish that the bile duct is connected to the gallbladder via the **cystic duct** (*Atlas, 142, 156*). Then, follow the bile passages toward the liver and identify the **common hepatic duct,** and the rather short right and left hepatic ducts. Be mindful of the possible variations of the cystic and hepatic ducts (*Atlas, 161 A and B*).

Note that the structures in the hepatoduodenal ligament are surrounded and accompanied by a substantial network of autonomic nerve fibers. Discard these nerves, and focus your attention on the bile passages and blood vessels. Using the scissor technique, carefully free the **hepatic artery,** which lies on the left side of the bile duct (fig. 3–27; *Atlas, 142, 147*). Proceed with intelligence. Be aware of the ramifications of the **common hepatic artery** and of its origin from the **celiac trunk** (fig. 3–28 or *Atlas, 132.1, 145*). Follow the common hepatic artery to the celiac trunk, a very short unpaired vessel which originates directly from the abdominal aorta immediately caudal to the diaphragm (*Atlas, 132.3, 188*). At the upper border of the first portion of the duodenum, the **common hepatic artery** divides into the **gastroduodenal artery** and the **hepatic artery proper.** Dissect the hepatic artery and its branches (fig. 3–28; *Atlas, 145*):

1. **Right gastric artery,** to the lesser curvature of the stomach.
2. **Left hepatic artery,** to the left lobe of the liver.
3. **Right hepatic artery,** to the right lobe of the liver.
4. **Cystic artery** (fig. 3–29), a slender branch, usually arising from the right hepatic artery.

Anatomical dissectors and surgeons alike must be aware of common variations in the hepatic and cystic arterial supply. If the arterial distribution in the cadaver does not conform with the usual pattern (fig. 3–28; *Atlas, 142*) consider alternate possibilities (*Atlas, 143, 144*). In about 12% of the cases, the right hepatic artery is aberrant and arises as a separate vessel from the superior mesenteric artery.

Next, dissect the two other branches of the celiac trunk:

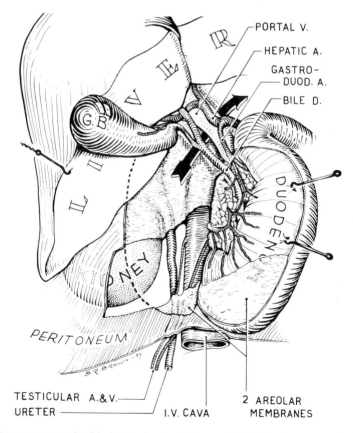

FIG. 3-27. Structures contained in hepatoduodenal ligament. Epiploic foramen marked by *arrow.*

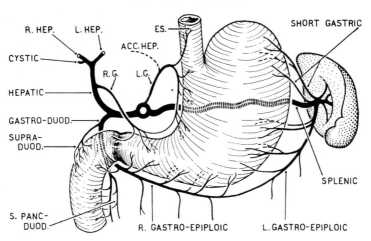

FIG. 3-28. Celiac trunk (artery) and its branches.

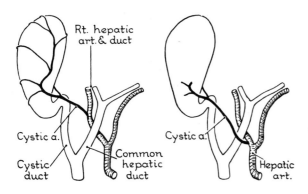

FIG. 3-29. Where to look for the cystic artery.

1. The large **splenic artery** (fig. 3–28; *Atlas, 158, 158.1*). Follow it for 2 to 3 cm along the superior border of the pancreas. Do not dissect it further at this time.
2. The **left gastric artery** (fig. 3–28; *Atlas, 132*). Follow it to the lesser curvature of the stomach. Observe that it anastomoses with the **right gastric artery** to form an arterial arch along the lesser curvature.

Along the greater curvature of the stomach, examine the arterial arch formed by the **right and left gastroepiploic arteries.** Clean the right **gastroepiploic artery** and follow it behind the first part of the duodenum where it arises from the gastroduodenal artery. Next, carefully clean the left gastroepiploic artery, and follow it through the fatty greater omentum toward the spleen. Leave the arterial arch attached to the greater curvature of the stomach, but sever the greater omentum (gastrocolic lig.) just inferior to the arterial arch. The greater omentum is still attached to the transverse colon. Understand why the detachment of the gastrocolic ligament from the stomach provides a wide access to the omental bursa (fig. 3–21 or *Atlas, 130.1*), particularly if the stomach is pulled cranially. Observe that the pancreas is readily accessible. Let your partner pull the spleen forward while you are tracing the **left gastro-epiploic**

artery to the hilus of the spleen and to the splenic artery (fig. 3–28; *Atlas, 132*). Next, complete the dissection of the splenic artery. Observe that it contributes branches to the body and tail of the pancreas (*Atlas, 158.1*). Look for short gastric branches from the splenic artery to the fundus of the stomach (fig. 3–28; *Atlas, 132*).

Carefully mobilize the tail and then the body of the pancreas. Note that the **splenic vein** lies caudal to the splenic artery (*Atlas, 149, 153*). Follow the splenic vein to the **portal vein** (*Atlas, 135*). Observe that the **superior mesenteric vein** is the largest tributary of the portal vein. The **inferior mesenteric vein** may empty into either the splenic vein or the superior mesenteric vein, or it may join the portal vein at the junction of the splenic and superior mesenteric veins (*Atlas, 132.2*). Look for the **gastric veins** which carry blood from the esophagus and the lesser curvature of the stomach to the portal vein. Review the portal system of veins (Fig. 3–30; *Atlas, 160.1*).

Portal hypertension (i.e. portal venous pressure above 20 cm of H₂O) may result from suprahepatic causes (e.g. heart failure), intrahepatic causes (e.g. cirrhosis), or infrahepatic causes (e.g. portal vein thrombosis; tumor compression of portal vein). As a consequence of portal venous hypertension, the esophageal and gastric veins become engorged, dilated, and eventually varicose. Rupture and extensive bleeding from these **esophageogastric varices** is an alarming and serious complication of portal venous hypertension. An understanding of the anatomy of the portal venous system is a prerequisite for intelligent diagnosis and treatment.

Superior and Inferior Mesenteric Vessels

The **superior mesenteric artery** is an unpaired vessel which arises from the abdominal aorta about 1 cm caudal to the celiac trunk. It has about the same diameter as the celiac trunk (*Atlas, 188*). The objective is to demonstrate the **extensive field of supply** of the superior mesenteric artery: Duodenum, except its superior portion; jejunum and ileum; cecum and

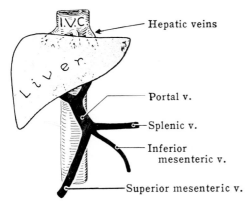

FIG. 3-30. Portal vein and its tributaries. (From *Grant's Atlas of Anatomy*.)

appendix; ascending colon; approximately one-half of the transverse colon (*Atlas, 162*). Reflect tail and body of the pancreas to the right, then carefully free the origin and initial portion of the superior mesenteric artery. Note the dense nervous network surrounding the vessel. This is the **superior mesenteric plexus of nerves.** Remove it to the necessary extent. Follow the artery to the point where it crosses anteriorly to the inferior part of the duodenum (*Atlas, 158.1*). Do not damage branches to the pancreas and duodenum. The **superior mesenteric vein** lies immediately to the right of the artery. It drains the same area supplied by the artery.

Next, follow the superior mesenteric vessels to the various parts of the small and large intestine. Use of the following approach: Throw the transverse colon, with the attached greater omentum, over the chest margin and retain it there. Draw the small intestine to the *left*, and have your partner stretch the mesentery taut. Palpate the superior mesenteric vessels just to the right of the duodenojejunal junction. Then, using the scissor technique or two pairs of blunt forceps, expose the vessels between the two layers of the mesentery (fig. 3-31). Now, identify and follow the **branches of the superior mesenteric artery:**

1. **Intestinal arteries,** 15 to 18 arteries to **jejunum** and **ileum.** Arteries unite to form loops or arches from which straight terminal branches arise. These are the **vasa recta** which pass alternately to opposite sides of the jejunum and ileum (figs. 3-31, 3-32, 3-33, or *Atlas, 166, 167*). The vasa recta do not anastomose within the mesentery; thus, 'windows' appear between the vessels (fig. 3-32). In the ileum, the arterial loops and arches become more complex, and the vasa recta become progressively shorter (fig. 3-33). Demonstrate a few arterial arches and vasa recta in the jejunum and ileum.
2. **Ileo-colic artery** (fig. 3-34; *Atlas, 162*). Passes to the right iliac fossa. Supplies cecum and appendix (appendicular artery). Anastomoses with ileal branches and with the right colic artery.

3. **Right colic artery** (*Atlas, 162*). Arises from either the superior mesenteric or the ileocolic artery. Supplies ascending colon. Anastomoses with neighboring arteries.
4. **Middle colic artery** (*Atlas, 162*). Supplies the

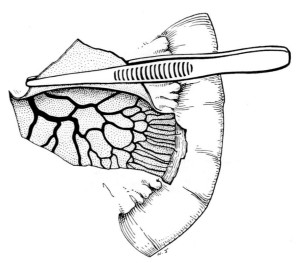

FIG. 3-31. Exposure of blood vessels contained in the mesentery.

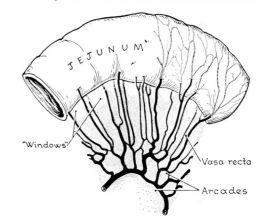

FIG. 3-32. Arteries of the jejunum. (From *Grant's Atlas of Anatomy*.)

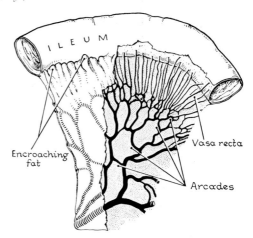

FIG. 3-33. Arteries of the ileum. (From *Grant's Atlas of Anatomy*.)

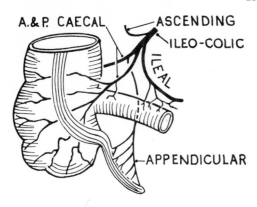

FIG. 3-34. Branches of the ileocolic artery. (From *Grant's Method of Anatomy.*)

right half of the transverse colon. Anastomoses with neighboring arteries.

The tributaries of the **superior mesenteric vein** correspond to the branches of the superior mesenteric artery. Identify the superior mesenteric vein, and trace it to the **portal vein.**

The **inferior mesenteric artery** is an unpaired vessel which arises from the abdominal aorta, about 3 cm cranial to the aortic bifurcation. The inferior mesenteric artery is much smaller than the superior mesenteric artery (*Atlas, 188*). The objective is to demonstrate the **field of supply** of this artery: Left half of transverse colon; descending colon; sigmoid colon; the greater part of the rectum (*Atlas, 163*). First palpate, and then dissect the origin of the inferior mesenteric artery. It is surrounded by the inferior mesenteric plexus of nerves. Trace the artery toward the large intestine, and identify its branches:

1. **Left colic artery** (*Atlas, 163*). Runs toward the left colic flexure. Supplies the descending colon and the left half of the transverse colon. Anastomoses with the middle colic artery.
2. Sigmoid arteries (fig. 3–35; *Atlas, 163*). Usually four branches which form arches.
3. Superior rectal artery (fig. 3–35 or *Atlas, 163.2*). Supplies proximal part of rectum. Divides into a right and a left branch which descends on either side of the rectum (*Atlas, 195*).

The branches of the superior and inferior mesenteric arteries form a series of anastomosing loops along the colon. The result is a continuous **marginal artery** (of Drummond) situated along the wall of the large gut (fig. 3–36). There are areas where the anastomoses are insufficiently developed, and hence there is little chance of effective collateral circulation (+ in fig. 3–36). This fact is of clinical importance in cases of mesenteric arterial occlusion (thrombosis; embolism).

The tributaries of the **inferior mesenteric vein** correspond to the branches of the inferior mesenteric artery. Identify the inferior mesenteric vein, and trace it to the **portal vein.**

Be aware that the **superior rectal vein** originates in the rectal venous plexus (*Atlas, 160.1*). The rectal venous plexus is also

drained by the middle and inferior rectal veins which, in turn, empty into the caval system of veins. In portal venous hypertension, blood flow in the superior rectal vein may be reversed: Portal blood may be carried to the rectal plexus and, from there, shunted into the caval system. The resulting increased blood flow and pressure in the rectal venous plexus leads to the development of hemorrhoids. Thus, in case of hemorrhoids, the physician must always evaluate the condition of the portal venous system.

The portal venous system has no valves. This fact explains why the blood flow in the portal system can be easily reversed.

Removal of the G.I. Tract

Next, remove the entire G.I. tract together with its 3 unpaired glands. Proceed with this *en bloc* extirpation in the following manner:

1. Tie two strings, about 2.5 cm apart tightly around the **rectum.** Cut the rectum between the two strings to prevent escape of its contents.
2. Cut the **inferior mesenteric artery** close to the abdominal aorta. Leave a 1 cm stump attached to the aorta for future reference.

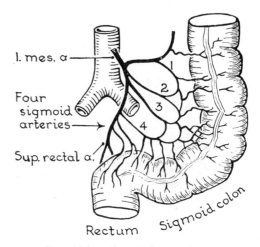

FIG. 3-35. Sigmoid branches of the inferior mesenteric artery. (From *Grant's Method of Anatomy.*)

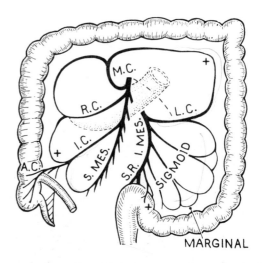

FIG. 3-36. Superior and inferior mesenteric arteries (+ denotes three weak points in the marginal anastomoses.

3. Cut through the V-shaped mesentery of the **sigmoid colon.** Keep to its lateral side in order *not* to damage the inferior mesenteric vessels or the left ureter.

4. With your fingers, detach the **descending colon** from the posterior abdominal wall. At the left colic flexure, cut through the phrenicocolic ligament.

5. Detach the **ascending colon** from the posterior abdominal wall. Keep to its lateral side in order *not* to damage the vessels supplying the colon.

6. Pull the transverse colon with the attached greater omentum caudally, and expose the origin of the **superior mesenteric artery.** Sever this vessel close to the abdominal aorta. If the right hepatic artery arises from the superior mesenteric artery (12%), be sure to include it in this section.

7. Sever the celiac trunk at its origin from the aorta. Make sure to include all its branches. Also, cut through autonomic nerve fibers that accompany the celiac trunk.

8. In the thorax, tie a string around the **esophagus** close to the diaphragm. Cut the esophagus and the vagal nerves superior to the string. Free the distal portion of the esophagus from the esophageal hiatus of the diaphragm (*Atlas, 191*) and from peritoneal reflections, and pull it into the abdominal cavity. Free the **stomach** completely so that it is only attached to the duodenum and blood vessels. Cut vagal branches to the celiac plexus of nerves.

9. With your fingers, detach the **duodenum** and **pancreas** from the posterior abdominal wall. Do *not* damage the bile passages or vessels of the pancreatico-duodenal region.

10. Identify the **inferior vena cava** as it approaches the dorsal surface of the liver (*Atlas, 147, 148*). Cut through this large vessel as close to the liver as possible.

11. The last organ to be mobilized is the **liver:** Incise the falciform ligament between diaphragm and diaphragmatic surface of the liver. Cut the left triangular ligament, and then the anterior portion of the coronary ligament (*Atlas, 130.3*). Pull the liver down forcibly with one hand, and cut the inferior vena cava at the point where it pierces the diaphragm (*Atlas, 191*). Cut along the remaining portion of the coronary ligament. Again, observe the hepatorenal ligament as you cut through it (*Atlas, 130.3*).

12. Finally, remove the detached G.I. tract together with liver, pancreas, and spleen. Carefully lift the organs out of the abdominal cavity. *Avoid* tearing the fragile inferior mesenteric vein; thus, support the weight of the sigmoid colon and the descending colon with one hand. Place the organs on a tray or table, and arrange them in their *characteristic anatomical config-*

uration (*Atlas, 124*). Review the branches of three unpaired arteries (celiac; superior mesenteric; inferior mesenteric).

13. Next, turn the viscera over, and arrange them in their *characteristic anatomical configuration* as seen from *behind*. Take care *not* to twist the structures of the porta hepatis (bile passages; hepatic artery; portal vein). This is an instructive exercise which will contribute greatly to your understanding of the disposition of the G.I. tract and its 3 unpaired glands (liver, pancreas, and spleen).

Posterior Aspect of G.I. Tract and its Unpaired Glands

Once again, identify the main **tributaries of the portal vein** (splenic; superior mesenteric; inferior mesenteric; fig. 3-30 or *Atlas, 132.2*). Using the scissor technique, clean these vessels and the portal vein. Make a special effort to trace **esophageal and gastric veins** to the portal vein. Review the clinical implications of esophageo-gastric varices.

Clean the **celiac trunk.** Observe strands of nerve fibers accompanying the celiac trunk and its branches. These fibers are derived from the celiac plexus of nerves. Review (fig. 3-28 or *Atlas, 132.1; 158.1*) and then clean all branches of the celiac trunk (splenic; left gastric; hepatic). Follow the gastroduodenal artery, and note a branch which supplies the posterior aspect of the pancreas and duodenum (posterior superior pancreaticoduodenal artery; *Atlas, 159*). Realize that the splenic artery gives branches to the body and tail of the pancrease (*Atlas, 158.1, 159*).

Pick up the severed end of the superior mesenteric artery (*Atlas, 159*). Clean and follow its branches to the head of the pancreas and the three distal portions of the duodenum. Review the relations of the duodenum, pancreas, and superior mesenteric vessels (fig. 3-37; *Atlas, 153–154*): The four portions of the duode-

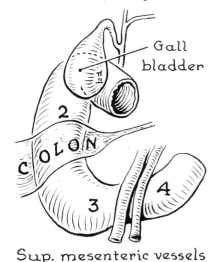

FIG. 3-37. Duodenum and superior mesenteric vessels (anterior view).

num are molded around the head of the pancreas. Near the junction of its 3rd and 4th portions, the duodenum is crossed (ventrally) by the superior mesenteric vessels (keep in mind that you view the G.I. tract from behind). Review the blood supply to duodenum and pancreas. (fig. 3–38; *Atlas, 158.1*). If present, identify and follow the right hepatic artery from the superior mesenteric artery to the porta hepatis.

Still working on the posterior aspect of the G.I. tract, review the **bile passages** (fig. 3–39 or *Atlas, 156*). Follow the (common) **bile duct** to a groove on the posterior surface of the head of the pancreas (*Atlas, 154, 159*). Using the scissor technique, carefully free the duct from surrounding pancreatic tissue. Follow it to the point where it passes obliquely through the coats of the descending (2nd) portion of the duodenum. The opening into the duodenum is the **major duodenal papilla** (of Vater). Take great care *not* to destroy the **main pancreatic duct** which (usually) joins the terminal portion of the (common)

bile duct (fig. 3–39). Notice that the wall of the common terminal portion of both ducts is thickened. This is due to a smooth sphincter muscle, the **sphincter of Oddi.** Follow the main pancreatic duct for 5 cm into the substance of the pancreas. Note numerous small ducts which drain into the main duct. In addition, an accessory duct may open separately into the duodenum (*Atlas, 156*). Variations of the duct system are common (*Atlas, 157*). Open the duodenum by a 5 cm incision just opposite to the entrance of the common bile duct. Observe the **major duodenal papilla** and the **hood-like plica** that covers it (*Atlas, 168*). If an accessory pancreatic duct is present, there may be a minor duodenal papilla about 2 cm superior to the major papilla (*Atlas, 168*).

Follow the cystic duct to the **gall bladder.** With probe and forceps, carefully remove part of the fundus of the gall bladder from its bed. Notice numerous small veins which plunge directly from the gall bladder into the liver (*Atlas, 146.1*). These small veins are of surgical importance. Immediately after chole-cystectomy (removal of gall bladder) the surgeon must overcome the problem of blood oozing from the gall bladder bed. Incise the gall bladder and observe its characteristic honeycombed mucous coat. Be aware of variations (*Atlas, 161 C and D*).

Next, examine the **liver.** Note that its sharp inferior border separates the visceral from the diaphragmatic surface. On the posterior aspect, observe the triangular, granulated **bare area.** Here, the liver was attached to the diaphragm (fig. 3–23; *Atlas, 130.3*). Around the bare area note the peritoneal reflections of the **coronary ligament.**

Observe the four lobes of the liver: *Right, left, quadrate,* and *caudate* (figs. 3–40, 3–41, or *Atlas, 139*). Note the H-shaped deep fissures and wide sulci, defining the four lobes (fig. 3–41; *Atlas, 136.1*):

1. **Right sagittal fossa.** Posteriorly forming a groove for the inferior vena cava (I.V.C.), and

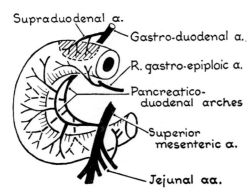

FIG. 3–38. Blood supply of duodenum. (From *Grant's Method of Anatomy*.)

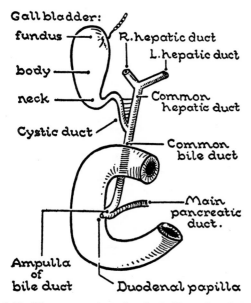

FIG. 3–39. Bile passages (anterior view). (From *Grant's Method of Anatomy*.)

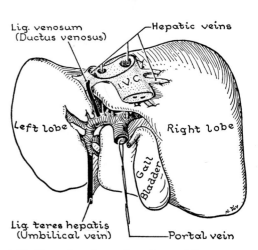

FIG. 3–40. Visceral and dorsal surfaces of liver as seen from behind. Portal vein and inferior vena cava (I.V.C.). (From *Grant's Method of Anatomy*.)

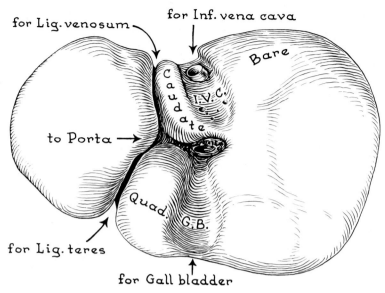

FIG. 3-41. H-shaped fissures and sulci of the liver (posteroinferior view).

inferiorly forming the shallow bed for the gall bladder.

2. **Left sagittal fissure.** Accommodates the ligamentum venosum posteriorly, and the round ligament (lig. teres) inferiorly.
3. **Transverse fissure,** the porta hepatis.

Review all structures passing through the porta hepatis. Examine the small segment of **inferior vena cava** (I.V.C.) which is attached to its groove. Note that the two or three large **hepatic veins** drain directly into it. Be fully aware of the difference between portal vein and hepatic veins (*Atlas, 132.2; 160.1*).

Section part of the left lobe of the liver. Observe:
1. Branches of portal vein, hepatic artery, and bile ducts (stained green) lying together.
2. Intrahepatic veins lying alone.

Spleen (*Atlas, 149, 150*). Sizes and weights vary considerably. Observe:
1. **Hilus.** For entrance and exit of splenic vessels.
2. **Borders.** Anterior and superior borders are sharp and often notched. Posterior and inferior borders are rounded.
3. **Visceral surface.** Divided according to contact areas with other viscera: Gastric, renal, pancreatic, and colic.
4. **Diaphragmatic surface.** Convex and smooth.

Place your hand into the (now empty) left hypochondriac region, where the spleen was located. Realize the topographical relationship of spleen to ribs 9, 10, and 11 (fig. 3-42). Push a probe horizontally through the 9th intercostal space, about 2 to 3 cm posterior to the midaxillary line. Realize that the instrument passes through the pleural cavity into the abdominal cavity and then into the spleen (fig. 3-43). These topographical relations are of great importance in evaluating stab wounds.

The interior of representative portions of the G.I.

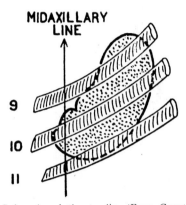

FIG. 3-42. Spleen in relation to ribs. (From *Grant's Method of Anatomy.*)

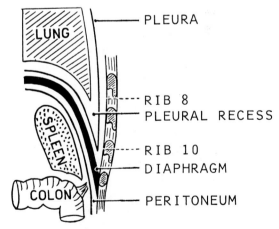

FIG. 3-43. Topographic relations of spleen. Coronal section in midaxillary line. (From *Grant's Method of Anatomy.*)

tract should be inspected. Study prosected specimens and specially prepared museum specimens. If these are not available, use the removed G.I. tract of the cadaver and observe the following:

1. **Stomach** (*Atlas, 128*). Longitudinal ridges along the lesser curvature. Pyloric sphincter and orifice (*Atlas, 168*).
2. **Duodenum** (*Atlas, 168*). Major and minor duodenal papillae (seen before). Pronounced plicae circulares.
3. **Jejunum** (*Atlas, 168*). Tall, closely packed plicae ciruclares.
4. **Ileum** (*Atlas, 168*). Few plicae circulares in upper part; absence of plicae in lower part. Look for Meckel's diverticulum, found in 2% of all cases (*Atlas, 170.1*).
5. **Ileocecal region** (*Atlas, 170*). Ileocecal orifice. Orifice of appendix. Section the appendix and examine its interior surface.
6. **Colon** (*Atlas, 170*). Haustra (sacculations). The crescentric folds between the haustra are called the plicae semilunares.

Store the detached G.I. tract with its 3 unpaired glands in a plastic bag for future reference.

Posterior Abdominal Viscera

General Remarks and Orientation

Work will be more pleasant if you sponge the posterior abdominal region and pouches. It is impossible to dissect nerves and vessels in a pool of liquified fat. Always keep the specimen moist with mold-deterrent preservative fluid.

Palpate the kidneys and the suprarenal (adrenal) glands. The suprarenal glands are friable and very easily torn. Note that the suprarenal glands are closely related to the cranial poles of the kidneys. Only a film of fatty tissue intervenes between kidney and suprarenal gland. Once again, identify the abdominal aorta and its bifurcation. To the right of the aorta observe the inferior vena cava (I.V.C.). Before continuing with the dissection, review the posterior abdominal viscera and their ventral relations (fig. 3-44; *Atlas, 176, 177*):

Point your finger to the caudal part of the **right kidney.** Here, it was in contact with the right colic flexure. About three-fourth of the ventral surface is still covered with parietal peritoneum. Here, the right kidney was in contact with the visceral surface of the liver (hepatorenal recess; compare *Atlas, 130.3*). Place your finger on the medial border of the right kidney. Here, it was in contact with the descending portion of the duodenum. Examine the **left kidney.** At about the middle of its ventral surface, it was in contact with the tail of the pancreas (fig. 3-44; *Atlas, 176, 177*). Caudal to this pancreatic area is a region which was in contact with the left colic flexure.

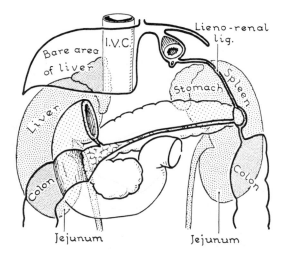

Fig. 3-44. Anterior relations of kidneys and suprarenal glands.

Plan for Dissection

The parietal peritoneal covering of the posterior abdominal wall will be removed. This procedure will completely expose the abdominal aorta and its branches, and the inferior vena cava and its tributaries. The kidneys will be shelled out of their fatty capsules. Next, their vessels and excretory ducts (ureters) will be studied. After ventral reflection of the kidneys and removal of the fatty renal capsule, the posterior abdominal wall will be accessible. Its muscles will be studied. Then, the lumbar plexus of nerves will be examined. Finally, the roof of the abdominal cavity, the diaphragm, will be studied.

Testicular and Ovarian Vessels

Testicular Arteries and Veins (*Atlas, 177*). See these vessels shining through the parietal peritoneal covering. They course obliquely between the great vessels at the level of the kidneys (*Atlas, 177*) and the deep inguinal ring (*Atlas, 179*). Realize that the testicular vessels cross the ureter (*Atlas, 177, 179, 210.1*). This structure must *not* be damaged during dissection. Pick up the testicular vessels at the deep inguinal ring. Using the scissor technique, follow them cranially. Observe (*Atlas, 177, 179*):

1. The **left testicular vein** drains into the **left renal vein.**
2. The **right testicular vein** drains directly into the **I.V.C.**
3. The **right** and **left testicular arteries** originate directly from the aorta, caudal to the origin of the renal arteries.

In the **female cadaver,** dissect the corresponding **ovarian vessels** (*Atlas, 233*). They cross the external iliac vessels very close to the ureter.

Kidneys and Suprarenal Glands

Kidneys [L., renes = kidneys]. The kidney is embedded in a substantial mass of fat, the **perirenal fat or adipose (fatty) capsule.** Observe that little fatty tissue lies in front of the kidney. Most of the fat lies lateral and posterior to the organ (*Atlas, 178*). The **renal fascia** (*Atlas, 178*) encloses both the kidney and its fatty capsule. Verify that the kidneys are *not* rigidly fixed to the posterior abdominal wall. In fact, they move slightly up and down during respiration.

With your fingers, shell out the kidneys from the renal fascia and fatty capsule. The upper pole is separated from the suprarenal gland by a thin layer of fat. Carefully pass your fingers between kidney and suprarenal gland and separate the two organs. Note the characteristic bean-shape of the kidney (*Atlas, 181*).

The approximate measurements of an adult kidney are: Length, 11 to 12 cm; breadth, 5 to 8 cm; thickness, 3 to 4 cm. The weight of each kidney varies from 120 to 170 grams. In one out of 400 cases, you may find a 'horseshoe' kidney. This is an anomaly (*Atlas, 187*).

Left kidney (*Atlas, 179*). Dissect the **left renal vein** from I.V.C. to the hilus of the left kidney. Observe and dissect two tributaries: **Left spermatic or ovarian vein** (already seen), and venous channels from the left suprarenal gland. In order to have full access to the renal artery, the left renal vein must be severed close to the I.V.C. and reflected toward the left. Now, find the **renal artery.** Follow this large vessel to the renal hilus. Usually, the artery divides into two branches before it enters the kidney (*Atlas, 189*). Accessory renal arteries are common (*Atlas, 187, 189*). Observe fine branches to the ureter (*Atlas, 189*) and to the suprarenal gland (Atlas, 180). The arteries are accompanied by autonomic nerve fibers.

The arterial distribution in the kidney is of surgical importance. Usually, the renal artery divides into an anterior and posterior branch. These branches supply the anterior and posterior halves of the kidney, respectively (*Atlas, 183.1, 184.1*). There are no anastomoses. Thus, there are no large vessels in the longitudinal plane of the kidney. Hence, surgical procedures along this plane (nephrotomy) offer the advantage of minimal hemorrhage.

Left Renal Pelvis and Ureter. Reflect the left kidney forward and toward the right. At the most posterior part of the hilus, identify the **renal pelvis** and its downward continuation, the **ureter** (*Atlas, 181–183*). Follow and dissect the ureter. Observe:

1. **Abdominal part of ureter** (*Atlas, 179*). Crosses the psoas major muscle. Runs obliquely posterior to the testicular (ovarian) vessels.
2. **Pelvic part of ureter.** Dissect it for a short distance along the wall of the pelvic cavity. Its junction with the urinary bladder (*Atlas, 182*) will be seen later.

Right Kidney. Dissect the relatively short right renal vein from I.V.C. to the hilus of the right kidney (*Atlas, 179*). Since the left renal vein was severed earlier, the I.V.C. can easily be reflected downward and slightly to the right. This procedure will expose the right renal artery (or arteries). Identify the renal pelvis, and follow the ureter caudally. Observe the relations between right ureter, right testicular (ovarian) vessels, and psoas muscle.

Next, remove the substantial fatty renal capsule and the renal fascia by forcibly pulling it off the posterior abdominal wall. Clean the posterior abdominal wall, and sponge the entire area clean. Identify the following muscles (fig. 3-45; *Atlas, 179*): **Transversus abdominis, quadratus lumborum, iliacus,** and **psoas major.** Also, identify the floating **12th rib** and the **diaphragm.** Now, study the topographic relations between kidneys and the posterior abdominal wall. Verify that the dorsal surface of each kidney is in contact with the diaphragm, psoas major, quadratus lumborum, and the posterior tendinous portion of the transversus abdominis. The superior pole of the right kidney lies at the level of the 12th rib. The left kidney is positioned somewhat higher; its upper pole lies at the level of the 11th rib (fig. 3-45). The liver seems to be responsible for 'pushing' the right kidney down (and the right lung up).

The traditional surgical approach to the kidney is the lumbar renal or retroperitoneal approach. Lumbar nephrectomy (extirpation of kidney via the retroperitoneal lumbar route) is indicated

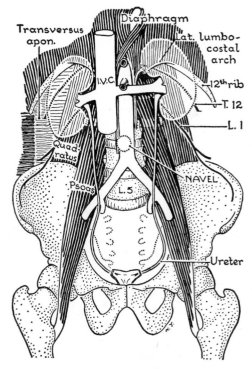

FIG. 3-45. Posterior relations of the kidneys. (From *Grant's Method of Anatomy.*)

when contamination of the peritoneal cavity is likely (inflammatory renal disease, calculi). The lumbar approach to the kidney (*Atlas, 173–175*) is an optional exercise described in the *Appendix* of this Dissector (p. 168). The transabdominal approach to the kidney is employed for surgery of the renal vessels.

Kidney on Section (fig. 3–46; *Atlas, 183*). Do *not* sever the kidneys from their vessels or ureters. Divide the left kidney into anterior and posterior halves by splitting it longitudinally along its convex, lateral border. Identify and observe:

1. **Fibrous capsule,** which can be easily stripped off.
2. **Renal cortex.** The outer one-third; of granulated appearance (Microanatomy: consists of glomeruli and convoluted tubules).
3. **Renal medulla,** consists of:
   a. **Renal pyramids** (Microanatomy: Loops of Henle; collecting ducts join a central tube which opens at a renal papilla).
   b. **Renal columns** (Microanatomy: interlobular arteries and veins.
4. **Renal papillae.** In groups of two or three, projecting into small cups, the calyces minores.
5. **Calyces minores,** unite to form two or three **calyces majores.** The major calyces unite to form the **renal pelvis,** which leads to the **ureter.**

As a clinical correlation, study an intravenous and retrograde pyelogram. Normally, the renal pelvis is found at the level of the spinous process of L_1. Be aware of anomalies (*Atlas, 187*).

Suprarenal (Adrenal) Glands (*Atlas, 180*). Realize that numerous arteries supply the suprarenal glands. These vessels are derived from the aorta, renal artery, or inferior phrenic artery. The venous blood is emp-

tied either into the renal vein or inferior vena cava. The suprarenals receive numerous sympathetic nerve fibers. Section one gland, and distinguish between cortex and medulla.

Review the abdominal aorta and its branches. Identify (*Atlas, 188, 188.1, 189.1*):
1. **Branches to the G.I. tract and its 3 unpaired glands** (celiac; superior and inferior mesenteric).
2. **Branches to the 3 paired glands** (suprarenal; renal; testicular or ovarian).
3. **Branches to walls** of abdominal cavity (phrenic; lumbar).
4. **Bifurcation of abdominal aorta,** at the level of L_4. The umbilicus projects just superior to the bifurcation (fig. 3-45 or *Atlas, 104.2 D*).
5. **Common iliac arteries,** which divide into internal and external iliac arteries (*Atlas, 189.1, 244*).

Review the **inferior vena cava** and its tributaries (*Atlas, 188.2*). Recapitulate the porta-caval system (*Atlas, 160.1*).

Posterior Abdominal Wall

Once again, identify the muscles of the posterior abdominal wall (*Atlas, 190*):
1. **Psoas major.** Arises from lumbar vertebrae (sides; intervertebral discs; transverse processes). Ventral to the psoas major, the long flat tendon of the psoas minor can be observed (*Atlas, 191.3*).
2. **Iliacus.** Occupies the extensive iliac fossa. Iliacus and psoas form a functional unit. Thus, they are referred to as **iliopsoas.** The iliopsoas is the most powerful flexor of the thigh.
3. **Quadratus lumborum.** Thick, rhomboidal muscular sheet, running from iliac crest to lumbar transverse processes and rib 12. Flexes vertebral column (fig. 3-47 or *Atlas, 104.2 B*).
4. **Transversus abdominis** (fig. 3-47). Running horizontally behind the oblique borders of the quadratus lumborum.

Nerves of the Posterior Abdominal Wall (*Atlas, 190*). These are ventral rami of T_{12} to L_5. Carefully remove the fascia from the posterior abdominal muscles and dissect the following nerves:
1. **Subcostal nerve** (T_{12}). About 1 cm caudal to rib 12.
2. **Iliohypogastric and ilioinguinal nerves** (L_1). Descending steeply in front of the quadratus lumborum. Positively identify the ilioinguinal nerve: Identify it again at the anterior abdominal wall. Trace it back from the superficial inguinal ring (*Atlas, 105*) to the plane between internal oblique and transversus abdominis (*Atlas, 110, 111*). Establish its continuity at the posterior abdominal wall.
3. **Genitofemoral nerve** (*Atlas, 190*), piercing the

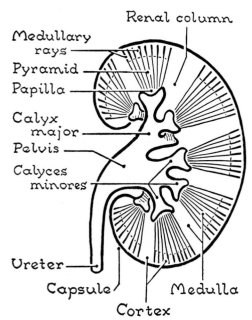

FIG. 3-46. Macroscopic structure of kidney on longitudinal section. (From *Grant's Method of Anatomy.*)

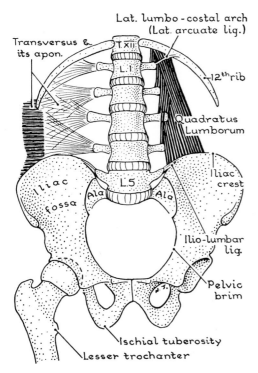

FIG. 3-47. Muscles of posterior abdominal wall.

anterior surface of the psoas. Supplies genito-femoral area (*Atlas, 248*).

4. **Lateral cutaneous nerve of the thigh** (*Atlas, 190*). It passes deep to the inguinal ligament. This sensory nerve supplies part of the thigh (*Atlas, 248, 256*).

5. **Femoral nerve** ($L_{2,3,4}$). Very large nerve lying in the angle between psoas and iliacus, and then deep to the inguinal ligament. Substantial motor supply to femoral muscles (*Atlas, 190, 250, 256*).

6. **Obturator nerve** ($L_{2,3,4}$). At the medial border of the psoas. Find the nerve in the following manner:
   a. Identify the obturator foramen in the skeleton. Palpate the obturator groove from inside the pelvis.
   b. Now, palpate the obturator groove from inside the pelvis in the cadaver. This is precisely the point where the obturator nerve passes from the pelvis into the thigh (*Atlas, 213, 217, 250*). Free the nerve with a probe, and follow it cranially to the medial border of of the psoas.

7. **Lumbosacral trunk** (*Atlas, 190, 213.1*). This large trunk consists of ventral rami of part of L_4 and all of L_5. The trunk runs caudally to the sacral plexus. The large and flat lumbosacral trunk is tightly applied to the ala of the sacrum. It is difficult to see with the psoas muscle in place.

The origin of the nerves of the posterior abdominal wall (1.–7.) from the lumbar plexus can only be studied after careful removal of the psoas muscle.

Since the nerves traverse the muscle at different depths, it is necessary to remove the psoas in a piecemeal fashion. Remove the psoas **on the right side only.** Using fingers and forceps, peel up the muscle and remove it gradually bit by bit. Study the **lumbar plexus** on the right side. Identify the right **lumbosacral trunk** (*Atlas, 190*).

Diaphragm

Diaphragm (*Atlas, 190, 191*). The diaphragm forms the roof of the abdominal cavity. Strip parietal peritoneum and areolar tissue off its fleshy fibers. Identify:
1. Sternal part.
2. **Costal part,** from last 6 ribs; interdigitating with transversus abdominis.
3. **Lumbar part** (*Atlas, 190, 191*).
   a. The **right crus** and **left crus** from the bodies of the lumbar vertebrae.
   b. Fleshy fibers from the arcuate ligaments (lumbocostal arches).
4. **Medial arcuate ligament** (*Atlas, 191*); a tendi-

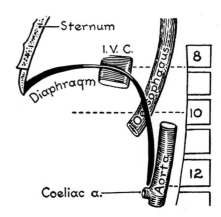

FIG. 3-48. Diaphragm. The higher the vertebral level, the more ventral the hiatus in the diaphragm. (From *Grant's Method of Anatomy.*)

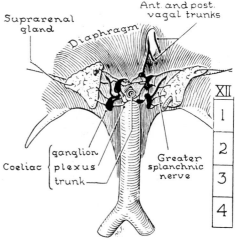

FIG. 3-49. Structures lateral to the celiac trunk.

nous arch providing a gap for the psoas muscle.

5. **Lateral arcuate ligament;** across the superior portion of the quadratus lumborum.
6. **Central tendon.**

Study the three large openings in the diaphragm (fig. 3-48; *Atlas, 191, 191.2*). Readily identify the two openings from which the traversing structures have been removed: **Vena cava foramen** and **esophageal hiatus.** The aorta (still in place) traverses the **aortic hiatus.** Note that this hiatus is formed by the union of the medial tendinous margins of the two crura. Identify the thoracic vertebral levels at which the openings in the diaphragm occur (fig. 3-48 or *Atlas,* *191.2*). Observe: The higher the vertebral level, the more ventral is the hiatus (opening) in the diaphragm.

The **greater splanchnic nerves** traverse the crura (*Atlas, 190*). To quickly find them, proceed in the following manner: In the thorax, identify the greater splanchnic nerve on one side. Follow it to the diaphragm. Parallel to the nerve, push a probe through the diaphragm. Pick up the probe and splanchnic nerve at the abdominal aspect of the crura (*Atlas, 190*). Note that the main portion of the splanchnic nerve runs toward the **celiac ganglion** (fig. 3-49 or *Atlas, 180.1*).

CHAPTER 4

PELVIS AND PERINEUM

General Remarks and Definitions

The **pelvis** [L., pelvis = basin] is divided into the greater pelvis and lesser pelvis. By definition, the **pelvic brim** is the circumference of a plane dividing the two pelvic portions (fig. 4-1 or *Atlas, 191.6 C*). The **greater pelvis** (pelvis major; false pelvis) is situated superior to the pelvic brim, and is bounded on either side by the ilium. The **lesser pelvis** (pelvis minor; true pelvis) is situated caudal to the pelvic brim.

The walls of the pelvic cavity are in part lined with muscles (fig. 4-8; *Atlas, 193.2*). No muscle crosses the pelvic brim (if muscles would cross the pelvic brim, they would interfere with childbirth by partially obstructing the pelvic inlet).

The floor of the pelvis is formed by muscles collectively called the **pelvic diaphragm** (fig. 4-1 or *Atlas, 191.6 C*).

The principal organs contained in the pelvic cavity have their outlet in the median plane (fig. 4-2). They pass through the **pelvic floor** and are anchored to it. The G.I. tract (rectum) lies posteriorly and passes through the 'anal triangle.' The urinary system lies anteriorly. The genital system takes an intermediate position. Both systems (urinary and genital) pass through the 'urogenital triangle' (of the pelvic floor).

The **peritoneal cavity** extends into the lesser pelvis (hence the term 'abdominopelvic cavity'). In the lesser pelvis, the peritoneum partially invests several pelvic organs, notably the rectum and bladder (fig. 4-6), and the uterus in the female (fig. 4-29).

The intrapelvic surfaces of the muscles lining the walls of the pelvic cavity are covered with the **pelvic fascia.** This fascia is firmly attached to the pelvic brim (fig. 4-8). The space between pelvic fascia and peritoneum (retropubic space) contains extraperitoneal fat and areolar tissue, blood vessels, and nerves.

The structures which fill the inferior aperture (outlet) of the pelvis are called the **perineum.** The perineum is a diamond-shaped area (fig. 4-3) extending from symphysis pubis to coccyx. A transverse line between the right and left ischial tuberosities divides the perineal region into two triangular areas, the urogenital region (triangle) and the anal region (triangle).

The dissections of the **male** and **female pelvis** will be covered separately. Students are urged to exchange information in the dissection of a specimen from the opposite sex.

Important Landmarks

Refer to an articulated pelvis, preferably one with intact ligaments. Observe the following (*Atlas, 218, 220*):

1. The bony pelvis is formed by:
   a. **Right hip bone** (os coxae), anteriorly and laterally on the right.
   b. **Left hip bone** (os coxae), anteriorly and laterally on the left.
   c. **Sacrum and coccyx,** parts of the vertebral column, interposed dorsally between the two hip bones.
2. **Pelvic brim** (*Atlas, 221*). Surrounds the **pelvic inlet or superior aperture** of the pelvis. Extends from the promontory of the sacrum dorsally to the **symphysis pubis** ventrally. Distinguish the three parts of the pelvic brim:
   a. Anterior border of ala of sacrum (sacral part)
   b. Arcuate line (iliac part)
   c. Pecten pubis and pubic crest (pubic part)
3. In the **erect posture** (anatomical position), the anterior superior iliac spines and the upper end of the symphysis pubis occupy the same vertical plane (*Atlas, 221.1*). In this position, the plane of the superior aperture (pelvic inlet) forms an angle of 50° to 60° with the horizontal plane. Verify this.
4. **Obturator foramen** (*Atlas, 242*). This foramen is closed by the obturator membrane (*Atlas, 217, 284*). Superiorly, the obturator canal (for obturator nerve and vessels) traverses the membrane.
5. **Ischial tuberosity** (*Atlas, 242, 243*).
6. **Ischial spine** (*Atlas, 222, 243*).
7. **Sacrospinous ligament** (dorsal view, fig. 4-4; medial view, *Atlas, 217*). From cocyx to ischial spine.
8. **Sacrotuberous ligament** (dorsal view, fig. 4-4; medial view, *Atlas, 217*). From sacrum to ischial tuberosity.

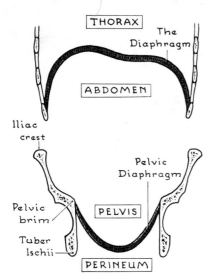

FIG. 4-1. Diaphragm and pelvic diaphragm, in coronal section. The perineum is the region caudal (inferior) to the pelvic diaphragm. (From *Grant's Atlas of Anatomy*.)

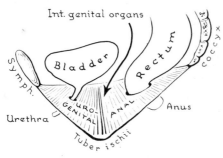

FIG. 4-2. Urinary system passing through 'urogenital triangle,' digestive system traversing 'anal triangle' of the diamond-shaped floor of pelvis (pelvic diaphragm). (From *Grant's Atlas of Anatomy*.)

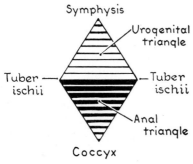

FIG. 4-3. Diamond-shaped perineal region. Urogenital and anal triangles. (From *Grant's Atlas of Anatomy*.)

9. The sacrospinous and sacrotuberous ligaments partially bound two foramina: **Lesser sciatic foramen** and **greater sciatic foramen** (fig. 4-4; *Atlas, 217*). Important vessels and nerves pass from the pelvis through the greater sciatic foramen into the gluteal region (for details see *gluteal region*, p. 75).

10. **Pubic arch** (*Atlas, 242*). Compare male and female pelves (*Atlas, 218, 220*). In the female, the pubic arch is much wider.

11. **Sacrum** [L., sacer = sacred]. On the ventral or pelvic surface observe (fig. 4-5; *Atlas, 373*): **Promontory, anterior sacral foramina** for the passage of ventral nerve rami S_1 to S_4. On the dorsal surface observe (*Atlas, 374*): **Dorsal sacral foramina** for the passage of dorsal nerve rami S_1 to S_4. Superiorly, observe the **sacral canal** which transmits spinal nerves S_1 to S_5 on their way to the sacral foramina.

12. **Sacroiliac articulation.** A joint (chondrosis type) between the auricular surfaces of sacrum and ilium (*Atlas, 222*). Held together by posterior sacroiliac (fig. 4-4) and anterior sacroiliac ligaments. Once the strong sacrospinous and sacrotuberous ligaments (fig. 4-4) are severed, the sacroiliac ligaments can be

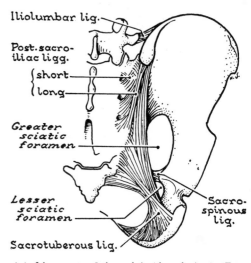

FIG. 4-4. Ligaments of the pelvis (dorsal view). (From *Grant's Method of Anatomy*.)

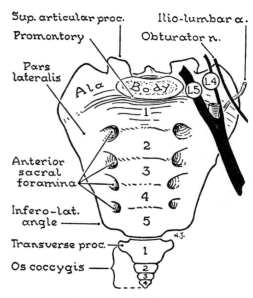

FIG. 4-5. Pelvic or ventral surface of sacrum and coccyx (the lumbosacral trunk, L_4 and L_5, is not labeled). (From *Grant's Method of Anatomy*.)

broken by force. Then, the sacrum and ilium can be separated to some extent. This procedure will be used during dissection to obtain greater access to the lesser pelvis.

13. Coccyx [Gk., kokkyx = cuckoo; resembling a cukoo's bill]. Three to five rudimentary vertebrae (Fig. 4-5; *Atlas*, *222*, *373*).

14. Realize that the hip bone (os coxae; innominate bone) consists of three parts: Ilium, ischium, pubis (*Atlas*, *351*). These three elements meet at the acetabulum, the cup-shaped cavity for the head of the femur. In the child, the three parts of the hip bone are not fused with each other. However, by age 16, fusion occurs.

Male Pelvis and Perineum

Plan for Dissection

The study of the male pelvis will begin with an examination of the peritoneal reflections. After removing the peritoneum and the subperitoneal fat, various pelvic structures (bladder, rectum, ductus deferens, ureter, blood vessels) will be dissected to a certain extent. However, complete and satisfactory dissection of all pelvic structures will be difficult because of limited access through the small pelvic inlet. Therefore, access to pelvic structures will be accomplished by partially disarticulating the right hip bone.

Subsequently, with the cadaver in the prone position, the anal region and the ischiorectal fossa will be dissected. The student will be encouraged to combine digital rectal examination with visual observations. Thus, the student will understand fully the topographical relations in the pelvis.

Finally, with the cadaver in the supine position, the external genitalia and the urogenital region will be studied in detail. Using a midsagittal section, the urethra will be followed from the glans penis to the bladder.

Peritoneum in the Male Pelvis

Examine the **peritoneum** in the male pelvis (fig. 4-6). The peritoneum passes from the anterior abdominal wall (*1*) to the level of the pubic bone (*2*) on to the superior surface of the urinary bladder (*3*). Next, it passes approximately 2 cm down the posterior surface of the bladder (*4*) to cap the seminal vesicles (*5*) (which cannot be seen at this time). Posteriorly, the peritoneum lines the **rectovesical fossa** (*6*) to the middle part of the rectum. At this level, it covers only the front of the rectum. However, at higher levels it gradually envelops the sides of the rectum (*7*). Finally, at the third sacral vertebra, the peritoneum becomes the sigmoid mesocolon (*8*). The **paravesical**

fossa, a peritoneal fossa, is apparent on each side of the bladder (*Atlas*, *205*). The peritoneal recess on each side of the rectum is called the **pararectal fossa** (Atlas, 202).

As the bladder fills, the peritoneal reflection is elevated above the level of the pubic bones, and raised from the anterior abdominal wall. Thus, a filled bladder can be surgically approached through an incision just above the pubic bones without entering the peritoneal cavity.

Structures Adhering to Peritoneum. With your fingers, detach the peritoneum from the pelvic wall and note the following structures which adhere to the peritoneum (fig. 4-7):
1. Rectum
2. Ureter
3. Ductus (vas) deferens
4. Bladder

Retropubic Space, Retrorectal Space, and Internal Iliac Vessels

Retropubic Space (Prevesical Space; Space of Retzius; fig. 4-8; *Atlas*, *203*). This U-shaped space lies

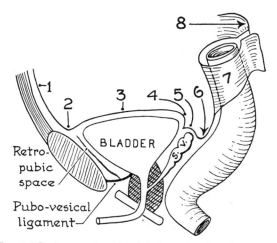

Fig. 4-6. Peritoneum in male pelvis, in paramedian plane.

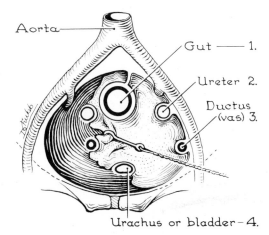

Fig. 4-7. Pelvic structures adhering to peritoneum.

between the symphysis pubis and the bladder and extends dorsally on each side of the bladder. Dorsally, the retropubic space is limited by the rectovesical fascia (fig. 4-9; *Atlas, 207*) which contains arteries and veins of the bladder and of the internal genital organs. The retropubic space is filled with fat and loose areolar tissue which accommodate the expansion of the bladder. Place your fingers between the symphysis pubis and anterior border of the bladder. Move the fingers to each side of the bladder (fig. 4-8). Inferiorly, the exploring finger is stopped by two cord-like thickenings of the pelvic fascia anchoring the neck of the bladder to the pubis: These are the **pubovesical** and **puboprostatic ligaments** (fig. 4-9).

Retrorectal Space or Presacral Space (fig. 4-10). The fused vertebrae S_3 to S_5 and the coccyx are covered with the rectum. Pass two fingers caudally behind the rectum and ease it off the sacrum and coccyx. Now, your fingers are in the deep retrorectal

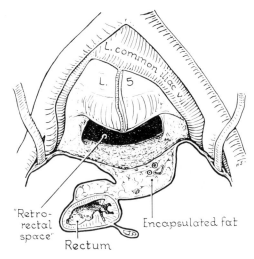

FIG. 4-10. The 'retrorectal space' between sacrum and rectum (viewed from above).

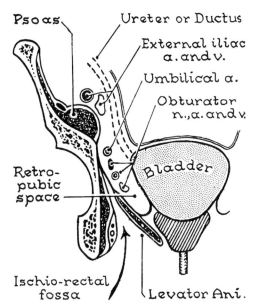

FIG. 4-8. Retropubic space extending laterally to bladder (coronal section). Ureter and ductus deferens are subperitoneal (*dotted lines*). (From *Grant's Method of Anatomy*.)

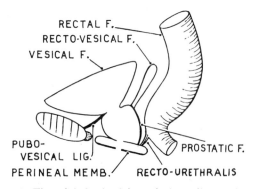

FIG. 4-9. The pelvic fascia of the male, in median section. (From *Grant's Method of Anatomy*.)

space. This space is limited inferiorly by a strong fascia investing the levator ani. As a result of this fascial arrangement, an infection in the retrorectal space (retrorectal abscess) is prone to rupture into the rectum. Feel strands of **pelvic splanchnic nerves** (sacral parasympathetic outflow; *Atlas, 204, 214*) on each side of the retrorectal space. These autonomic nerves branch off the ventral rami S_{2-4} after traversing the corresponding anterior sacral foramina.

Follow the **internal iliac artery** and its branches as far as possible (fig. 4-11; *Atlas, 211*). Complete dissection of these vessels will be done when the pelvic cavity is more accessible. Usually, the obturator artery arises directly from the internal iliac artery (70%). There is a slender anastomosis between obturator artery and inferior epigastric artery (*Atlas, 212 A*). However, commonly the obturator artery may receive the bulk of its blood supply from the inferior epigastric artery (*Atlas, 212 B*). Identify the **internal iliac vein** and some of its tributaries (*Atlas, 210*). Follow the vein to its junction with the external iliac vein. Here the common iliac vein is formed. Note that the left common iliac vein lies directly below the bifurcation of the aorta (*Atlas, 213*). On each side, follow the ureter and the ductus deferens toward the bladder and the prostate, respectively. Remove fat and areolar tissue surrounding vessels and ducts (figs. 4-8, 4-12). Clean the accessible parts of the bladder wall, but do *not* destroy its blood supply. Cleaning of the bladder will be facilitated by attaching a hemostat at its apex and pulling it taut. If in doubt whether or not the (collapsed) organ is really the bladder, make a small incision at the median plane, and observe the lumen of this hollow organ. If the rectum interferes with the field of dissection, have your partner pull it to the left side. Frequently sponge the area to keep it clean. Moisten the dissecting field with mold-deterrent preservative fluid.

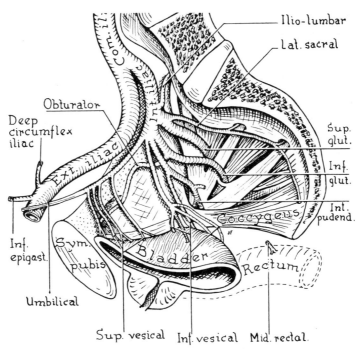

FIG. 4-11. Internal iliac artery and its branches.

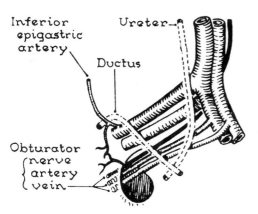

FIG. 4-12. The structures on the side wall of the male pelvis. Note the medial positions of the ureter and the ductus deferens. (From *Grant's Method of Anatomy*.)

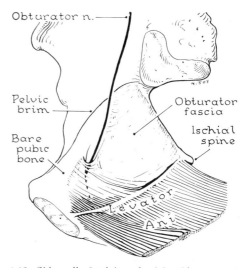

FIG. 4-13. Side wall of pelvis and origin of levator ani.

Pelvic Diaphragm

Lateral Wall of Pelvic Cavity. Once again identify the **obturator foramen** and the **obturator nerve and vessels** passing through the obturator canal. The obturator foramen is closed internally by the **obturator internus** muscle. Realize that only the most superior portion of the muscle can be seen (*Atlas*, *193.2*): Superiorly, the fascia of the obturator internus is thickened and forms a **tendinous arch** stretching from ischial spine to pubic bone. The **levator ani** arises in part from this tendinous arch (figs. 4-8, 4-13; *Atlas*, *209*).

Realize that the **pelvic diaphragm** is funnel-shaped. The rectum is anchored to it in the middle

(*Atlas*, *193.2*). Identify the **three portions of the pelvic diaphragm** (*Atlas*, *209*):

1. **Pubococcygeus,** arising from the pubic bone.
2. **Iliococcygeus,** arising from the tendinous arch.
   } Levator ani
3. Coccygeus (Ischiococcygeus), arising from the ischial spine.

The **pubococcygeus** is the thickened and most important part of the pelvic diaphragm. Observe fibers of the right and the left pubococcygeus uniting *behind* the rectum. This union of fibers creates a U-shaped 'puborectal sling' (fig. 4-14 or *Atlas*, *204.1*; *196*). This sling is responsible for the curvature at the

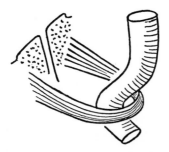

FIG. 4-14. The 'puborectal sling.' (From *Grant's Method of Anatomy*.)

anorectal junction. During defecation, the puborectal sling relaxes, the anorectal junction is straightened, and defecation is facilitated.

Anal Region (Triangle)

The *next objective* is the study of the **anal region** (triangle) and its nerve and blood supply. This is best accomplished by placing the cadaver into the prone position. By reflecting the gluteus maximus and partially exposing the gluteal region, it will be easier to trace nerves and blood vessels to the perineal region.

Skin Incisions. Turn the cadaver into the prone position (face down). Make skin incisions according to figure 4-15:

1. A median vertical cut from the lower lumbar region to coccyx (A to B).
2. From point A lateralward just above the iliac crest, until stopped by the table (A to C).
3. From the medial aspect of the thigh about 2.5 cm below the gluteal fold, to the lateral part of the thigh about 15 cm below the greater trochanter (D to E).
4. From points B to D.

To save time, remove skin and subcutaneous fat in one piece (from skin down to deep fascia enveloping both gluteus maximus and the thigh). This approach will destroy some of the cutaneous nerves of the gluteal region. Realize however, that these cutaneous nerves do exist (*Atlas, 249*). Do not cut too deeply across the posterior aspect of the thigh (D to E), otherwise the posterior cutaneous nerve of the thigh (*Atlas, 249*) will be injured.

Dissection. Remove skin and subcutaneous tissue. Expose the gluteus maximus (*Atlas, 267*). Define the superior and inferior borders of this vast rhomboidal muscle. Reflect the gluteus maximus in the following manner:

1. Detach its upper portion close to the ilium.
2. With a scalpel, cut through its fibers very close to their origin from the posterior surface of the sacrum and coccyx.
3. Place your fingers under the inferior portion of the muscle. Realize that it is attached to the sacrotuberous ligament. Now, carefully detach

the gluteus maximus from the sacrotuberous ligament, using a pair of scissors. Do *not* cut the ligament.

4. It is not necessary to reflect the muscle completely. Thus, reflect the muscle laterally to the point where the inferior gluteal nerve and vessels enter it (i.e. near its 'center').

Refer to an articulated pelvis, preferably one with its ligaments intact. Once again, identify the **greater and lesser sciatic foramina.** Palpate the **ischial spine** and **ischial tuberosity.** Now, coming from the gluteal region, palpate the same structures in the cadaver. Force your finger through the greater sciatic foramen. Observe that your finger passes along with the piriformis muscle and the sciatic nerve (*Atlas, 273*).

Next, push your finger through the lesser sciatic foramen into the ischiorectal fossa of the anal triangle. The finger runs in the same direction as the pudendal nerve and the inferior pudendal vessels (fig. 4-16). These vessels and nerve fibers supply the perineal structures.

The **ischiorectal fossa** (figs. 4-8, 4-17; *Atlas, 192*) is a large wedge-shaped space on either side of the anus. Its surfaces are formed by the fasciae of the obturator internus and levator ani. Its base is the skin of the perineum. The ischiorectal fossa is filled with soft fat. This tissue accommodates the distended rectum. Incise the fat of the ischiorectal fossa (fig. 4-17): With the blade directed toward the anus, start the incision roughly midway between ischial tuberosity and coccyx. Insert the blade approximately 4 cm deep. As the anus is approached, gradually withdraw the scalpel. Insert your finger into the incision. Palpate the **inferior rectal** (hemorrhoidal) **vessels and nerve.** Enlarge the opening with your finger. In a piecemeal fashion, remove the fat with a forceps. Dry the area with paper towels. Observe vessels and nerves travers-

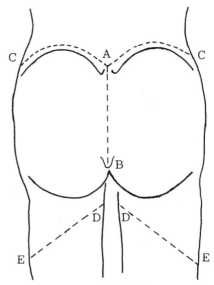

FIG. 4-15. Skin incisions.

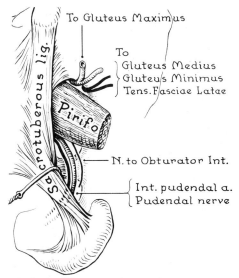

FIG. 4-16. Pudendal nerve and internal pudendal vessels leaving the gluteal region through the lesser sciatic foramen.

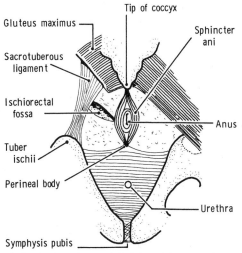

FIG. 4-17. Anal region and ischiorectal fossa. Cadaver in the prone position.

ing the fossa from the lateral wall toward the anus (*Atlas, 192*).

Infections of the ischiorectal fossa may result in the formation of an abscess. The abscess may spontaneously open into the rectum or through the skin into the perineal region. Surgeons must be aware of the fact that the right and left ischiorectal fossae communicate via the deep postanal space (which lies posterior to the anus between superficial and deep external sphincter). As a result, an infection in one ischiorectal fossa may eventually involve a semicircular area around the posterior aspect of the anus.

Clean the **sphincter ani externus** (*Atlas, 192*). It consists of three parts (*Atlas, 193*):

1. Subcutaneous part, delicate, encircling the anal orifice.
2. Superficial part, anchoring the anus to the **perineal body** ventrally and to the coccyx posteriorly.

3. Deep part, forming a wide encircling band. It is fused with the levator ani (puborectal sling). During defecation the puborectal sling and all parts of the sphincter ani externus relax.

With a gloved hand, insert your middle finger into the rectum. At the same time, place the fingers of your other hand on the sphincter ani externus within the ischiorectal fossa. Appreciate the thickness of this muscle.

Clean the fascia of the **obturator internus** within the ischiorectal fossa. The inferior portion of the obturator fascia is thickened. It splits to form a fibrous canal, the **pudendal canal** (*Atlas, 192, 194.1*). The canal contains the **pudendal nerve** and the **internal pudendal vessels.** These structures run along the ischiopubic ramus toward the urogential diaphragm (*Atlas, 215*). Carefully incise the obturator fascia along the ischiopubic ramus and just ventral to the sacrotuberous ligament. With a probe, pick up the contents of the pudendal canal. Carefully push the probe into the canal. Then, push forward along the ischiopubic ramus toward the inferior portion of the symphysis pubis. This is the course of the pudendal nerve and inferior pudendal vessels to the urogenital diaphragm and the dorsum of the penis (clitoris).

Partial Disarticulation of Right Hip Bone

While the cadaver is still in the prone position, preparations will be made for partial disarticulation of the **right hip bone.** *Important:* Only the **right** hip bone will be partially disarticulated. The following two steps are preparatory to disarticulating the right sacroiliac joint. On the **right side only** cut the following ligaments (fig. 4-4):

1. **Sacrotuberous ligament.** Cut it close to the ischial tuberosity.
2. **Sacrospinous ligament.** Cut it close to the ischial spine. Be aware of the close relationship of the ischial spine and pudendal structures (fig. 4-16; *Atlas, 215*). Do *not* damage the nerve or vessels.

Next, turn the cadaver into the supine position (face up). Place a wooden block, 15 to 20 cm high, under the small of the back. Now, once again examine the **levator ani:** Place the middle finger of one hand in the ischiorectal fossa and touch its roof (levator ani). Place the middle finger of the other hand into the lesser pelvis so that both fingers approach each other. The intervening muscular sheet is the funnel-shaped levator ani. Again, place your finger into the rectum. At the same time, with the other hand in the pelvis, appreciate:

1. The length and direction of the anal canal from external sphincter to pelvic diaphragm (*Atlas, 196*).
2. The position of the prostate gland lying anterior to the rectum and inferior to the bladder (*Atlas, 203*).

Now, prepare to disarticulate the right hip bone. The hip bone will be forced laterally. This ensures widened access to the lesser pelvis. Logically, structures holding the hip bone in position must be severed. *Before taking any action*, refer to appropriate illustrations and an articulated pelvis. Understand the logic of the *intended procedures:*

1. On the right side, the strong sacrotuberous and sacrospinous ligaments must be cut (already done).
2. On the right side, the levator ani (pubococcygeus and iliococcygeus) must be detached from the pubic bone and the tendinous arch of the obturator internus fascia, respectively (*Atlas, 209*).
3. Structures attached to the symphysis pubis and pubic arch must also be severed on the right side. These include:
   a. Suspensory ligament of penis (*Atlas, 198.1*);
   b. Urogenital (U.G.) diaphragm (fig. 4-18; *Atlas, 201*).
4. The pubic part of the two hip bones must be separated at their joint, the symphysis pubis (*Atlas, 242*).
5. The *right* iliopsoas muscle was removed earlier, during dissection of the lumbar plexus.
6. Other smaller ligaments holding the sacroiliac joint together (fig. 4-4), must be severed by force.
7. All other structures connecting the pelvis with the lower extremity (nerves, vessels, piriformis muscle) are suitably positioned and will withstand the stress of partial disarticulation of the right hip bone.

Now, **carry out the five necessary procedures** in the following manner:

1. Make sure that the **sacrotuberous** and **sacrospinous ligaments** were severed on the right side (as specified earlier; p. 55).

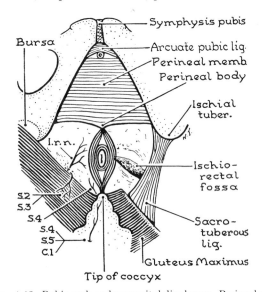

FIG. 4-18. Pubic arch and urogenital diaphragm. Perineal membrane, inf. fascia of U.G. diaphragm. Perineal body, central tendon of perineum.

2. On the right side, detach the **levator ani** (*Atlas, 209*): Place a probe deep to the muscle fibers. Then, cut the relatively thick pubococcygeal part. Next, detach the iliococcygeal part from the tendinous arch.
3. On the right side, free the **symphysis pubis** and **ischiopubic ramus**:
   a. With blunt dissection, expose **suspensory ligament of the penis** (*Atlas, 198.1*). It anchors the root of the penis to the symphysis pubis. Cut the ligament.
   b. Carefully detach the **U.G. diaphragm** from the ischiopubic ramus (figs. 4-18, 4-19; *Atlas, 201*). Begin your cut at the symphysis pubis, and carry it toward the ischial tuberosity. Cut as close to the bone as possible. Be extremely careful to avoid injuring the vessels and nerves (*Atlas, 201*). Keep in mind that you see only the **perineal membrane**, i.e. the inferior fascia of the U.G. diaphragm. At a deeper level, there are a muscular sheet and the superior fascia of the U.G. diaphragm (*Atlas, 216*). By detaching the U.G. diaphragm, you are cutting through all three components (fascia, muscle, fascia).
4. Prepare to **disarticulate the symphysis pubis.** First, find and partially dissect the unpaired deep dorsal vein of the penis. It passes underneath the symphysis pubis (fig. 4-19). To protect this vein from injury, push the handle of a forceps between the symphysis pubis and dorsum of penis. Now, push the handle all the way into the pelvis. Next, with a saw or sturdy knife, cut the symphysis pubis in the midline down to the handle of the forceps. Do *not* cut into the urinary bladder.
5. Now, the **right sacroiliac joint** is ready for partial disarticulation: Forcibly, abduct both extended lower limbs to such a degree that the feet are about 2 to 3 feet (up to 1 meter) apart. As a result, the two pubic bones will pull apart about 10 cm. The cracking noise that your hear is caused by tearing the anterior and posterior sacroiliac ligaments. *On the right side*, palpate the 2 cm gap between sacrum and ilium. Keep the extended lower limbs widely abducted (with the aid of a wooden board or with ropes). The lesser pelvis is now wide open. Access to pelvic structures will be even more convenient if you remove a 3 cm wedge of right pubic bone. Make sure that a block, 15 to 20 cm high, is positioned under the small of the back.

Complete Dissection of Male Pelvis and Perineum

With the pelvic girdle widened, the pelvic structures are now readily accessible, particularly on the right side. In the following manner, examine and

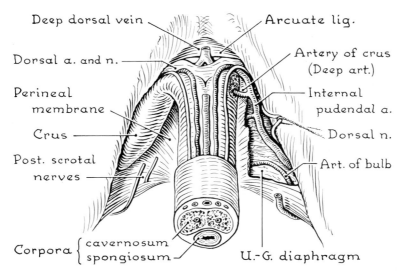

Deep dorsal vein

Arcuate lig.

Dorsal a. and n.

Artery of crus
(Deep art.)

Perineal
membrane

Internal
pudendal a.

Crus

Dorsal n.

Post. scrotal
nerves

Art. of bulb

Corpora { cavernosum
spongiosum

U.-G. diaphragm

FIG. 4-19. U.G. diaphragm and penis. Deep dorsal vein of penis (cut) passing underneath symphysis pubis.

dissect these structures, noting their topographical relations:

1. **Levator ani** (*Atlas, 205*). On the right side, pick up the muscular slips with a pair of forceps. Observe the relatively thick pubococcygeal portion and the thin iliococcygeal part. Note that the prostate rests on the pelvic diaphragm (*Atlas, 205*). Review the levator ani (*Atlas, 209*).

2. **Ureter** (fig. 4-20; *Atlas, 182, 207*). Follow the ureter to the posterolateral portion of the urinary bladder. Here, the ureter travels obliquely through the bladder wall.

3. **Ductus (vas) deferens** (*Atlas, 205–207*). Once again, observe that the ductus deferens hooks around the inferior epigastric vessels (*Atlas, 202, 216*). To facilitate dissection, cut through the medial aspect of the right inguinal ring. Now, the right testis and its attached duct and vessels can be placed into the abdominal cavity. Next, follow the ductus deferens toward the bladder. Near the posterolateral angle of the bladder, it crosses anterior to the ureter. Subsequently, follow the duct along the posterior aspect of the bladder. Here it expands to form the **ampulla.** Lateral to each ampulla lies a **seminal vesicle.** Each seminal vesicle is a convoluted tube. Using a probe, carefully expose the union of the ampulla and the duct of the seminal vesicle (figs. 4-20, 4-21; *Atlas, 207*). This is the beginning of the **ejaculatory duct,** which traverses the posterior half of the prostate gland (*Atlas, 207.1*).

4. Again, place your gloved finger into the anal canal and perform a **digital rectal examination.** Palpate structures topographically related. At the same time, make visual observations (fig. 4-22). Palpate the muscular wall formed by the sphincter ani externus. Higher up, at the anorectal junction, feel the puborec-

talis (puborectal sling; part of levator ani). Anteriorly, feel the prostate and the seminal vesicles.

Rectal examination is an important part of every physical examination. The size and consistency of the prostate gland can be assessed. Normally, the wall of the rectum can be moved against the prostate because of the intervening areolar tissue (fig. 4-22; *Atlas, 203*). If this is not possible, one should suspect malignant tumor infiltration from prostate into rectum.

Posteriorly, the anterior surface of sacrum and coccyx can be palpated. Laterally, the ischiorectal fossa can be examined. Thus, pathological processes (e.g. abscess) may be detected by digital examination.

Appreciate this unique opportunity to combine digital palpation with visual observation.

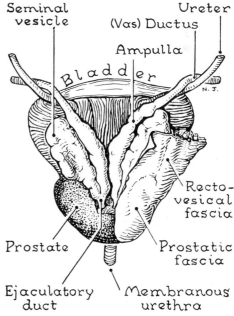

Seminal
vesicle

Ureter
(Vas) Ductus

Ampulla

Bladder

Recto-
vesical
fascia

Prostate

Prostatic
fascia

Ejaculatory
duct

Membranous
urethra

FIG. 4-20. Ureter, ductus deferens, and seminal vessels (dorsal view). Note the rectovesical fascia which limits the retropubic space dorsally.

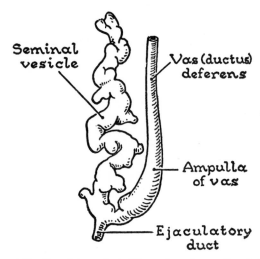

FIG. 4-21. Ejaculatory duct: The union of ampulla of ductus deferens and seminal vesicle (unraveled). (From *Grant's Method of Anatomy*.)

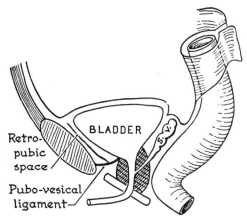

FIG. 4-22. Topographic relations of rectum, prostate, and seminal vessels.

5. Observe the **rectal venous plexus.** Note the numerous veins on the surface of the rectum. The importance of this plexus in cases of portal venous hypertension has been stressed earlier (*Atlas, 160.1*).

6. Observe the **vesical venous plexus** at the base of the bladder. It receives blood from the **prostatic venous plexus,** which lies ventral and lateral to the prostate. Note that the **deep dorsal vein of the penis** empties into the prostatic plexus. The venous plexuses in the pelvis intercommunicate. This is of considerable clinical importance (e.g. transportation of tumor cells along vascular channels). Do not attempt to dissect these complex pelvic plexuses. Remove all tributaries of the internal iliac vein so that the arterial distribution can be clearly demonstrated.

7. **Internal iliac artery and branches** (fig. 4-11 or *Atlas, 211*). Demonstrate the important branches of the internal iliac artery. Carefully dissect the **internal pudendal artery** as far as

possible. Note that it lies medial to the sciatic nerve and is accompanied by the pudendal nerve (fig. 4-23 or *Atlas, 213.1*). On the right side of the cadaver, observe the internal pudendal artery in relation to the levator ani: Note **middle rectal** and **inferior rectal branches** (*Atlas, 192, 195*). Review the blood supply to the rectum. Observe branches of the internal pudendal artery to the perineum and scrotum.

8. **Piriformis muscle** (*Atlas, 213*). Observe its origin from the pelvic or ventral surface of the sacrum at segments S_2, S_3, and S_4. Note that the muscle fibers converge and pass through the greater sciatic foramen. The ventral nerve rami S_2 and S_3 emerge between the digitations of the piriformis.

9. **Sacral plexus.** The sacral plexus is closely related to the anterior surface of the piriformis. In the cadaver, verify the following (fig. 4-23; *Atlas, 213, 213.1*):

   a. The **lumbosacral trunk** (L_4, L_5) contributes to the sacral plexus.

   b. The ventral rami of S_2 and S_3 emerge between the digitations of the piriformis.

   c. Ventral rami from L_4 through S_3 converge and form the large **sciatic nerve.** It passes through the greater sciatic foramen together with the piriformis.

   d. Usually, the **gluteal arteries** (branches of the internal iliac artery) pierce the sacral plexus: The lumbosacral trunk and rami S_1 are separated by the superior gluteal artery. The inferior gluteal artery usually separates ramus S_1 from S_2.

   e. Ventral rami S_2, S_3, and S_4 contribute to

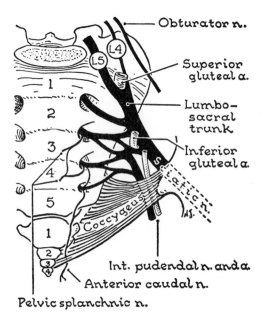

FIG. 4-23. Sacral plexus and related vessels. (The student may consider coloring the 3 arteries that pierce the sacral plexus.) (From *Grant's Method of Anatomy*.)

the pudendal nerve (fig. 4-23; *Atlas, 215*). Remember, ventral rami S$_2$, S$_3$, and S$_4$ contain preganglionic parasympathetic fibers (sacral parasympathetic outflow; pelvic splanchnic nerves; *Atlas, 214*). These autonomic nerves supply pelvic organs and the distal portion of the G.I. tract from left colic flexure to rectum.

    f. Note the **sympathetic chain** and its **ganglia** medial to the sacral foramina (*Atlas, 213*). These ganglia give off gray rami communicantes to the ventral rami forming the sacral plexus.

10. **Penis** [L., penis = tail]. **Fascia, vessels, and nerves.** Remove the skin of the penis leaving the glans intact. The **superficial fascia** is devoid of fat. It contains superficial veins which drain to the inguinal region. Deep to the loose superficial fascia is the tight tubular investing sheath, the **deep fascia of the penis** (*Atlas, 199*).

The fascial arrangements of penis and scrotum are of clinical importance. If the urethra is injured and perforated (penetrating injuries; faulty passage of catheter or cytoscope) urinary extravasation can occur. In most cases, urine (usually infected urine) invades the space between superficial and deep fascia. The superficial fascia of the penis is continuous with Dartos' fascia of the scrotum and Scarpa's fascia of the lower abdominal wall. Thus, urinary extravasation leads to inflammation with sizable swelling of penis, scrotal sac, and lower abdominal wall.

Carefully incise the deep fascia between the glans and the symphysis pubis. On the dorsum of the shaft note:

    a. The unpaired **deep dorsal vein of the penis;** most of the blood from the penis drains through it into the prostatic venous plexus (fig. 4-19).

    b. The paired **dorsal arteries of the penis,** branches of the internal pudendal artery (fig. 4-19, *Atlas, 199, 201*).

    c. The paired **dorsal nerves of the penis,** branches of the pudendal nerve (fig. 4-19, *Atlas, 199, 215*).

If you have not done so, follow the deep dorsal vein underneath the symphysis pubis to the prostatic venous plexus. Next, on the right side pick up the internal pudendal artery and the pudendal nerve in the pelvic cavity. Clean these structures. Follow them through the greater and lesser sciatic foramina. Establish the continuity of artery and nerve with those on the dorsum of the penis.

11. **Superficial perineal muscles** (*Atlas, 192*). On the right side, the structures of the urogenital triangle were detached from the ischiopubic ramus. Therefore, the *left side* of the urogenital triangle is best suited for studying the superficial perineal muscles. Identify and dissect:

    a. **Central tendon of perineum** (perineal body; fig. 4-18). It is the central fibromuscu-

lar area where most perineal muscles are in part attached.

    b. **Bulbospongiosus** (bulbocavernosus) (*Atlas, 192*). Arises from the perineal body and a median raphe below the bulb of the penis. Raise the thin anterior free border of the muscle. *Function:* The paired bulbospongiosi form a sphincter that empties part of the spongy urethra. Also, assists in erection by compressing the deep dorsal vein.

    c. **Ischiocavernosus** (*Atlas, 192*). Covers crus of corpus cavernosum. *Function:* Compresses veins and thus retards blood flow from erectile tissue.

    d. Superficial transverse perineal muscle (*Atlas, 192*). Narrow muscular slip from ischial tuberosity to central tendon.

When separating these three muscles (bulbospongiosus, ischiocavernosus, superficial transverse perineal) from each other, note a small triangular area of exposed perineal membrane. This membrane is the inferior fascia of the U.G. diaphragm (*Atlas, 192*).

12. **Urethra** (fig. 4-24; *Atlas, 203*). The male urethra begins at the neck of the bladder and extends to the external urethral orifice (on the glans penis). The urethra is divided into three portions: **Prostatic, membranous,** and **spongy.** The **spongy portion** (penile urethra) will be demonstrated first. The objective is to open the entire penile urethra in a longitudinal direction: Push a probe into the navicular fossa of the glans (*Atlas, 199.1*). With a sharp scalpel, cut longitudinally through the ventral part of the glans until stopped by the probe. Push the probe deeper into the spongy urethra. Continue to split it until reaching the bulb of the corpus spongiosum. Here the urethra bends at almost a right angle and passes through the U.G. diaphragm (fig. 4-24). Examine the mucous membrane of the spongy urethra. Note the orifices of tiny mucous glands (*Atlas, 199.1*).

Now, split the penis in the midsagittal plane into right and left parts. Do *not* destroy the dorsal artery and nerve of the penis. In the section, include the bulb of the corpus spongiosum. Observe the dark red cavernous structure of the erectile tissue of the corpus spongiosum and corpus cavernosum penis (*Atlas, 197, 198, 199.1*). Note the right and left crus of the corpus caverosum (*Atlas, 193*). Expose one crus by removing the overlying ischiocavernosus (*Atlas, 192*).

Next, explore the **membranous urethra** (fig. 4-24; *Atlas, 197*). It is only 1 to 2 cm long and traverses the U.G. diaphragm. Within the U.G. diaphragm, it is surrounded by a sphincter muscle, the **sphincter urethrae** (*Atlas, 203*). With sharp scissors in the membranous urethra, slit open the wall of the urethra, and cut through the surrounding sphincter urethrae.

Examine the inferior and superior fascia of the U.G. diaphragm (fig. 4-24). Appreciate the functional importance of the sphincter urethrae. Note the prostate resting on the U.G. diaphragm. Push the probe through the **prostatic urethra** into the bladder. Cut through the ventral portion of the prostate until stopped by the probe. With scissors, extend the cut through the anterior border of the urinary bladder. Examine the interior of the prostatic urethra (*Atlas, 208*):

a. Approximate length: 3 cm.
b. On the posterior wall, observe a median ridge, the **urethral crest.** The ovoid enlargement of the crest is the **colliculus seminalis.**
c. In the midline of the colliculus find a small blind opening, the **utricle.**
d. On each side of the utricle, find the minute **orifice of the ejaculatory duct.**
e. On each side of the urethral crest, observe a groove, the **prostatic sinus.** Here, the numerous ducts of the prostate open into the urethra.

13. **Urinary bladder** (fig. 4-25; *Atlas, 208*). The anterior border of the urinary bladder was already incised. With scissors, carry the incision all the way to the apex. Open the bladder completely. Examine the **muscular coat** of the organ. It consists of bundles of smooth muscle. (This muscular coat is collectively called the *detrusor urinae* [L., detrudere = to thrust out]). Examine the **interior of the bladder** (*Atlas, 208*):

a. The **trigone** is an equilateral triangle on the posterior wall. Its angles are formed by the **two orifices of the ureters** and the **internal urethral orifice.** The internal urethral orifice is situated at the lowest point of the bladder.

b. Note that the mucous membrane over the trigone is smooth. Over the other parts of the bladder, it lies in folds, when the bladder is empty.
c. Pass a fine probe into one of the two orifices of the ureters. Verify that the ureters traverse obliquely the muscular wall of the bladder (*Atlas, 208.1*).

14. **Anal canal** (fig. 4-26; *Atlas, 203*). Slit the anal canal; clean it thoroughly. Examine the interior features (this may be difficult to demonstrate in some cadavers):

a. 5 to 10 **anal columns.** These are longitudinal ridges of mucosa in the upper part of the anal canal. The terminal 'branches' of the superior rectal vessels are contained in the anal columns. Here, the superior rectal veins anastomose with the portacaval system (*Atlas, 160.1*). Abnormal increase in pressure in the valveless portal system leads to an

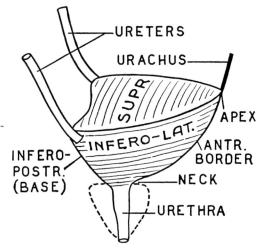

FIG. 4-25. The urinary bladder: Its 4 surfaces, 4 angles, and 4 ducts. (From *Grant's Method of Anatomy.*)

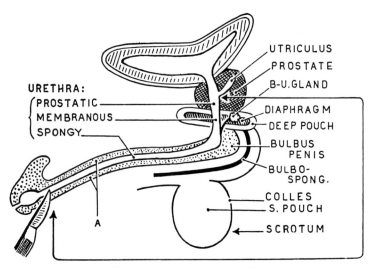

FIG. 4-24. The male urethra. (From *Grant's Method of Anatomy.*)

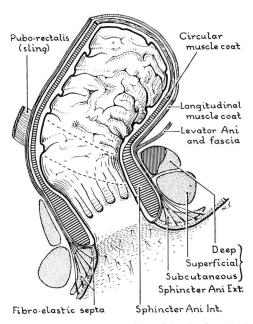

Fig. 4-26. Rectum and anal canal (sagittal section).

enlargement of the veins contained in the anal columns, resulting in 'internal hemorrhoids.'

b. **Anal valves,** semilunar folds uniting the lower ends of the anal columns. If these anal valves are torn by hard fecal material, an infection could spread from here into the wall of the anal canal.

Review the **sphincter muscles** of the anus and the puborectal sling (fig. 4-26 or *Atlas, 196*).

Female Pelvis and Perineum

General Remarks and Orientation

Review the important landmarks of the pelvis (p. 49–51). Familiarize yourself with some measurements of the female pelvis. These measurements are of obstetrical importance. Obtain an articulated female pelvis and observe the following (fig. 4-27):

1. A line connecting the upper end of the symphysis pubis with the coccyx lies in the horizontal plane.
2. **Anteroposterior or conjugate diameter** (10.5 to 11 cm). A midsagittal line connecting the upper end of the symphysis pubis with the promontory of the sacrum. This line indicates the plane of the pelvic inlet or brim.
3. **Transverse diameter** (13.5 cm). Across greatest width of superior aperture.
4. The plane of the pelvic inlet forms an angle about 60° with the horizontal plane.
5. A line connecting the lower end of the symphysis with the tip of the coccyx indicates the **pelvic outlet** (anteroposterior diameter, 9 to 11 cm).

The plane of the pelvic outlet forms an angle of about 15° with the horizontal plane.
6. The transverse diameter (11 cm) of the pelvic outlet is measured between the two ischial tuberosities.
7. The pubic arch in the female is wide. The subpubic angle measures about 90° (in the male, only about 60°; *Atlas, 220*).

Understand the general arrangement of the *soft parts* of the female pelvis (fig. 4-28):

1. The **urethra** is short (3.5 to 4 cm). It pierces the anterior portion of the U.G. diaphragm.
2. The **vagina** is about 7 to 8 cm long. The vagina also traverses the U.G. diaphragm. The anterior wall of its middle part is in contact with the bladder. Its posterior wall is in contact with the rectum.
3. The **uterus** is about 7 cm long. It intervenes between bladder and rectum. The longitudinal

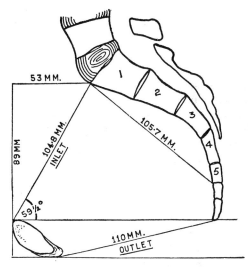

Fig. 4-27. Outlines of female bony pelvis, in median section. (From *Grant's Method of Anatomy.*)

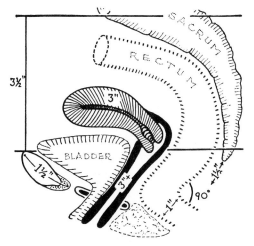

Fig. 4-28. The soft parts inserted in figure 4-27. (From *Grant's Method of Anatomy.*)

axes of uterus and vagina are at almost a right angle.

4. **Fornix** of vagina [L., fornix = arch]. The circular gutter surrounding the intravaginal part of the cervix uteri. It is divisible into *anterior*, *posterior*, and *lateral parts*. Posteriorly, the fornix is larger than anteriorly.

5. **Rectum** and **anal canal** are constructed as in the male (p. 60).

Plan for Dissection

The study of the female pelvis will begin with an examination of the peritoneal reflections. After removing the peritoneum and subperitoneal fat, various pelvic structures (bladder, rectum, uterus, ovaries, ovarian tubes, blood vessels, ureter) will be dissected to a certain extent. However, complete and satisfactory dissection of all pelvic structures will be done after partially disarticulating the right hip bone (as described for the male pelvis).

Subsequently, with the cadaver in the prone position, the anal triangle and the ischiorectal fossa will be dissected. The student will be encouraged to combine digital rectal and vaginal examinations with visual observations.

Finally, with the cadaver in the supine position, the external genitalia and the U.G. diaphragm will be studied. Using a midsaggital section, the urethra will be followed to the bladder. The birth canal will be examined from the uterus to the external orifice of the vagina.

Peritoneum in the Female Pelvis

Examine the peritoneum in the female pelvis (fig. 4-29). The peritoneum descends from the anterior abdominal wall (*1*) to the level of the pubic bone (*2*) on to the superior surface of the urinary bladder (*3*).

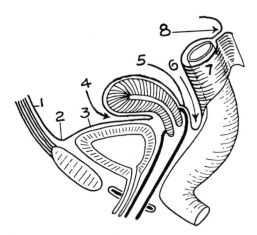

FIG. 4-29. Peritoneum in female pelvis, on median section.

Next, it passes from bladder to uterus (*4*). Here it forms the **vesico-uterine pouch** (fig. 4-29; *Atlas, 233, 236*). The peritoneum covers the fundus and body of the uterus. It extends over the posterior fornix and the wall of the vagina (*5*). Between the uterus and the rectum, the peritoneum forms the deep **recto-uterine pouch** (*6*). From the bottom of the rectouterine pouch (*Atlas, 233*) the peritoneum passes on to the front and sides of the rectum (*7*). Finally, at the third sacral vertebrae, the peritoneum becomes the sigmoid mesocolon (*8*). The **paravesical fossa,** a peritoneal fossa, is apparent on each side of the bladder (*Atlas, 205*). The peritoneal recess on each side of the rectum is called the **pararectal fossa** (*Atlas, 202*).

Broad Ligament of the Uterus (fig. 4-30; *Atlas, 232–233*). At the sides of the uterus, two layers of peritoneum (from the back and front of that organ) come together to form a broad fold, the broad ligament of the uterus. The 'ligament' extends to the side wall of the pelvis. The **uterine tube** is contained within its free margin. The peritoneal fold (meso) that surrounds the uterine tube is called the **mesosalpinx** [Gk., salpinx = tube]. The **ovary** is attached to the posterior aspect of the broad ligament (*Atlas, 232*). The peritoneal fold (meso) that contains the ovary is the **mesovarium.** Observe the ovary on the side wall of the pelvis. The loose fatty and areolar tissues enclosed between the two layers of the broad ligament are collectively called **parametrium** [Gk., para = beside; metra = womb, uterus].

Round Ligament of Uterus (Ligamentum Teres; *Atlas, 232.1, 233*). Visible through the anterior layer of the broad ligament. Observe its subperitoneal course over the pelvic brim, around the lateral side of the inferior epigastric artery, and toward the deep inguinal ring. It terminates in the labium majus.

Ligament of Ovary (*Atlas, 232, 233*). Lateral part of the upper border of the broad ligament.

Suspensory Ligament of Ovary (*Atlas, 232.1, 233*). The most lateral part of the upper border of the broad ligament. Contains the ovarian vessels (*Atlas, 232, 236*).

Recto-uterine Fold (*Atlas, 233*). A sharp fold curving dorsally from the isthmus of the uterus (*Atlas, 233.1*) past the side of the rectum to the sacrum. It forms the brim of the recto-uterine pouch. The rectouterine fold contains the **sacro-uterine ligament** which anchors the uterus to the sacrum. The rectouterine folds and the sacro-uterine ligament can be palpated by digital rectal examination.

Structures Adhering to the Peritoneum. With your fingers detach the peritoneum from the pelvic wall (*Atlas, 232.1*). Note the structures that adhere to the peritoneum:

1. Rectum
2. Bladder
3. Ureter
4. Ovarian vessels
5. Round ligament of uterus

Retropubic Space, Retrorectal Space, and Internal Iliac Vessels

Identify and explore the **retropubic space** and the **retrorectal space** (compare 'male pelvis,' p. 51–52). In the female, the pelvic fascia is substantially thickened at the side of the cervix and vagina. This is the important **transverse cervical ligament** (lateral cardinal lig.; cardinal lig.; lig. of Mackenrodt). The ligament is triangularly shaped and holds the uterus in position by anchoring it to the lateral wall of the pelvis. The uterine vessels run on its upper aspect.

Explore the **retrorectal space** (see 'male pelvis' p. 52).

Follow the **internal iliac artery** and its branches as far as possible (compare 'male pelvis,' p. 52). Trace the **uterine artery** to the lateral margin of the uterus. Give special attention to the fact that the uterine artery crosses above the **ureter** near the lateral fornix of the vagina (fig. 4-30; *Atlas, 234, 235*). At this location, the ureter may be accidentally clamped and severed during hysterectomy (extirpation of uterus). The **ureter** is also in danger when the ovarian vessels are being tied during surgery. The ovarian vessels and the ureter lie very close to each other where they cross the pelvic brim (*Atlas, 233*). The uterine artery becomes sizable during pregnancy.

Identify the **vaginal artery** (fig. 4-31, *Atlas, 234, 235*). Dissect the ovarian vessels, and review their course (fig. 4-31; *Atlas, 188, 188.2*). Demonstrate the anastomoses of ovarian artery with the corresponding uterine artery. This can be done later when access to the pelvis is widened. Review all structures that cross the pelvic brim (ureter, ovarian vessels, round ligament of uterus, possibly vermiform appendix (fig. 4-32).

Pelvic Diaphragm

Lateral Wall of Pelvic Cavity. Identify the **obturator foramen, obturator nerve and vessels, obtur-**

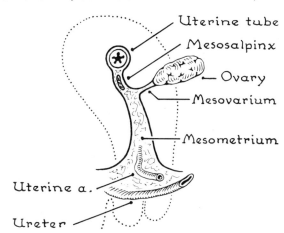

FIG. 4-30. Broad ligament of uterus, its subdivisions and chief relations (paramedian section).

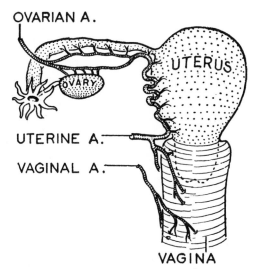

FIG. 4-31. Arterial supply of uterus, ovary, and vagina. (From *Grant's Method of Anatomy*.)

ator internus muscle, and the **pelvic diaphragm** (compare with 'male pelvis,' p. 53–54). In the female, portions of the pubococcygeus muscle are inserted into the terminal portion of the vagina. Review the puborectal sling (*Atlas, 204.1*).

The pubococcygeus, particularly the portions supporting the vagina and rectum, are frequently injured during childbirth. The supporting ligaments of the pelvic fascia may also be torn during parturition. As a consequence, the pelvic viscera are no longer adequately supported by the pelvic diaphragm. Pelvic organs may push downward and prolapse through the weakened vaginal wall (prolapse of bladder = cystocele; prolapse of rectum = rectocele), or the uterus may descend down the vaginal canal (prolapse of uterus).

Anal Region (Triangle)

The *next objective* is the study of the **anal region** (triangle) and its nerve and blood supply. Place the female cadaver into the prone position (face down). Follow the same procedures prescribed earlier for the male cadaver (p. 54–55).

Be aware of the close relationship of sacrospinous ligament, ischial spine, and pudendal nerve. Local anesthesia of the pudendal nerve is of great obstetrical and gynecological importance. Bilateral pudendal nerve block anesthetizes the skin and musculature of the perineum. To achieve effective results, the needle is aimed toward the ischial spine through the ischiorectal fossa.

Partial Disarticulation of Right Hip Bone

While the cadaver is still in the prone position, preparations will be made for partial disarticulation of the **right hip bone.** *Important:* Only the **right** hip bone will be partially disarticulated. The following two steps are preparatory to disarticulating the right sacroiliac joint. On the **right side only** cut the following ligaments (fig. 4-4):

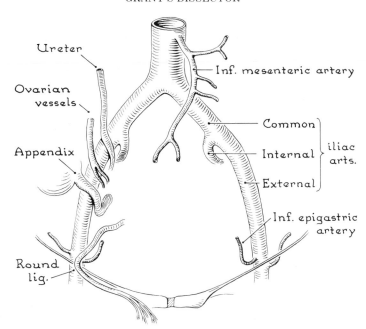

FIG. 4-32. Iliac arteries and certain structures crossing them to enter or leave the pelvis. Sigmoid colon and mesocolon (left side only) are not shown.

1. **Sacrotuberous ligament.** Cut it close to the ischial tuberosity.
2. **Sacrospinous ligament.** Cut it close to the ischial spine. Be aware of the close relationship of the ischial spine and pudendal structures (fig. 4-16). Do *not* damage the nerve or vessels.

Next, turn the cadaver into the supine position (face up). Place a wooden block, 15 to 20 cm high, under the small of the back. Now, once again examine the levator ani: Place the middle finger of one hand in the ischiorectal fossa and touch its roof (levator ani). Place the middle finger of the other hand into the lesser pelvis so that both fingers approach each other. The intervening muscular sheet is the funnel-shaped levator ani. Again, place your finger into the rectum. At the same time, with the other hand in the pelvis, appreciate:

1. The length and direction of the anal canal from external sphincter to pelvic diaphragm (*Atlas, 196*).
2. The position of the vagina and the cervix of the uterus (*Atlas, 236*).

Now, prepare to disarticulate the right hip bone. Follow the same procedures prescribed earlier for the male cadaver (p. 56). Substitute the term 'clitoris' for 'penis.' For example, the 'suspensory ligament of the penis' will become the 'suspensory ligament of the clitoris.'

Complete Dissection of Female Pelvis and Perineum

With the pelvic girdle widened, the pelvic structures are readily accessible, particularly on the right side. In the following manner, examine and dissect these structures, noting their topographical relations:

1. **Levator ani** (*Atlas, 231*). On the right side, pick up the muscular slips with a pair of forceps. Observe the relatively thick pubococcygeal portion with some of its fibers extending toward the vagina and rectum, and anus. Once again, note that the female pelvic diaphragm is traversed by three structures: Urethra, vagina, and rectum.
2. **Ureter.** Follow the ureter to the posterolateral portion of the urinary bladder (fig. 4-25; *Atlas, 232.1*). Of special interest is the region where the uterine artery crosses over the ureter (*Atlas, 234, 235*).
3. **Ovary** (*Atlas, 232, 236*). In nulliparous women, each ovary lies in a shallow depression bounded by ureter, external iliac vein, and uterine tube. If not already done, dissect the ovarian vessels throughout their course. Incise one ovary. The structure of the ovary varies with age. If the age of subject is under 40 to 50 years, look for follicles.
4. **Digital examination of rectum and vagina.** Again, place the gloved finger into the rectum. Perform digital examination of pelvic organs *per rectum*. At the same time, make visual observations (*Atlas, 236*). Palpate the muscular wall formed by the sphincter ani externus. Higher up, at the anorectal junction feel the puborectalis (puborectal sling; part of levator ani). Anteriorly, feel the posterior wall of the vagina and cervix of the uterus. Place one finger of the other hand in the recto-uterine fossa and

note that the anterior wall of the rectum intervenes between the two fingers. Laterally, feel the sharp recto-uterine fold.

Next, perform digital examination of the pelvic organs *per vaginam*. Place one or two gloved fingers in the vagina. Place the fingers of the other hand in the pelvis. Between the two hands, palpate and observe: Urinary bladder, cervix of uterus, recto-uterine pouch, and uterus.

Digital rectal and vaginal examinations are very important procedures in assessing the disposition and condition of pelvic organs. Under pathological conditions, one can palpate the enlarged or displaced broad ligament, enlarged ovaries, and uterine tubes (inflammatory processes, tumors, cysts, ectopic pregnancies, etc.).

Note that only the posterior fornix of the vagina intervenes between the peritoneal cavity (rectouterine pouch of Douglas) and the outside (fig. 4-29; *Atlas, 236*). Therefore, a needle can be pushed through the posterior vaginal fornix to aspirate pathological contents from the rectouterine pouch. Also, a culdoscope can be introduced through the posterior vaginal fornix into the abdominal cavity. The culdoscope allows visual observations of uterine tubes, ovaries, posterior surface of uterus, and anterior surface of rectum.

5. Observe the **rectal venous plexus.** Note numerous small veins on the surface of the rectum. The importance of this plexus in cases of portal venous hypertension has been stressed earlier (*Atlas, 160.1*).

6. Observe **venous plexuses** lying on each side of the vagina and uterus, and surrounding the neck of the bladder. The clitoris drains into the vesical plexus. Usually, the venous plexuses intercommunicate. This fact is of clinical importance (e.g. transportation of tumor cells or inflammatory processes along vascular channels).

Do not attempt to dissect the complex pelvic venous plexuses. Remove all tributaries of the internal iliac vein so that the arterial distribution can be clearly demonstrated.

7. **Internal iliac artery and branches.** Follow instructions given for male cadaver (p. 58). In addition, dissect the vaginal and uterine arteries. At the lateral wall of the uterus, establish anastomotic connections between uterine and ovarian vessels (fig. 4-31; *Atlas, 232.1, 233.3*).

8. Identify the **piriformis** muscle. Follow instructions given for the male cadaver (p. 58).

9. Dissect the **sacral nervous plexus.** Follow instructions given for the male cadaver (p. 58).

10. **Clitoris.** Identify the glans which lies between two folds formed by labia minora. The anterior folds form the right and left sides of a hood over the glans clitoridis, the **prepuce** of the clitoris (fig. 4-33). The clitoris is homologous to the penis. It consists mainly of erectile tissue. Distinguish between its subdivisions: Glans,

body, and crura (*Atlas, 224*). Each crus is attached to the ischipubic ramus.

If you have not done so, pick up the right internal pudendal artery and the pudendal nerve in the pelvis. Clean and follow the nerve and artery. Establish the continuity of these structures to the U.G. diaphragm and to the clitoris (*Atlas, 226*).

11. **Superficial perineal muscles** (fig. 4-33; *Atlas, 227*). The structures of the urogenital triangle were detached from the ischiopubic ramus on the right side. Therefore, the *left side* of the urogenital triangle is best suited for studying the superficial perineal muscles. Remove the labia majora and minora: Lateral to the labium majus, make a longitudinal cut through the superficial perineal fascia. Next, on both sides of the symphysis pubis cut longitudinally down to the bone (*Atlas, 226*). This procedure will leave exposed the *suspensory ligament of the clitoris* (*Atlas, 227*). Identify and dissect (fig. 4-33; *Atlas, 227*):

a. **Central tendon of perineum** (perineal body; fig. 4-18). It is the central fibromuscular area where most perineal muscles are in part attached.

b. **Bulbospongiosus** (bulbocavernosus). Blends with sphincter ani externus at central tendon. Surrounds orifice of the vagina, and dimishes the vaginal orifice.

c. **Ischiocavernosus.** Arises from inner surface of ischial tuberosity and covers crus of clitoris. Retards venous return. Thus, keeps the erectile tissue engorged with blood.

d. Superficial transverse perineal muscle (fig. 4-33). Narrow muscular slip from ischial tuberosity to central tendon. Holds central tendon in place.

When separating these three muscles (b,c,d) from each other, note a small triangular area of exposed perineal membrane (asterick in fig. 4-33). This perineal membrane is the inferior fascia of the U.G. diaphragm.

The muscles of the female perineal region are of great obstetrical importance. Perineal lacerations during childbirth are common. Frequently, the external orifice of the birth canal is prophylactically widened by episiotomy (surgical incision when laceration seems imminent during delivery). Intelligent repair of either lacerations or episiotomy wounds requires sufficient knowledge of the female perineal region.

Deep to the bulbospongiosus are two paired structures (fig. 4-34; *Atlas, 228*): The **bulb of the vestibule** which is an elongated mass of erectile tissue, and the **greater vestibular glands.** Each gland has a 2.5 cm duct which opens into the lateral groove between labium minus and vaginal orifice. On the right side, where the U.G. diaphragm was detached from the ischiopubic ramus, search for the greater vestibular

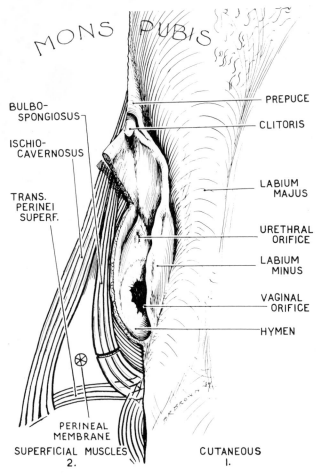

MONS PUBIS

BULBO-SPONGIOSUS

ISCHIO-CAVERNOSUS

TRANS. PERINEI SUPERF.

PREPUCE

CLITORIS

LABIUM MAJUS

URETHRAL ORIFICE

LABIUM MINUS

VAGINAL ORIFICE

HYMEN

PERINEAL MEMBRANE

SUPERFICIAL MUSCLES 2.

CUTANEOUS I.

FIG. 4-33. Female perineum: (2) superficial muscles; (1) external genitalia.

gland and the bulb of the vestibule. Use forceps and the handle of a scalpel (fig. 4-34).

12. **Urethra** (*Atlas*, 236). The female urethra is about 3.5 to 4 cm long. It entends from the neck of the bladder to the **urethral orifice,** lying about 2 cm posterior to the clitoris and anterior to the vaginal orifice (fig. 4-33; *Atlas*, 227). Place a probe into the urethral orifice and push it into the bladder. Palpate the probe (which represents the urethra) through the anterior vaginal wall. Next, make a midsagittal section through the clitoris down to the probe. Examine the urethra in relation to the U.G. diaphragm. Note the musculature surrounding the membranous urethra, the **sphincter urethrae.**

13. **Urinary bladder.** The interior of the female urinary bladder does not differ from that of the male. Follow instructions outlined on p. 60.

14. The next objective is to expose the **vagina** and the interior of the **uterus.** Proceed as follows: Complete the midsagittal section through the bladder. Cut through the anterior vaginal wall and extend the midsagittal section through the

uterus. Do *not* damage the posterior vaginal wall or the rectum.

15. **Vagina** [L., vagina = sheath]. Observe that the anterior vaginal wall is about 7.5 to 8 cm long. The posterior wall is slightly longer to accommodate the posterior vaginal fornix. Once again, examine the relationship of posterior fornix to rectouterine pouch (*Atlas*, 236). Observe the close topographical relations of lateral vaginal fornix and uterine artery (*Atlas*, 233.3). In the living, particularly in the pregnant woman, the pulsations of the uterine artery may be felt through the lateral fornices. Realize that the vagina is so distensible that it can accommodate head and shoulders of a baby passing through the birth canal.

16. **Uterus** (*Atlas*, 236). Note its normal anteverted position. Observe that the longitudinal axes of uterus and vagina are at an angle of approximately 90°. Realize that the position of the uterus must change when the bladder is full or in pregnancy. Identify the following features of the uterus (*Atlas*, 233.1):

a. **Cervix,** protruding into the vaginal canal. The cervical canal opens through the **ostium** uteri (external os) into the vagina. Review

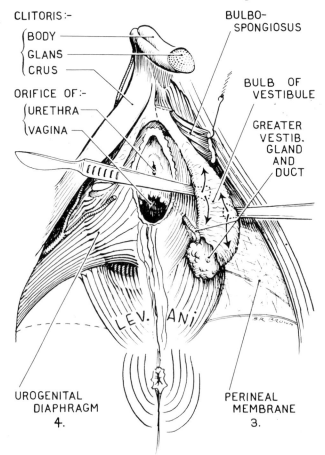

CLITORIS:-

BODY

GLANS

CRUS

ORIFICE OF:-

URETHRA

VAGINA

BULBO-SPONGIOSUS

BULB OF VESTIBULE

GREATER VESTIB. GLAND AND DUCT

LEV. ANI

UROGENITAL DIAPHRAGM 4.

PERINEAL MEMBRANE 3.

FIG. 4-34. Female perineum: Bulb of vestibule and U.G. diaphragm.

the strong ligamentous attachments that hold the cervix in place (sacro-uterine ligament; transverse cervical or cardinal ligament).

b. **Body of uterus.** Identify the **vesical surface** facing the vesico-uterine pouch, and the **superior surface** facing the recto-uterine pouch. Note that the lateral surfaces are attached to the **broad ligament** (*Atlas, 232*). Structures to and from the uterus are contained in the loose areolar tissue between the two layers of the broad ligament. This tissue is the **parametrium.** Identify the **uterine cavity.** In sagittal section, it is a mere slit (*Atlas, 236*). In coronal section, it is triangular in shape (*Atlas, 233.1*). The uterine mucosa is called **endometrium.** Observe the thick uterine wall composed of smooth musculature, the **myometrium.** Understand clinically important terms: *Endometrium* [Gk., endon = within; metra = uterus]; *myometrium* [Gk., mys = muscle]; *parametrium* [Gk., para = beside]. The **fundus** is the rounded part of the uterus which lies above the entrances of the tubes (*Atlas, 233.1*).

17. **Uterine tube** (Fallopian tube; oviduct). With a pair of scissors, open one uterine tube longitudinally. Note the funnel-shaped **infundibulum** with its **fimbriae** (*Atlas, 232*). Observe the narrow medial one-third of the uterine tube, the **isthmus.** Realize that the uterine tubes provide an open channel from the outside into the peritoneal cavity. With a probe follow this channel from vagina via cervical canal, uterine cavity, and uterine tubes into the abdominal cavity.

18. **Rectum.** In order to preserve the relations of vagina, uterus, bladder, and rectum, study the anal canal in the male cadaver (p. 60–61).

CHAPTER 5

LOWER EXTREMITY

Introductory Remarks

The essential functional requirements of the lower extremity are: (1) weight bearing; (2) locomotion; and (3) maintenance of equilibrium. Anatomically, the lower extremity is divided into three segments:
1. Thigh; the segment between hip and knee;
2. Leg; specifically the segment between knee and ankle; and
3. Foot.

It is advantageous to dissect the lower extremity in the following sequence: First, the front and the medial region of the thigh. Subsequently, with the cadaver in the prone position, the gluteal region, back of thigh, and popliteal fossa. Finally, the three crural compartments of the leg will be dissected, and their contents will be followed onto the dorsum and into the sole of the foot.

Front and Medial Region of Thigh

Bony Landmarks

Refer to the skeleton and study the following landmarks (*Atlas, 242, 243*):
1. **Anterior superior iliac spine.**
2. **Anterior inferior iliac spine.**
3. *Inguinal ligament*, stretching from anterior superior iliac spine to pubic tubercle.
4. **Greater trochanter** of femur.
5. **Lesser trochanter** of femur.
6. **Lateral condyle** and **epicondyle** of femur.
7. **Medial condyle** and **epicondyle** of femur.
8. **Adductor tubercle** located on the medial epicondyle. The adductor tubercle is close to the *epiphyseal plate*, where most of the growth in length of the femur takes place.
9. **Linea aspera.**
10. **Patella.**
11. **Tuberosity** (tubercle) **of tibia.**

Plan for Dissection

After reflecting the skin, the saphenous opening and its relation to the saphenous vein will be studied.

Subsequently, the femoral sheath, canal, and ring will be explored. The femoral triangle will be defined, and some of its contents will be followed into the adductor canal. The muscles of the anterior and medial regions of the thigh will be displayed.

Skin Incisions

Make skin incisions according to figure 5-1.
1. If not already done, make a skin incision from the anterior superior iliac spine along the inguinal ligament to the pubic tubercle. From there carry the incision toward the ischial tuberosity (*F* to *G*).
2. Make a horizontal incision about 5 cm below the tibial tuberosity (*H* to *I*).
3. Join the two incisions by a vertical one on the middle of the front of the thigh (*K* to *L*). Reflect the skin (but not the superficial fascia) medially and laterally.

Superficial Veins and Nerves

Observe the **great saphenous vein,** the longest vein in the body [Gk., saphenous = manifest; visible].

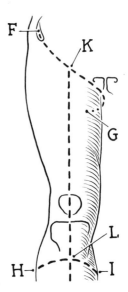

FIG. 5-1. Skin incisions.

Realize that it begins at the medial aspect of the foot and terminates about 3 cm below the inguinal ligament (*Atlas, 245*). Here, the vein passes through an oval aperture in the deep fascia, the **saphenous hiatus** or **saphenous opening** or fossa ovalis, to end in the femoral vein (fig. 5-3, *Atlas, 254, 258*). Trace the great saphenous vein obliquely up the thigh to the saphenous opening. Pass the handle of the knife behind the cleaned vein. Carry it upward until arrested by the vein hooking over the lower sharp margin of the saphenous opening (fig. 5-2). Do not dissect the tributaries of the vein, but realize that they exist (*Atlas, 245*).

One of its tributaries, the superficial epigastric vein, is of clinical importance. It is a potential collateral channel in patients with obstruction of the inferior vena cava or the portal vein (compare p. 24).

Slit open the proximal portion of the *great saphenous vein* and observe one or two of its valves. There are 10 to 20 valves along the entire course of the vein (*Atlas, 255*). Note the *small saphenous vein* at the back of the leg (*Atlas, 246*). Valve incompetency in the saphenous veins and their tributaries leads to the condition of 'varicose veins.'

Look for **superficial inguinal lymph nodes** (fig. 5-3; *Atlas, 251*). A horizontal group lies about 2 cm below the inguinal ligament. A vertical group is applied to both sides of the great saphenous vein.

The cutaneous nerves supplying the anterior and lateral aspects of the thigh are the **lateral, intermediate,** and **medial cutaneous nerves of the thigh** (*Atlas, 248*). These cutaneous nerves pierce the deep fascia along the line of the **sartorius,** the slender strap-like muscle crossing the front of the thigh obliquely from the anterior superior iliac spine to the medial side of the knee (fig. 5-4 or *Atlas, 258*). Make a brief attempt to identify the nerves and to determine their cutaneous distribution. It is relatively easy to follow the **lateral cutaneous nerve:** Identify it on the posterior abdominal wall above the inguinal ligament (*Atlas, 256*), hold it taunt, and trace it distally into the thigh (fig. 5-4; L.C.).

Remove the remains of the superficial fascia from

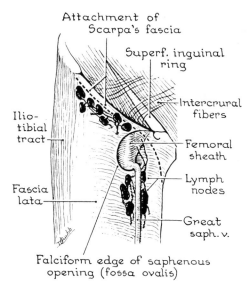

FIG. 5-3. Femoral sheath and inguinal lymph nodes.

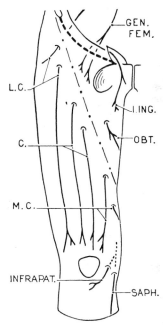

FIG. 5-4. Anterior cutaneous nerves of thigh (*L.C., I.C.,* and *M.C.:* lateral, intermediate, and medial cutaneous nerves of thigh).

the front of the thigh down to the level of the upper border of the patella. Use a sponge to blot dry the exposed *fascia lata.*

If time permits, make a vertical incision on the patella down to the bone. Prolong the incision to the tibial tuberosity. Do not cut through the patellar ligament. Explore the **prepatellar bursa** (*Atlas, 301*). The bursa, which is lined with synovial membrane and contains some synovial fluid, may become inflamed and distended by chronic and repeated irritation.

Femoral Sheath and Contents

Femoral sheath, canal, and ring (*Atlas, 253, 254, 256*). This delicate sheath envelops the femoral artery, femoral vein, and some lymph vessels. Realize that

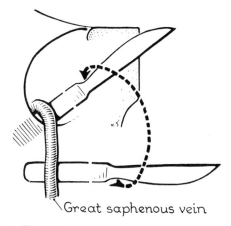

FIG. 5-2. To find lower margin of saphenous opening.

the sheath is formed by a prolongation of the fasciae lining the abdomen, and that it extends under the inguinal ligament into the thigh (*Atlas, 256*). Notice that the femoral sheath is shaped like a short cone (fig. 5-6). The sheath is subdivided by two delicate vertical partitions into three compartments (figs. 5-5, 5-6; *Atlas, 256.1*).

1. The *lateral compartment* is occupied by the **femoral artery** (*A* in fig. 5-5).
2. The *middle compartment* is occupied by the **femoral vein.**
3. The *medial compartment* contains lymph vessels, a small lymph node, and areolar tissue. This small medial compartment is also known as the **femoral canal,** which is conical in shape. The **femoral ring** is the mouth of the femoral canal.

Knowledge of the femoral ring and canal is important in understanding the mechanism of **femoral hernia.** A femoral hernia is a protrusion of parts of abdominal viscera through the femoral

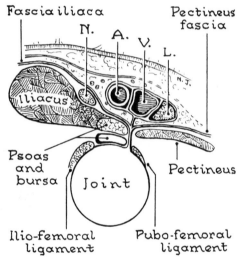

FIG. 5-5. Femoral sheath on cross section.

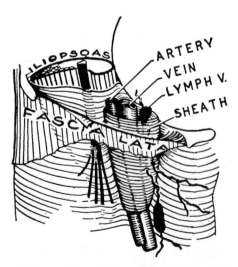

FIG. 5-6. Femoral sheath. (From *Grant's Method of Anatomy.*)

ring into the femoral canal. Study figure 5-6. Understand the following: A femoral hernia (1) is relatively small since it is contained in the limited femoral canal; (2) can usually be palpated below the inguinal ligament; (3) is frequently strangulated due to tightness of the inguinal ligament.

Clean the fascia lata in the vicinity of the **saphenous opening.** Insert the handle of the knife into the opening and ease back the underlying femoral sheath without injuring it. With the handle of the knife clean the pectineal fascia medial to the saphenous opening and behind it (*Atlas, 254*). Appreciate that the vein and lymph vessels lie behind the opening itself, whereas the artery lies behind the lateral edge of the opening (*Atlas, 254*).

Now, the objective is to expose the entire femoral sheath. Therefore, carefully incise the lateral edge of the saphenous opening. Reflect the flap of deep fascia, and remove it (*Atlas, 254*). Next, place a block under the knee in order to flex the hip joint. This procedure will render the femoris sheath lax. Subsequently, separate the femoral sheath from the underlying fasciae, the pectineal fascia and the fascia iliaca (fig. 5-5 or *Atlas, 256.1*). Sever the septum that passes backward from the sheath. Detach the front of the sheath from the inguinal ligament. Establish the continuity of the femoral sheath with the fasciae lining the abdomen (*Atlas, 256*).

The next objective is the examination of the **three compartments** of the femoral sheath. In the midline of each compartment, make a vertical cut (*Atlas, 254*). In the **lateral compartment** observe the femoral artery. In the **middle compartment** identify the femoral vein. The **medial compartment** is the **femoral canal,** which contains lymphatics and loose areolar tissue. Pass a probe up into the femoral canal and study topographical relations of its mouth, the **femoral ring.** These are (*Atlas, 254, 256.1*):

1. Anteriorly, the inguinal ligament.
2. Posteriorly, the pectineus and its fascia separate the ring from the superior ramus of the pubic bone (*Atlas, 109.1*).
3. Laterally, the femoral vein.
4. Medially, the sharp lateral edge of the lacunar ligament (*Atlas, 109.1*).

Femoral Triangle

The **femoral triangle** is bounded by the **inguinal ligament, sartorius,** and **adductor longus** (fig. 5-7 or *Atlas, 258, 258.1*). Clean the **femoral artery and vein** within the limits of the femoral triangle. Just below the inguinal ligament, the artery gives rise to superficial branches to the abdominal wall and scrotum or labium majus (*Atlas, 254, 225*). Pay particular attention to the following three substantial arteries; these may arise from a large common stem, or may arise independently (*Atlas, 244*):

1. **Profunda femoris** artery. It pursues the same

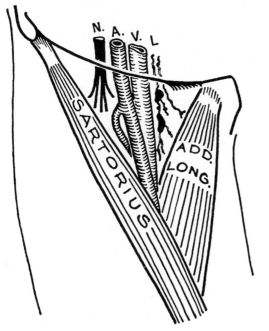

Atlas, 263). Pass a probe into the canal and study its walls. It is bounded laterally by the **vastus medialis,** posteromedially by the **adductor longus and magnus,** and anteriorly by the **sartorius.** Verify these relations on a cross section (*Atlas, 264*).

Lift the **sartorius** out of its bed. Slit open the fascial roof of the adductor canal. Now, the whole length of the femoral vessels is exposed. The vein lies posterior to the artery. Trace the femoral artery to the point where it passes through the **hiatus** in the adductor magnus (fig. 5-8; *Atlas, 244*). Here, the artery changes its name to popliteal artery. Note that the **saphenous nerve** does *not* pass through the adductor hiatus. Instead, it runs in front of the adductor magnus tendon (*Atlas, 263*) toward the medial aspect of the knee (*Atlas, 248*). Follow the saphenous nerve until it becomes superficial between the sartorius and the tendon of the **gracilis.**

Fascia Lata

In the lateral region of the thigh, the **fascia lata** (deep fascia) is strong and dense (*Atlas, 258*). Immediately behind and below the anterior superior iliac spine, the fascia lata encases a muscle, the **tensor fasciae latae** (*Atlas, 259*). Identify it. Verify that it pulls on a strap-like, longitudinal thickening of the fascia lata, the **iliotibial tract** (*Atlas, 260*). Split the fascia lata longitudinally between rectus femoris and vastus lateralis. Retract the iliotibial tract from the underlying vastus lateralis (*Atlas, 264*). With your fingers and the handle of the knife, follow the fascia

Fig. 5-7. Contents of femoral triangle. (From *Grant's Method of Anatomy*.)

general direction as the femoral artery, but on a more posterior plane.

2. **Lateral femoral circumflex** artery.
3. **Medial femoral circumflex** artery. This artery is clinically important since it supplies the bulk of blood to the head and neck of the femur (*Atlas, 244, 279*).

Cut vertically through the fascia iliaca and expose the **femoral nerve** just lateral to the femoral artery (*Atlas, 258*). Notice the numerous branches of the nerve. Once again, identify the **intermediate** and the **medial cutaneous nerve of the thigh.** These nerves follow the medial border of the sartorius in front of the femoral artery. Also, identify **motor branches** to the **sartorius** and to the **rectus femoris.**

Preserve the femoral, profunda femoris, and the great saphenous veins. In order to clarify the dissection field, remove all other smaller veins (compare *Atlas, 257*). Display the floor of the femoral triangle by removing fat and fascia, particularly from the pectineus and adductor longus (*Atlas, 258*). Open the interval between the contiguous borders of psoas and pectineus. The medial femoral circumflex vessels pass dorsally between these two muscles (M.F.C. in fig. 5-8; *Atlas, 259*).

Adductor Canal

In the middle third of the thigh, the femoral vessels and the saphenous nerve are contained in the **adductor canal** (Hunter's canal). The adductor canal is a narrow fascial tunnel which begins at the **apex of the femoral triangle** (*Atlas, 259*) and ends at the **opening or hiatus of the adductor magnus** (fig. 5-8;

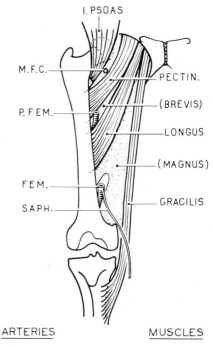

Fig. 5-8. Iliopsoas and adductors, and the arteries passing between them (*M.F.C.,* med. fem. circumflex; *P.FEM.,* profunda femoris; *FEM.,* femoral artery).

lata posteriorly. Here, it is continuous with a very strong **intermuscular septum** which is attached to the **linea aspera** on the posterior aspect of the femur (*Atlas, 262, 264*).

Muscles of Front of Thigh

Define the **rectus femoris** in the middle of the anterior thigh (*Atlas, 260*). If possible, follow its two tendinous heads to their origins (*Atlas, 284*): A straight tendon to the anterior inferior iliac spine; and a reflected tendon to the region above the acetabulum. Observe that the flattened tendon of the muscle is inserted into the patella.

Identify and examine the **three vasti muscles** (*Atlas, 260, 261*). The **vastus lateralis** lies on the lateral side of the femur. The **vastus medialis** covers the medial aspect of the thigh. Between the vastus medialis and lateralis is the **vastus intermedius.** Expose the vastus intermedius in the following manner: Section the overlying rectus femoris close to its tendinous insertion into the patella. Then, reflect the rectus femoris upward. Identify the nerve branches supplying the vasti (*Atlas, 250*). Study the vasti on cross section (*Atlas, 262, 264*). Realize that their origins include large parts of the shaft of the femur (*Atlas, 265, 266*).

The four muscles (vastus lateralis, medialis, intermedius, and rectus femoris) are collectively known as the **quadriceps femoris.** Observe that the tendons of all four heads of the quadriceps unite to form a strong tendon. This tendon is inserted into the patella, and continues downward to the tibial tuberosity as the **ligamentum patellae or patellar tendon.**

Tapping the **patellar tendon** (distal to the patella) normally leads to the elicitation of the **quadriceps reflex** (patellar reflex; knee jerk). The tapping activates muscle spindles in the quadriceps. Afferent impulses from these muscle spindles travel in the femoral nerve to spinal segments L_2, L_3, and L_4 (*Atlas, 250*). From here, efferent impulses are mediated in motor fibers of the femoral nerve to the quadriceps, resulting in a jerk-like contraction of this muscle. Obviously, intelligent clinical evaluation of the quadriceps reflex depends on thorough knowledge of the underlying anatomical substrate.

Medial Side of Thigh

Remove any remaining deep fascia from the medial side of the thigh in order to display the **adductors.** Observe that **pectineus, adductor longus,** and **gracilis** originate from a curved line on the pubic bone (fig. 5-8; *Atlas, 260*). Follow the slender, strap-like **gracilis** down the medial aspect of the thigh to its insertion into the tibia (fig. 5-8; *Atlas, 262*). Trace the **pectineus** and **adductor longus** as they fan out to their insertions along the **linea aspera** on the posterior aspect of the femur (*Atlas, 266*). Note that the **profunda femoris vessels** pass between the two muscles (*Atlas, 259*). Now, separate the adjacent

borders of pectineus and adductor longus. Cut the adductor longus 5 cm from its origin and reflect it (*Atlas, 263*). The adductor brevis can now be seen. On cross section, verify that the brevis lies posterior to the longus (*Atlas, 264*).

Examine the **adductor brevis.** Realize that part of it is covered by the pectineus (*Atlas, 261*). Therefore, carefully cut the pectineus close to its origin, and reflect it. Clean the adductor brevis. Do not damage nerves and vessels anterior to the muscle. Now, it should be easy to identify the **obturator nerve.** If in doubt, gently pull on the nerve within the pelvis, or pass your probe along the nerve through the obturator foramen (*Atlas, 216*). Realize that the obturator nerve is motor to the adductor muscles (*Atlas, 250*).

Examine a cross section of the thigh (*Atlas, 262, 264*), and verify that some branches of the obturator nerve run anterior, others posterior to the adductor brevis. First, examine the *anterior* nerve branches in your cadaver specimen (*Atlas, 263*). Next, verify that the *posterior* nerve branches pass between **adductor brevis** and **adductor magnus.** With your fingers, separate the two muscles.

Now, study the **profunda femoris artery** and its distribution (*Atlas, 244*). To clarify the dissecting field, sacrifice the accompanying veins. Note that the profunda artery arises from the femoral artery 2 to 5 cm below the inguinal ligament. Clean the artery and some of its branches. Identify one or two of the **perforating arteries,** which encircle the femur and supply the adjacent musculature.

Cut and reflect the adductor brevis in order to display the whole length of the **adductor magnus.** Once again, define the **hiatus** in the adductor magnus through which the femoral vessels pass to become the popliteal vessels (*Atlas, 244, 269*). Medial to the hiatus, trace the adductor tendon to its insertion into the **adductor tubercle** on the medial epicondyle. Realize that the bulk of the adductor magnus is inserted, by means of a broad aponeurosis, into the **linea aspera.**

Review the **obturator nerve.** Study its motor branches (*Atlas, 250*) and its cutaneous branches (*Atlas, 248*). Observe that the proximal portion of the obturator nerve is accompanied by branches of the obturator artery (*Atlas, 244*).

Gluteal Region

General Remarks

The gluteal (buttock) region was considered in part during the dissection of the perineum and pelvis (pp. 54–55). The gluteus maximus was partially reflected so that: (1) the greater and lesser sciatic foramina could be defined; (2) the nerve and blood supply to the perineal region could be traced; and (3) the right sacroiliac joint could be disarticulated.

If the prescribed dissections of your gross anatomy course conform with the particular sequence of chapters in this Dissector, the above mentioned procedures have been already performed.

If you have not as yet dissected the perineum and pelvis, the gluteal region will be completely intact.

Time does not permit dissection of the superficial nerves. However, realize that the cutaneous nerve supply of the gluteal region is extensive. It involves branches from several lumbar and sacral segments (fig. 5-9; *Atlas*, 249, 663).

Important Landmarks

Refer to the skeleton and an articulated pelvis with intact liagments. Identify the following landmarks:
1. **Greater sciatic notch** (*Atlas*, 243).
2. **Lesser sciatic notch.**
3. **Ischial spine** separating the greater and lesser sciatic notches.
4. **Ischial tuberosity.**
5. **Sacrotuberous ligament** (fig. 5-10).
6. **Sacrospinous ligament.**
7. Understand how these two ligaments (5 and 6) contribute to the formation of the **greater sciatic foramen** and the **lesser sciatic foramen.**

Plan for Dissection

If not already done during the dissection of the pelvis and perineum, the skin and superficial fascia overlying the gluteal region will be removed in one piece.

The large gluteus maximus will be studied. The muscle will be divided and reflected to allow access to the deeper plane of the gluteal region. The greater and

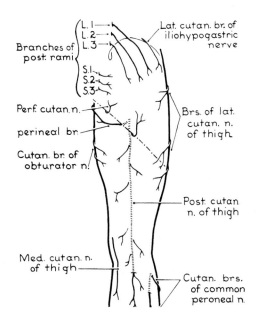

FIG. 5-9. Cutaneous nerves of gluteal region.

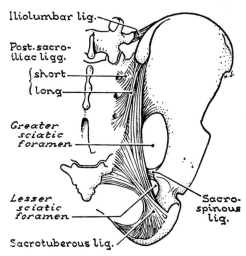

FIG. 5-10. Ligaments of pelvis (posterior view). (From *Grant's Method of Anatomy*.)

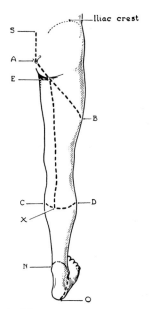

FIG. 5-11. Skin incisions.

lesser sciatic foramina are key areas. It will be demonstrated that these foramina are traversed by important nerves, vessels, and muscles.

Skin Incisions

Turn the subject into the prone position (face down). To steady the limb, put blocks under the anterior iliac spines and under the ankles. Make skin incisions according to fig. 5-11. If not already done **during dissection of pelvis and perineum, make skin incisions S to A and A to B.** At this time, it is advantageous to make additional skin incisions for the back of the thigh and the popliteal fossa:
1. Make a horizontal cut across the back of the leg, about 12 to 15 cm below the level of the patella (*C* to *D*).

2. Make a vertical cut down the middle of the back of the thigh (*E* to *X*), and beyond point *X* half way down to the heel.
3. Reflect the skin medially and laterally. Remove the superficial fascia from the back of the thigh, but not from the popliteal fossa.

Dissection

If not already done during the dissection of the pelvis, expose the thin deep fascia covering the **gluteus maximus.** Define the superior and inferior borders of this vast, rhomboidal muscle (*Atlas, 267*). If you cut too deep below the inferior border, you will severe the **posterior cutaneous nerve of the thigh** (fig. 5-9 or *Atlas, 249*). Avoid this by carefully cleaning and defining the inferior border of the gluteus maximus. Then, by using the scissor technique, the nerve in danger can be picked up midway between ischial tuberosity and greater trochanter. A portion of the **gluteus medius** can be seen superior to the gluteus maximus (*Atlas, 267, 268*). Identify it. Coming from above, push your fingers into the space between gluteus medius and maximus.

If the pelvis and perineum were already dissected, you will find the gluteus maximus reflected from its origin. *On the right side*, the sacrospinous and sacrotuberous ligaments were cut to make partial disarticulation of the sacroiliac joint possible. Thus, the gluteus maximus is already well reflected laterally.

On the left side, the gluteus maximus is only partially reflected form its origin. Place this muscle into its original position. On the left side, as well as in the heretofore undissected gluteal region, proceed as follows (fig. 5-12):
1. Divide the **gluteus maximus** into upper and lower halves by separating its fibers. Start the incision over the **greater trochanter,** which can be easily palpated.
2. Cut down to the bony trochanter. In doing so,

you open the large **bursa** between greater trochanter and gluteus maximus.
3. Rotate the thigh laterally in order to render the gluteus maximus lax. Pass a finger through the incision, and sweep it around circularly in the plane deep to the muscle.
4. With your finger in this deep plane, palpate the following: Fatty, areolar tissue; and **inferior gluteal nerve and vessels** entering the gluteus maximus.

Retract the borders of the incision (fig. 5-12). Identify the **sciatic nerve,** the largest nerve in the body. Avoid its medial side. Rapidly clean the region lateral to the nerve, where there is nothing to damage ('Safe Side'). Trace the nerve up to the **inferior border of the piriformis.** The piriformis occupies a key position in the gluteal region. Realize that the described approach to the gluteal region is also an effective surgical approach to the back of the hip joint and to structures in the gluteal region.

Now, the gluteus maximus should be detached from its sites of origin. If not already done during dissection of the perineum and pelvis (p. 54), proceed as follows:
1. Detach the posterosuperior portion of the gluteus maximus close to the ilium (*Atlas, 266*).
2. With a scalpel, cut through its fibers very close to their origin from the posterior surfaces of the sacrum and coccyx.
3. Place your fingers under the inferior portion of the muscle. Realize that it is attached to the sacrotuberous ligament. Using a pair of scissors, carefully detach the muscle from this ligament.
4. Reflect the muscle slightly. Observe the inferior gluteal nerve and vessels entering its substance near its center. Leave a small button of the maximus attached to the nerve. Now, completely reflect the muscle laterally (*Atlas, 268*).

Observe the insertions of the gluteus maximus: The lower deeper ¼ of the muscle is attached to the gluteal tuberosity of the femur (*Atlas, 276.1*); ¾ of the muscle is inserted into the iliotibial tract (*Atlas, 271*).

The gluteus maximus slides over the greater trochanter of the femur. Therefore, this bony landmark is separated from the muscle by a **bursa.** Open this trochanteric bursa which is the largest in the body (*Atlas, 270*). Observe another smaller bursa between the gluteus maximus and the ischial tuberosity.

Now, the deeper structures of the gluteal region are suitably exposed for examination. Identify the **sciatic nerve,** the largest nerve in the body. Verify that the nerve is located midway between the ischial tuberosity and the greater trochanter (*Atlas, 268*). Follow the nerve proximally to the point where it appears in the gluteal region from under cover of the **piriformis muscle** (*Atlas, 268, 270, 271, 273*). Be aware of the fact that a different relationship between piriformis and sciatic nerve may exist (*Atlas, 323 A*).

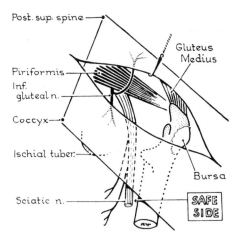

FIG. 5-12. Incision through gluteus maximus to expose piriformis and related structures.

The sciatic nerve has two sides: (1) A side of safety, its lateral side (fig. 5-12); and (2) a side of danger, its medial side (fig. 5-12;

Atlas, 250). Anatomists and surgeons must be extremely careful on the medial side of the sciatic nerve. Here, the nerves to the hamstring muscles are easily severed.

The **piriformis occupies** a *key position* in the gluteal region. Verify that this muscle passes through the greater sciatic foramen and divides it (fig. 5–13; *Atlas, 273*). A number of vessels and nerves traverse the greater sciatic foramen and reach the gluteal region. Some of these structures enter the gluteal region *above* the piriformis; others enter *below* the piriformis (fig. 5-14).

At the *upper border* of the piriformis (fig. 5-14) identify the stems of the **superior gluteal nerve and vessels.** These structures are more or less covered by the **gluteus medius** (*Atlas, 270*).

At the *lower border* of the piriformis (fig. 5-14; *Atlas, 270, 271*) identify the following structures:

1. **Inferior gluteal nerve and vessels** (which were cut during the reflection of the gluteus maximus.
2. **Sciatic nerve,** the largest nerve in the body.
3. **Posterior cutaneous nerve of thigh,** running parallel to the sciatic nerve.
4. **Pudendal nerve** and **internal pudenal vessels.**

The **pudendal nerve** and **internal pudenal vessels** appear only briefly in the gluteal region, entering through the greater sciatic foramen. They exit through the **lesser sciatic foramen** (fig. 5-15) to reach structures in the anal and urogenital regions (*Atlas, 215*). If you have difficulties finding the nerve and vessels, carefully cut the sacrotuberous ligament close to the sacrum. Then reflect the ligament and expose

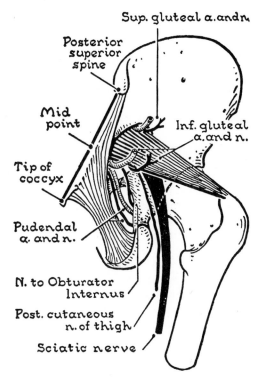

FIG. 5-14. Structures passing through the greater sciatic foramen superior and inferior to the piriformis. (From *Grant's Method of Anatomy.*)

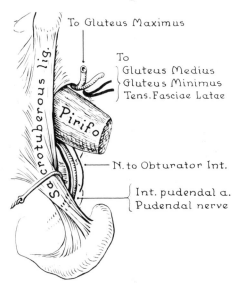

FIG. 5-15. Pudendal nerve and internal pudendal artery entering gluteal region via greater sciatic foramen and leaving it via lesser sciatic foramen.

nerve and vessels. Push a probe along these structures through the lesser sciatic foramen into the **pudendal canal.**

Identify the **obturator internus** which issues through the lesser sciatic foramen (*Atlas, 271, 272*). Clean the broad tendon of the obturator internus. Notice that the tendon lies between the fleshy **gemelli.** The *superior gemellus* arises from the ischial

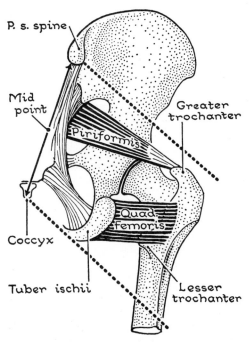

FIG. 5-13. The reference line in the gluteal region is the readily defined lower border of the piriformis. The position of the gluteus maximus is indicated by *dotted lines.* (From *Grant's Method of Anatomy.*)

spine; the *inferior gemellus* from the ischial tuberosity. Below the inferior gemellus, identify the **quadratus femoris** which stretches from ischial tuberosity to intertrochanteric crest of femur (fig. 5-13; *Atlas, 271*). With a probe, locate the **obturator externus** tendon, where it is inserted into the trochanteric fossa of the femur. Find it between the inferior gemellus and the quadratus femoris (*Atlas, 271*).

Identify the dense deep fascia covering the fan-shaped **gluteus medius** (*Atlas, 268*). Most muscle fibers arise from this fascia (*Atlas, 272.1*). Verify this fact by vertically incising the deep fascia overlying the gluteus medius.

Once again, identify the **superior gluteal nerve and vessels** above the piriformis. Follow these vessels by sweeping your fingers deep to the gluteus medius. Your fingers are now in the plane between gluteus medius and minimus (*Atlas, 272.1*). Sever the **gluteus medius** about 3 cm above its insertion into the **greater trochanter** of the femur (*Atlas, 271*). Reflect the muscle and see the underlying **gluteus minimus.** Occasionally, the medius and minimus are not well differentiated. Now, clean the superior gluteal nerve and vessels, including branches to the **tensor fasciae latae.**

Refer to a skeleton and your dissected specimen at the same time. Study the **functions of muscles in the gluteal region.** *Extend* the femur of the skeleton; this movement is accomplished by the gluteus maximus. *Abduct the femur;* this movement depends on the functional integrity of the three abductors of the hip joint: Gluteus medius, gluteus minimus, and tensor fasciae latae.

Intragluteal Injections. The gluteal region is commonly used for intramuscular injections of drugs. These injections should always be made superolaterally in the *upper outer quadrant*. Why? Divide the gluteal region into four quadrants. Realize that injections into the two lower quadrants will endanger and possibly paralyze the important sciatic nerve, or nerves and vessels entering the gluteal region below the piriformis muscle (*Atlas, 271*). Injections into the upper inner (medial) quadrant may injure the stems

of the superior gluteal nerve and vessels (*Atlas, 271*), or the peroneal division of the sciatic nerve (*Atlas, 323 A*). Intragluteal injections into the *upper outer quadrant* are relatively safe since the superior gluteal nerve and vessels are well ramified in this region. Be sure the needle never deviates downward or medially toward the greater sciatic foramen with its important structures.

If time permits, study the continuity of nerves, vessels, and muscles observed in the gluteal region. Within the pelvis (*Atlas, 213, 213.1*) review the gluteal vessels, the piriformis muscle, and essential components of the sacral plexus. Identify the fleshy part of the obturator internus covering the obturator foramen and membrane.

Popliteal Fossa and Back of Thigh

Plan for Dissection

It is advantageous to dissect the popliteal fossa (i.e. back of knee) before the back of the thigh. In this manner, the boundaries of the diamond-shaped popliteal fossa will not be disturbed. After identifying the important contents of the popliteal fossa (nerves, vessels), the muscular boundaries of the fossa will be established. Subsequently, the dissection will be extended into the back of the thigh. The hamstring muscles will be identified, and the sciatic nerve and its branches will be explored.

Popliteal Fossa

If time permits, dissect superficial nerves and veins. At any rate, be aware of the following:
1. The **posterior cutaneous nerve of the thigh** extends as far as the lower limit of the popliteal fossa (*Atlas, 249*).
2. The **small saphenous vein** (*Atlas, 246*) occupies the midline of the calf region and enters the popliteal fossa at its lower half. Note its communications with the greater saphenous vein. In line with the small saphenous vein lies the **medial sural cutaneous nerve** [L., sural = calf of leg].

In the **popliteal fossa**, identify this **medial sural cutaneous nerve.** Find it between the two bellies of the gastrocnemius (*Atlas, 285*). Incise the fascia. Free the nerve and trace it proximally to the **tibial nerve.** In the lateral portion of the popliteal fossa find and clean the **common peroneal nerve** which runs along the medial border of the biceps femoris (fig. 5-16; *Atlas, 285–287*). Find a large branch of the common peroneal nerve, the **lateral sural cutaneous nerve.** This cutaneous nerve sends a **communicating branch** to the medial sural nerve which, thereafter, is called the **sural nerve.** The level of branching and communicating varies substantially from specimen to specimen.

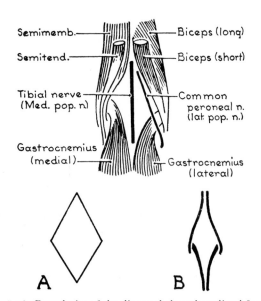

Semimemb.   Biceps (long)

Semitend.   Biceps (short)

Tibial nerve   Common
(Med. pop. n)   peroneal n.
                       (lat. pop. n.)

Gastrocnemius
(medial)   Gastrocnemius
                     (lateral)

A   B

Fɪɢ. 5-16. Boundaries of the diamond-shaped popliteal fossa.

Define the upper angle of the popliteal fossa (fig. 5-16): On the lateral side is the **biceps femoris.** On the medial side, identify the round **semitendinosus** and the fleshy **semimembranosus.** Define the lower angle of the popliteal fossa: Here, the two bellies of the **gastrocnemius** are closely applied to each other.

Place a block under the dorsum of the foot to relax the **gastrocnemius.** Incise the deep fascia at the medial and lateral borders of this muscle. Insert your two index fingers between the contiguous bellies of the gastrocnemius, raise them, and pull them widely apart (fig. 5-17). For a successful exposure, the two heads of the muscle must be freed and separated down to the **tendo calcaneus** (Achilles tendon). Now, the underlying **soleus, popliteus,** and **plantaris** muscles can be seen (*Atlas, 286*).

Trace the **tibial nerve** to the lower limit of the popliteal fossa. Notice that it passes through a gap in the origin of the soleus muscle (*Atlas, 286, 288*). Displace the nerve, and observe a very dense **vascular sheath** which envelops the **popliteal artery** and **popliteal vein.** Push a probe through the adductor hiatus, and establish the continuity of the femoral with the popliteal vessels (*Atlas, 244, 264.1*). Open the vascular sheath. Separate artery from vein. Cut away tributaries of the vein.

Spend a few minutes studying the elaborate anastomoses around the knee (*Atlas, 289–291*). If time permits, identify one or two of the genicular arteries.

Back of Thigh

Remove the deep fascia covering the course of the posterior cutaneous nerve of the thigh. Turn the nerve

up. Clean the **sciatic nerve** and its branches to the hamstring muscles (*Atlas, 250, 270*).

Clean and separate the **hamstring muscles** from one another (*Atlas, 268*). These muscles are the **semitendinosus, semimembranosus,** and the long head of the **biceps femoris.** Verify that these muscles have a **common site of origin: the ischial tuberosity.**

On the medial side of the thigh, identify the **semitendinosus** (meaning 'half tendon') with its round and remarkably long tendon of insertion. Separate the semitendinosus from the **semimembranosus** (meaning 'half membrane') with its substantial membranous tendon of origin.

On the lateral side of thigh, identify the **long head of the biceps femoris.** Verify that the **short head** of this muscle arises from the shaft of the femur (*Atlas, 266, 269*), *not* from the ischial tuberosity. For this reason and the fact that it also has a different nerve supply (*Atlas, 250*), the short head of the biceps femoris does not belong to the hamstring muscles.

Understand that the hamstring muscles span two joints: the hip joint and the knee joint. Verify that the biceps femoris tendon is inserted into the head of the fibula (*Atlas, 295, 296*). The semimembranosus has its insertion into the medial condyle of the tibia. The semitendinosus is inserted into the medial aspect of the tibia (*Atlas, 297, 298*). Understand that the principal actions of the hamstrings are flexion of the leg and extension of the thigh, especially during walking.

Look for arteries supplying the hamstring muscles (*Atlas, 270*). Most of the blood is derived from the *perforating branches* of the profunda femoris artery (*Atlas, 244*).

Leg (or Crus)

General Remarks

The morphological organization and function of the leg will be best understood if a cross section is studied and analyzed (fig. 5-18 or *Atlas, 304.1, 310*). Before attempting dissection, understand the following facts:
1. The two bones of the leg are unequal in size. The larger **tibia** lies medial; its medial surface is subcutaneous. The smaller **fibula** is deeply placed. Tibia and fibula are connected by an interosseous membrane.
2. The investing deep fascia reaches the fibula by means of septa, the **anterior and posterior crural septa.**
3. The two bones, their interosseous membrane, and the crural septa serve to divide the leg into **three compartments: anterior, lateral or peroneal,** and **posterior.** Each compartment contains a synergistic muscle group. A nerve supplying these muscles runs in each compartment.

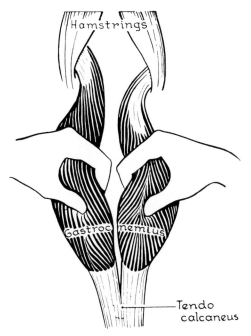

FIG. 5-17. Raise and separate the two bellies of the gastrocnemius to expose adequately the popliteal fossa.

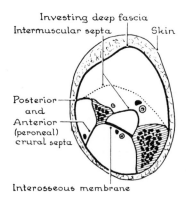

FIG. 5-18. The leg on cross section showing intermuscular septa. The large tibia lies medial; its medial surface is subcutaneous.

4. The muscle in the **anterior crural compartment** are mainly concerned with dorsiflexion of the foot (turning of the foot upward) and with extension of the toes. The nerve within this compartment is the **deep peroneal nerve** (*Atlas, 310*). It is a branch of the common peroneal nerve which passes around the lateral side of the neck of the fibula (*Atlas, 305.1, 306*). The nerve is accompanied by the **anterior tibial artery** which enters the anterior compartment through a gap above the proximal border of the interosseous membrane (*Atlas, 244, 306*).

5. The **lateral crural compartment or peroneal compartment** contains two muscles for plantar flexion and eversion of the foot. The nerve within this compartment is the **superficial peroneal nerve** (*Atlas, 310*). It is a branch of the common peroneal nerve (*Atlas, 250*).

6. The **posterior crural compartment** contains several muscles whose principal function is plantar flexion of the foot and toes (turning foot downward). The muscles are divided into a superficial and a deep group by an intermuscular septum. Note that the nerve of the posterior compartment runs between the superficial and deep group (*Atlas, 310*). This nerve is the **tibial nerve.** Study its ramifications (*Atlas, 250*). The nerve is accompanied by the **posterior tibial artery** (*Atlas, 244, posterior view*).

Important Landmarks

Refer to an articulated lower extremity of a skeleton. Identify the following landmarks:
1. **Medial condyle** and **lateral condyle of tibia** (*Atlas, 243*).
2. **Anterior border of tibia,** descending from the tibial tuberosity (*Atlas, 242*). Note that its proximal portion is sharp and prominent.
3. **Head of fibula** (*Atlas, 242, 243, 303*).
4. **Medial malleolus,** the large medial prominence at the ankle (*Atlas, 315*).

5. **Lateral malleolus,** the lateral prominence at the ankle (*Atlas, 315*).
6. In the articulated foot (*Atlas, 311–314*), identify the **tarsus** which consists of seven tarsal bones: **Talus** [L., = ankle bone]; **calcaneus** [L., calx = heel]; **navicular** [L., = little ship]; **cuboid** [Gk., = cube-shaped]; and the **three cuneiformes** [L., = wedge-shaped].
7. On the **calcaneus** identify the **tuber calcanei** (tuberosity) for attachment of the tendo calcaneus (*Atlas, 315*), and a groove below the **sustentaculum tali** for the passage of a tendon (*Atlas, 311, 315*).
8. Identify the **five metatarsals** (*Atlas, 313*), and the tuberosity of the 5th metatarsal.
9. Note that the first toe has two **phalanges,** whereas the other toes have three (*Atlas, 312, 313*).

Plan for Dissection

After reflecting the skin, the crural compartments (anterior; lateral; posterior) will be dissected. The derivation and course of blood vessels and nerves will be explored, and their continuation onto the dorsum or into the sole of the foot will be demonstrated. The muscles of the crural compartments will be followed to their insertions in the foot.

Skin Incisions

Turn the subject into the supine position (face up). Place a block under the popliteal fossa to steady the limb. Make skin incisions according to figure 5–19:
1. Make a vertical cut along the medial surface of the tibia (*L* to *M*).
2. Carry a curved incision from the medial mal-

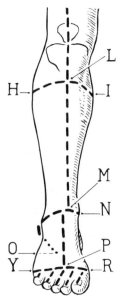

FIG. 5-19. Skin incisions; leg and dorsum of foot.

leolus across the ankle to the point of the heel (*N* to *O*).

3. Cut along the midline of the dorsum of the foot (*M* to *P*).
4. Cut transversely across the foot at the webs of the toes (*R* to *Y*). Cut along the midline of each toe.
5. Make all skin incisions at the sole of the foot according to fig. 5-20.
6. Remove all skin. Do not destroy the deep fascia or the extensor retinacula (compare, *Atlas*, *307–309*).

Anterior Crural Compartment and Dorsum of Foot

Briefly review but do not dissect the superficial veins (*Atlas*, 246, 247). The sural nerve runs with the small saphenous vein toward digit 5.

Find the **superficial peroneal nerve** or musculocutaneous nerve (fig. 5-21 or *Atlas*, 248). It emerges from the lateral crural compartment and runs medial to the fibula onto the dorsum of the foot. If time permits, trace this cutaneous nerve to its terminations on the toes.

The **deep peroneal nerve** of the anterior crural compartment sends only a small cutaneous twig to the foot. This small branch may be found (and clinically tested) between the first and second toe (fig. 5-21 or *Atlas*, 248).

Expose and clean the **deep fascia.** Demonstrate that muscle fibers of the **tibialis anterior** arise from this deep fascia: Make a vertical cut through the fascia just below the lateral tibial condyle, lift the edges of the deep fascia, and see the muscle fibers arising (fig. 5-22). Since the muscle takes origin from the fascia, this fascia must be strong and thick, the direction of its fibers vertical. The fascia is attached to the sharp anterior border of the tibia.

The **superior** and **inferior extensor retinacula** are transversely directed thickenings of the deep fascia that hold tendons in place (fig. 5-23; *Atlas*, 307–309).

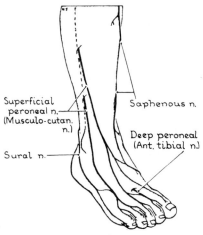

FIG. 5-21. Cutaneous nerves on dorsum of foot.

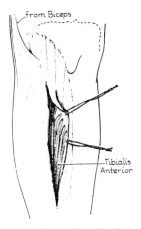

FIG. 5-22. Deep fascia (incised) giving in part origin to tibialis anterior. Therefore, the fascia is aponeurotic, thick, and creates lines on the tibia.

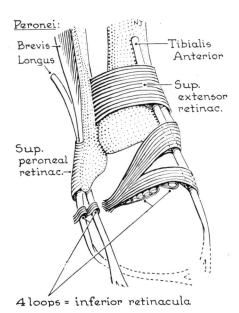

4 loops = inferior retinacula

FIG. 5-23. Retinacula.

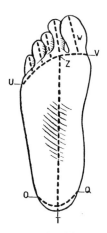

FIG. 5-20. Skin incisions; sole of foot.

The superior extensor retinaculum extends across the tendons above the ankle joint. The inferior extensor retinaculum is Y-shaped. The stem of the Y is fixed to the calcaneus in front of the lateral malleolus. Laterally, the stem of the inferior extensor retinaculum is in broken continuity with the **inferior peroneal retinaculum.** Define these retinacula and understand their function. Subsequently, cut vertically through the deep fascia over the anterior crural compartment.

The structures of the anterior crural compartment cross **in front of the ankle** (*Atlas, 307*). From the medial to the lateral side they are: **Tibialis anterior, extensor hallucis longus, deep peroneal nerve** together with **anterior tibial vessels,** and **extensor digitorum longus.** The lateral lower fleshy part of the extensor digitorum longus is the **peroneus tertius** (*Atlas, 307–309*). Separate the muscles from each other and trace them to their origins. Correlate your observations with a cross section through the anterior crural compartment (*Atlas, 310*). Trace the tendons down to their insertions (*Atlas, 307*).

Study the **anterior tibial artery** and the **deep peroneal nerve** (*Atlas, 305*). Observe that artery and nerve occupy the median plane and have two tendons on each side of them. Trace the artery upward to the point where it passes over the proximal border of the interosseous membrane. Verify that the nerve is a branch of the common peroneal nerve: Pull the common peroneal nerve behind the head of the fibula (fig. 5–24 or *Atlas, 305.1, 306*).

Review the **anterior tibial artery** and its ramifications (*Atlas, 244*). Understand the course and connections of the **perforating branch** of the peroneal artery which passes distal to the interosseous membrane. Occasionally, this perforating branch is large and may replace the dorsalis pedis artery. Usually, the **dorsalis pedis artery** [L., pes, pedis = foot] is the continuation of the anterior tibial artery onto the dorsum of the

foot. Note the **arcuate artery** across the base of the metatarsal bones. The **dorsal digital arteries** originate from it (*Atlas, 244, anterior view*). A deep plantar branch connects to the plantar arch in the sole of the foot (*Atlas, 244, posterior view*). In the cadaver specimen, demonstrate the various branches of the anterior tibial artery (*Atlas, 306, 306.1*). Note that the dorsalis pedis artery and its branches lie on the skeletal plane. There, they remain intact even if all muscles are torn away.

Examine the **deep peroneal nerve** and its muscular branches (*Atlas, 250, 305, 306*). Note the twigs to the two short extensors of the toes: The **extensor digitorum brevis** and the **extensor hallucis brevis.** Examine these muscles. They originate from the calcaneus and are inserted into the extensor expansions of the toes (*Atlas, 307*).

Lateral Crural Compartment

Open the **deep fascia** overlying the **lateral (peroneal) compartment.** This compartment contains two muscles, the **peroneus longus** and **peroneus brevis** (*Atlas, 310*). Distinguish these two muscles from each other. The brevis is inserted into the tuberosity of the 5th metatarsal bone (*Atlas, 304, 306*). Examine how the tendons of the two muscles are held in place. The **superior peroneal retinaculum** (*Atlas, 308*) retains the tendons behind the lateral malleolus; the **inferior peroneal retinaculum** holds them to the calcaneus. Follow the **peroneus longus tendon** to the point where it disappears into the sole of the foot. Realize (without dissection) that this tendon is indeed long: it reaches as far as the undersurface of the 1st metatarsal bone (*Atlas, 341*). Pull on the peroneal muscles. Understand that they evert the foot.

Identify the nerve of the lateral crural compartment, the **superficial peroneal nerve.** It lies along the anterior border of the peroneus brevis (*Atlas, 306, 310*). Follow the nerve distally. Its cutaneous branches to the dorsum of the foot were already seen (fig. 5–21 or *Atlas, 248*). Trace the nerve proximally and verify that it is a branch of the **common peroneal nerve** (fig. 5–24; *Atlas, 306*). Push a probe parallel to the nerve underneath the peroneus longus. You may carefully divide this muscle over the probe to establish continuity of the common, superficial, and deep peroneal nerves.

Of all nerves in the body, the **common peroneal nerve** is the most frequently injured. Once again, observe the superficial position of the nerve in relation to the head and neck of the fibula (fig. 5–24 or *Atlas, 305.1, 306*). The nerve may be readily damaged by superficial wounds, prolonged pressure by hard objects during sleep, anesthesia, and chronic illness, or by compression against the opposite patella, whilst sitting with the knees crossed.

What are the pathological findings on physical examination? The nerves of the lateral and anterior crural compartments are affected. Consequently, eversion, extension (dorsiflexion) of the

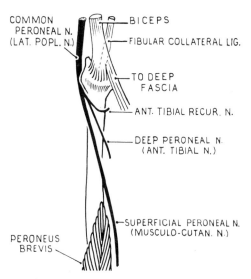

FIG. 5-24. Common peroneal nerve and branches in contact with fibula.

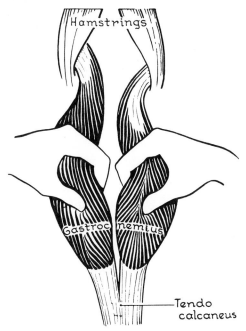

FIG. 5-25. Pull the two bellies forcibly apart to expose the underlying soleus, nerves, and vessels.

foot, and extension of the toes will be impaired. There is a 'foot drop' resulting in a characteristic 'steppage gait.' There may be some sensory loss on the dorsum of the foot and toes (compare *Atlas, 248*).

Posterior Crural Compartment (Back of Leg)

Review the contents of the **posterior crural compartment** on cross section (*Atlas, 310*). Turn the cadaver on its face (prone position). Clean the deep fascia, cut it vertically from popliteal fossa to calcaneus, and reflect it.

Once again, pull the two bellies (heads) of the **gastrocnemius** apart (fig. 5–25). Follow them to the **tendo calcaneus** (tendon of Achilles), the common tendon for the gastrocnemius and underlying **soleus.** Cut across the two bellies of the gastrocnemius well below the entrance of their nerves (*Atlas, 318*). Reflect the bellies up and down, and expose the underlying soleus. Verify that the two heads of the gastrocnemius originate from the medial and lateral condyles of the femur (*Atlas, 316*).

An **intermuscular septum** (*Atlas, 310*) separates the superficial from the deep muscles of the posterior compartment. The **tibial nerve** and **posterior tibial vessels** are closely related to the intermuscular septum. To obtain access to the plane of this septum, the **soleus** must be reflected. Proceed as follows:

Cut the **tendo calcaneus** about 5 cm above its insertion into the tuber calcanei. Lift the tendon upward together with the fleshy parts of gastrocnemius and soleus. Pass two fingers upward between soleus and the loose intermuscular septum. Palpate the horseshoe-shaped origin of the soleus from tibia and fibula (*Atlas, 316*).

Carefully detach the soleus from its tibial origin, but leave it attached to the fibula. Turn the muscle laterally. Now, the intermuscular septum is in full view. Using the scissor technique, slit the loose layer vertically to expose the **posterior tibial vessels** and the **tibial nerve** (*Atlas, 319*).

Three muscles comprise the **deep group** of the posterior crural compartment. To aid in identification, it is useful to correlate a cross section (*Atlas, 310*) with a figure showing the origin of the muscles (*Atlas, 316*). Note:

1. The **flexor digitorum longus** lies medial. It is closely attached to the tibia.
2. The **flexor hallucis longus** lies lateral. It is closely attached to the fibula.
3. The **tibialis posterior** lies in the middle. It takes origin from the tibia and the interosseous membrane.

Identify the three muscles (*Atlas, 319, 320*). Their insertions will be demonstrated later during dissection of the sole of the foot (*Atlas, 328, 329*). Without dissection, realize the following facts: The **flexor digitorum longus** lies *medial* in the posterior compartment; it is inserted into the four *lateral* toes. The **flexor hallucis longus** lies *lateral* in the posterior compartment; it is inserted into the most *medial* (1st) toe. Therefore, by necessity, the two tendons must cross each other (*Atlas, 328*).

Understand the arterial distribution in the back of the leg (fig. 5–26; *Atlas, 244, posterior view*). Clean the

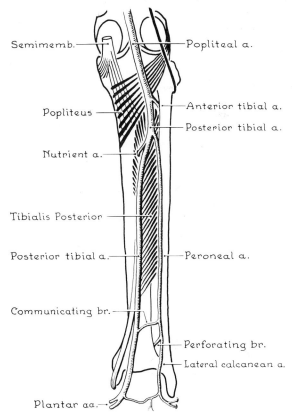

FIG. 5-26. Arteries of back of leg.

posterior tibial artery and the accompanying **tibial nerve** (*Atlas, 319, 320*). Remove the veins. The largest branch of the posterior tibial artery is the **peroneal artery.** Identify it. Briefly search for its *communicating branch* and its *perforating branch* (fig. 5-26 or *Atlas, 319.1*). Note the motor branches of the tibial nerve to the three deep muscles of the posterior compartment.

Sole of Foot (Planta)

General Remarks

Understand the following important facts:
1. The **foot is arched longitudinally** (fig. 5-27). Viewed from the medial side, the arch appears high. Viewed from the lateral side, the longitudinal arch is low. Can these facts be recognized in a foot print?
2. The **bearing points** of the foot are the calcaneus posteriorly, and the heads of the five metatarsal bones anteriorly (figs. 5-27, 5-28). These bearing points are the ends of the longitudinal arches.
3. The **plantar aponeurosis** (fascia) acts as a strong tie for the maintenance of the longitudinal arches. Therefore, it is logical that the plantar aponeurosis stretches from the calcaneus posteriorly to the five digits anteriorly (*Atlas, 325*). The plantar aponeurosis must be of considerable *strength* to perform its function. The aponeurosis is covered with thick skin.
4. Deep to the plantar aponeurosis are **four layers of muscles.** These will be described later.
5. The posterior tibial vessels are continuous with the **plantar vessels** in the sole of the foot (*Atlas, 244, 321, 326*).
6. The tibial nerve sends two branches into the the sole: The **medial plantar nerve** and the **lateral plantar nerve** (*Atlas, 321, 330*).

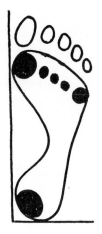

Fig. 5-28. The bearing points of the foot. (From *Grant's Method of Anatomy.*)

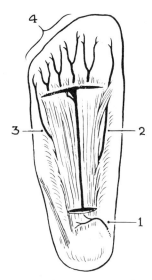

Fig. 5-29. Incisions in plantar aponeurosis.

Dissection

When dissecting the **plantar aponeurosis,** certain cutaneous nerves and vessels are easily cut. Therefore, attempt to secure these structures (fig. 5-29; *Atlas, 325, 326*). In a longitudinal direction, cut through the thick fatty fascia and a film of deep fascia. Find the:
1. **Digital branch of the medial plantar nerve** (and artery); to the medial side of the great toe.
2. **Digital branch of the lateral plantar nerve** (and artery); to the lateral side of the little toe. Other digital nerves (*4* in fig. 5-29) may be traced now or later.
3. If time permits, look for the medial calcanean nerve (*1* in fig. 5-29; *Atlas, 249, 325*), which supplies the skin of the heel.

Plantar Aponeurosis (fig. 5-29; *Atlas, 325*). Peel the superficial fascia off the plantar aponeurosis. Note its proximal attachment to the calcaneus. Define the

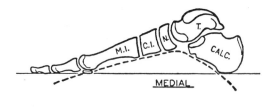

Fig. 5-27. Medial and lateral longitudinal arches. (From *Grant's Method of Anatomy.*)

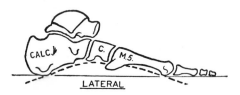

five diverging aponeurotic bands that pass to each
toe. To expose the underlying muscles, split the
plantar aponeurosis longitudinally throughout its
length (fig. 5-29). Then, carefully cut it transversely
close to the calcaneus and in the anterior third of the
foot. Reflect the flaps medially and laterally (*Atlas,
327*). Separate the flaps from the **flexor digitorum
brevis** which originates in part from the central
portion of the plantar aponeurosis.

First Layer of Muscles (fig. 5-30; *Atlas, 327*).
Medial to the plantar aponeurosis, expose the **abductor hallucis.** Note its origin from the calcaneus.
Understand its function. Be careful not to destroy the
plantar digital nerve and artery to the medial side of
the big toe.

On the lateral side, expose and clean the **abductor
digiti minimi.** Free the muscle to its origin and
insertion. Understand its function.

In the middle between the two abductors, identify
the **flexor digitorum brevis.** Trace its tendons forward to digits 2, 3, 4 (and 5). In doing so, remove
piecemeal the remaining and interfering distal part of
the plantar aponeurosis. Subsequently, cut the flexor
digitorum brevis close to the calcaneus and reflect it
forward.

Establish the continuity of the posterior tibial
artery and the tibial nerve with plantar structures.
Follow nerve and artery into the sole by pushing a
probe deep to the abductor hallucis (*Atlas, 330*).
Carefully cut the muscle overlying the probe, and
demonstrate the distribution of the **plantar nerves
and arteries** (fig. 5-30; *Atlas, 326, 330*).

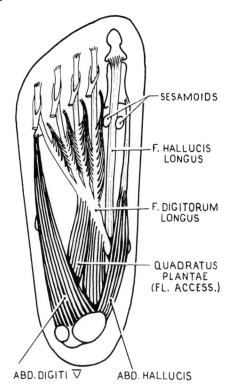

FIG. 5-31. Second layer of muscles displayed by removal of
flexor digitorum brevis.

Second Layer of Muscles (fig. 5-31 or *Atlas, 328,
328.1*). Reflect the flexor digitorum brevis as described above. To make reflection easier, you may
sacrifice some of the digital nerves and vessels.
Identify the **quadratus plantae** (flexor accessorius), a
sheet of fleshy muscle in the posterior half of the foot.
Note that the muscle arises from the calcaneus and is
inserted into the tendon of the **flexor digitorum
longus.** The flexor digitorum longus tendon divides
into four slips for toes 2, 3, 4, and 5. Four delicate
lumbricals arise from the tendinous slips. Note that
these slips perforate the tendons of the flexor digitorum brevis. A similar arrangement can be observed
in the hand.

Third Layer of Muscles (fig. 5-32 or *Atlas, 330,
330.1*). Cut through the flexor digitorum longus tendon where it is joined by the quadratus plantae.
Reflect the distal part of the tendon forward together
with the lumbricals. Thus, expose the short muscles
that lie in the anterior half of the foot. Identify the
flexor hallucis brevis. The muscle covers the first
metatarsal. With a probe or the handle of a knife,
separate it from the tendon of the flexor hallucis
longus. Observe the **flexor digiti minimi.** Identify the
adductor hallucis consisting of short adductor slips
for the big toe.

Identify the **plantar arterial arch.** Understand the
essentials of the blood supply to the foot (*Atlas, 244,
326, 327.1*). Attempt to identify the **perforating
branch** which connects the plantar arch with the
dorsalis pedis artery.

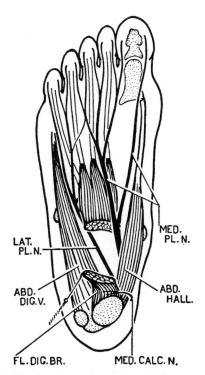

FIG. 5-30. The first layer of muscles and plantar nerves. (From
Grant's Method of Anatomy.)

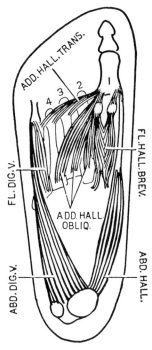

FIG. 5-32. Third layer of muscles displayed by reflection of flexor digitorum longus, quadratus plantae, and lumbricals. (From *Grant's Method of Anatomy.*)

Fourth Layer of Muscles (*Atlas, 331*). This layer consists of a compact muscular mass, the **interossei.** Time does not permit dissection of these muscles; but realize that they exist. The four dorsal interossei are abductors, the three plantar interossei are adductors of the toes. The reference axis for abduction and adduction passes through the second toe. The arrangement and action of the interossei is similar to that in the hand. Adduction and abduction of digits is more important in the hand than in the foot. Therefore, the interossei are more thoroughly discussed in the section for the hand.

Ankles

Medial Side of Ankle

If not already done, sever the **abductor hallucis** close to the calcaneus. Once again, identify the **quadratus plantae** (fig. 5-33; *Atlas, 328, 329*).

Identify the **flexor hallucis longus** in the posterior compartment of the leg. Follow its tendon distally until it disappears in an *osseofibrous tunnel.* Push a probe into the tunnel, then open it. Temporarily lift out the tendon of the flexor hallucis longus. Verify that it runs in a **groove** below the **sustentaculum tali,** using the sustentaculum as a pulley. The **flexor digitorum longus** tendon passes along the medial border of the sustentaculum. The **tibialis posterior** passes above this bony landmark. Trace the three

deep muscles of the posterior crural compartment in their continuity.

Lateral Side of Ankle

Review the **peroneus longus** and **peroneus brevis** (*Atlas, 308, 309*). Push a probe parallel to the peroneus longus tendon deep into the sole of the foot. Follow the probe and tendon along a groove in the cuboid bone to the first metatarsal bone (*Atlas, 331, 341*). Feel free to sever the long plantar ligament which covers the tendon.

Pull on the peroneal muscles and observe that the foot is everted. Review the motor nerves in the lower extremity (*Atlas, 250*).

Joints of the Lower Extremity

General Remarks

It is advantageous to dissect the joints only in one lower extremity. Keep the soft structures of the other limb intact for review purposes.

Refer to the articulated bones of the lower extremity. Identify the following joints:
1. Sacroiliac joint (*Atlas, 223*).
2. **Hip joint** (*Atlas, 282*).
3. **Knee joint** (*Atlas, 288*).
4. **Ankle joint** (*Atlas, 315*).
5. Tibiofibular joints (proximal; distal; *Atlas, 315*).
6. Various joints between the tarsal bones (talus; calcaneus; navicular; etc.; *Atlas, 311–314*).
7. Joints of the digits

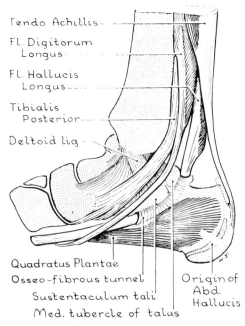

FIG. 5-33. Deep structures on medial side of ankle.

If time permits, refer to the appendix for a detailed text on the dissection of all joints (p. 170). If time is limited, dissect at least the following joints: **hip joint, ankle joint,** and **joints of inversion and eversion.**

The joints may be dissected in any order. Since the memory of anatomical details in the leg and foot is fresh, the ankle joint and the joints of inversion and eversion will be discussed first.

Ankle Joint

Cut and reflect the structures crossing the front of the ankle joint. However, leave the tibialis anterior tendon intact.

Medial Side of Ankle Joint (*Atlas, 321.2*). To display the medial aspect of the joint, cut and reflect the flexor digitorum longus. Displace forward (but do *not* cut) the tibialis posterior. Now, clean and define the **deltoid ligament.** It is a triangular ligament which attaches the medial malleolus to the tarsus. Note that the superficial fibers of this ligament are inserted into the whole length of the sustentaculum tali (*Atlas, 321.2; 339*). The most anterior fibers radiate toward the navicular bone. The deep portion of the ligament anchors the medial malleolus to the talus. This fact is best appreciated on vertical section (*Atlas, 334*).

Lateral Side of Ankle Joint. Displace forward (but do *not* cut) the peroneus longus and peroneus brevis tendons (*Atlas, 308*). Clean and define the ligaments that hold the lateral malleolus of the fibula to the tarsus (*Atlas, 338*): The **calcaneofibular ligament** and the **talofibular ligaments.**

Plantarflex the foot. Incise transversely the articular capsule of the ankle joint (*Atlas, 340*). Push the handle of the knife between body of talus and tibia (*Atlas, 338*). To display the articular surfaces, sever the ligaments that connect the fibula to the talus. Dislocate the foot by swinging it medially. The deltoid ligament, which remains intact, acts as a hinge. Study the articular surfaces (*Atlas, 303, 313, 334, 335*).

Joints of Inversion and Eversion

Study the movements of inversion and eversion of the foot in the articulated skeleton of the lower extremity. With one hand, immobilize the ankle joint, i.e. hold the talus tightly between tibia and fibula. With the other hand, invert and evert the foot. Observe the following:
1. The talus remains fixed in the ankle joint.
2. The entire foot rotates about the inferior and anterior surfaces of the talus.
3. This movement is augmented at the joint between calcaneus and cuboid.

Turn to the cadaver specimen. Produce **eversion** by pulling on the tendons of the peroneus longus and peroneus brevis. Follow the tendons to their insertions (*Atlas, 308, 341*). Produce inversion by pulling on the tendons of the tibialis anterior and tibialis posterior. Follow the tendons clearly to their insertions (*Atlas, 329, 341*).

Study the complex articular interactions between the talus on the one hand, and the calcaneus and navicular on the other (*Atlas, 311, 313*). The objective is to disarticulate the talus from the rest of the tarsus. Proceed as follows (*Atlas, 338, 340*):
1. If not already done, sever the ligaments that hold the lateral malleolus to the tarsus.
2. Cut the interosseous talocalcanean ligament.
3. Cut the posterior part of the subtalar joint capsule.
4. Force the handle of the knife between talus and calcaneus.
5. Swing the calcaneus and the foot medially. The deltoid ligament, which remains intact, acts as a hinge (*Atlas, 334*).

Identify the posterior talar facet of the calcaneus for the subtalar joint (fig. 5-34; *Atlas, 337*). Inspect the socket for the head of the talus. The articular components of this socket are formed by the **middle talar facet, anterior talar facet,** and **posterior articular surface of the navicular bone.** The floor of the socket is formed by the important **spring ligament** (*Atlas, 337*). Force a probe or needle through the floor of the socket. Next, approach the probe and ligament from the sole of the foot (fig. 5-35; *Atlas, 341, 342*). Identify the **spring ligament or plantar calcaneonavicular ligament.** Understand that this ligament and the tibialis posterior tendon are necessary for the support of the head of the talus. The socket for the head of the talus is of great importance to the integrity of the foot.

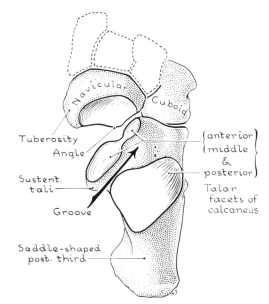

FIG. 5-34. Bones of foot on dorsal view; talus removed: To show where inversion and eversion take place.

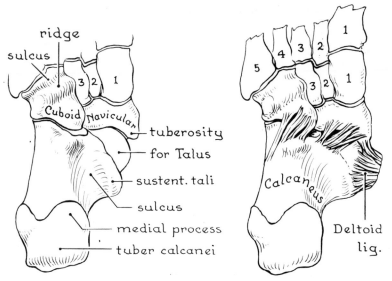

FIG. 5-35. Bones of foot on plantar view. Plantar ligaments of joints of inversion and eversion.

The socket supports the 'keystone' of the high medial arch.

Knee Joint

Review the bony landmarks related to the knee joint (*Atlas, 242, 243*).

Front and Sides of Knee Joint. On the **medial aspect,** detach the tendons of the sartorius, gracilis, and semitendinosus from their insertions (*Atlas, 262, 298*). Reflect muscles and tendons. Remove the deep fascia. Deep to the tendons of the three muscles identify the **tibial collateral ligament** (medial lig.) of the knee (*Atlas, 298*). With a probe, explore the relations between the ligament and the **medial meniscus.** Realize that the deeper portion of the ligament is firmly attached to the meniscus (*Atlas, 293*).

On the **lateral aspect** of the knee joint, identify the **iliotibial tract.** It is about 2 to 3 cm wide. The tract is inserted into the front of the lateral tibial condyle (*Atlas, 294, 296*). Cut the biceps tendon close to its insertion into the head of the fibula (*Atlas, 296*). Subsequently, define the **fibular collateral ligament** (lateral lig.) of the knee. Notice that it does *not* blend with the underlying meniscus (*Atlas, 293*), in contrast to the tibial collateral ligament.

On the **anterior aspect** of the knee joint, identify the expansions of the **vasti** muscles and the **ligamentum patellae.** Palpate the patella. Detach the quadriceps tendon from the patella. Be careful not to damage the underlying synovial capsule of the knee joint (fig. 5-36 or *Atlas, 301; synovial capsule shown in blue*). Make a transverse cut immediately above the patella through the synovial capsule into the joint cavity. With a blunt instrument, carefully explore the extent of the capsule. Gently pack the superior recess of the joint cavity with moist cotton. The established

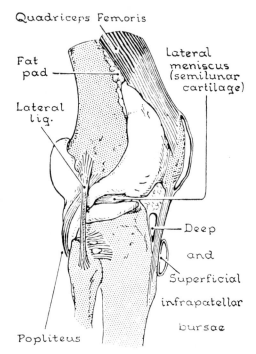

FIG. 5-36. Distended synovial capsule of knee joint on lateral view.

sac-like recess is the **suprapatellar or quadriceps bursa.**

Make a wide horseshoe-shaped incision through the vasti from epicondyle to epicondyle, rising just above the stuffed quadriceps bursa. Identify the bursa. Observe a layer of fat between bursa and femur.

Back of the Knee Joint. Sever and remove the vessels and nerves of the popliteal fossa (*Atlas, 287*). Cut the semimenbranosus and other hamstring muscles well above the knee joint. Free the plantaris and both heads of the gastrocnemius from the joint capsule. Then, remove these muscles from their bony origins (*Atlas, 288*). Cut through the fleshy fibers of the popliteus and remove this muscle (*Atlas, 287, 288*). During this procedure, the synovial capsule will be opened posteriorly. Observe that the capsule extends inferior to the lateral meniscus (*Atlas, 301*).

Clear away the back of the joint capsule. Remove any fat. Identify the **posterior cruciate ligament** (*Atlas, 293*). By means of transverse and vertical incisions, open the synovial cavity behind each femoral condyle. With a probe, explore the limits of the synovial cavity (*Atlas, 302*). Verify that the cruciate ligaments are entirely outside the synovial capsule.

Interior of Knee Joint. Turn to the front of the knee joint and open the synovial capsule widely by a transverse incision. Carry the incision around the sides and the back of the knee (*Atlas, 299*).

During development, the medial and lateral halves of the knee joint were originally two independent joint cavities separated by the membranes of the **intercondylar septum.** This septum partially broke down in front of the anterior cruciate ligament. Examine the anterior part of the septum, the **infrapatellar synovial fold** (*Atlas, 299*). Posterior to the infrapatellar fold, the septum is complete. Here, the synovial membranes are reflected across both sides of the cruciate ligaments. Therefore, the cruciate ligaments are situated outside the synovial cavity (*Atlas, 302*). However, they lie inside the fibrous capsule.

Snip through the infrapatellar fold. Verify that the femur and tibia remain attached to each other by four ligaments: The two **collateral ligaments** and the two **cruciate ligaments.** Rotate the femur medially. Note that the **fibular collateral ligament** becomes taut and stops the movement. Sever it. Note that medial rotation of the femur is now free and results in untwisting of the cruciate ligaments (*Atlas, 300*).

Verify that the strong cruciate ligaments cross each other. The **anterior cruciate ligament** attaches the femur to the tibia *anteriorly* (*Atlas, 300*). The **posterior cruciate ligament** attaches the femur to the tibia *posteriorly* (*Atlas, 293, 294*). Study the functions of the cruciate ligaments (fig. 5-37 or *Atlas, 292*):

Extend the leg (knee joint) maximally. In this position, observe:

1. The articular surfaces of femur and tibia are in maximal contact.
2. The joint is 'locked' in its most stable position.
3. The anterior cruciate ligament is taut and prohibits further extension.

Flex the leg (knee joint). Observe:

1. There is less contact between the articular surfaces.
2. Some rotation occurs in the knee joint (at the expense of its stability).
3. The posterior cruciate ligament prevents forward displacement of the femur; i.e. it prevents the femur from sliding forward off the 'tibial plateau.'
4. With the leg (knee joint) flexed to a right angle,

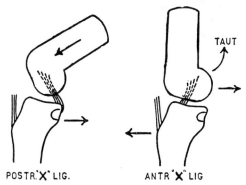

POSTR.'X' LIG.   ANTR.'X' LIG

FIG. 5-37. The posterior cruciate ligament prevents forward displacement of the femur or backward displacement of the tibia. The anterior cruciate 'X' ligament prevents backward displacement of the femur and hyperextension. (From *Grant's Method of Anatomy*.)

the tibia cannot be pulled forward; it is held back by the anterior cruciate ligament.

Cut the **anterior cruciate ligament** (*not* the posterior one!). Flex the leg to a right angle. Now, you will be able to pull the tibia forward. This forward movement is an important clinical sign in cases of a ruptured anterior cruciate ligament (see below).

Study the **menisci** or semilunar cartilages (*Atlas, 294, 301*). Test the mobility of the menisci. The *C-shaped* **medial meniscus** is firmly attached to the tibia by the coronary ligament. Once again, examine its attachment to the tibial collateral ligament. The small *o-shaped* **lateral meniscus** is distinctly mobile. Remember, it has no attachments to the collateral ligament (*Atlas, 293*).

The medial meniscus is injured about 6 to 7 times as often as the lateral meniscus. Why? The medial meniscus is firmly attached to the tibial collateral ligament and the underlying tibia (*Atlas, 300, 300.1*). It is virtually immobile. During forceful abduction of the leg, the tension exerted by the tibial collateral ligament can result in tearing of the medial meniscus. In contrast, the slightly mobile lateral meniscus is not attached to the fibular collateral ligament.

Forced abduction and lateral rotation of the leg may result in the simultaneous rupture or damage of three structures: (1) Tibial collateral ligament; (2) anterior cruciate ligament; and (3) medial meniscus. This injury is typical for football players. It has been named the 'unhappy triad.'

Hip Joint

Review the essential bony features of the hip joint and its vicinity (*Atlas, 242, 243, 276, 282*).

Anterior Relations of the Hip Joint. Realize (*Atlas, 258.1*) that the **sartorius** projects across the neck of the femur. The **femoral artery** and the inguinal ligament project in relation to the head of the femur or the acetabulum.

Cut and reflect the sartorius, rectus femoris, pectineus, and the femoral nerve and vessels. Identify the **iliopsoas** muscle (*Atlas, 261*). Trace its tendon to the lesser trochanter, and sever it close to this bony landmark. Reflect it upward.

Moisten the capsule of the hip joint to make it more pliable. Study the ligaments that contribute to the formation of the fibrous capsule. Identify the exceedingly strong **iliofemoral ligament** (*Atlas, 274*). Verify that the base of this triangular ligament is attached to the intertrochanteric line of the femur; its apex is attached to the anterior inferior iliac spine (*Atlas, 276, 276.1*).

Open the **joint capsule** by making a vertical incision along a line indicated by the former position of the psoas tendon. Inside the capsule, observe the extensive **articular area of the head** of the femur. Rotate the limb laterally: Note that you can see more of the articular surface. Rotate the limb medially: Observe that the articular surface disappears in the acetabulum.

At this stage, define the **obturator externus** (*Atlas, 274*). Once again, examine the obturator nerve as it enters the thigh.

Posterior Relations of the Hip Joint. Turn the cadaver into the prone position (face down). Review the essential features of the gluteal region (*Atlas, 268–273*). Cut and remove all muscles that hold the femur close to the hip bone: Piriformis, obturator internus with gemelli, quadratus femoris, gluteus medius and minimus. Cut and reflect the obturator externus tendon.

Clean the posterior aspect of the fibrous joint capsule. Identify the **ischiofemoral ligament** (*Atlas, 275*). Relax the capsule by rotating the lower limb in the appropriate direction. Open the joint cavity by incising the capsule vertically. Insert a probe, and explore the limits of the synovial cavity. Appreciate the thickness of the capsule.

The next objective is to dislocate the hip joint, i.e. to remove the head of the femur from its socket. Proceed as follows:

1. Have the cadaver in the prone position (face down).
2. Position the pelvis at the end of the table. Let the lower extremity hang over the end of the table.
3. Let your partner hold the pelvis steady.
4. Simultaneously, flex the hip joint and forcibly turn the femur medialward (medial rotation). Persist in this maneuver until the *ligament of the head of the femur* ruptures (*Atlas, 282*). Subsequently, the head of the femur will pass out of the acetabulum onto the dorsum of the ilium.

Examine the head and neck of the femur. Observe the articular surface and the reflections of the synovial membrane (*Atlas, 282*). Note the pit for the ligament of the head.

Socket for Head of Femur or Acetabulum (*Atlas, 276, 281–284*). Identify the smooth **lunate articular surface.** Observe that the **acetabular fossa** contains a fat pad which is lined with synovial membrane. Identify the torn ligament of the head of the femur.

Turn the cadaver over (supine position). Notice that the strong **iliofemoral ligament** is still intact in spite of the dislocation. Palpate its substantial thickness.

BACK

Muscles of the Back

General Remarks

The muscles of the back are divided into three groups: superficial, intermediate, and deep. The **superficial group** acts on the upper extremity. These muscles anchor the upper limb to the axial skeleton. This anchorage extends from the skull to the pelvic girdle. The *intermediate group* functions in respiration. The **deep group** consists of intrinsic or 'native' muscles of the back (dorsum). These are supplied by dorsal nerve rami (*Atlas, 405*). Embryologically, the superficial and intermediate groups migrated from the ventrum and hence are supplied by ventral nerve rami.

Bony Landmarks

Refer to the skull, the skeleton, and to the cadaver which must be in the prone position (face down). Identify the following bony landmarks:
1. **Occipital bone** (fig. 6-1 or *Atlas, 485*). Note the **external occipital protuberance or inion** and the **nuchal lines.**
2. **Mastoid process** (fig. 6-1 or *Atlas, 461, 485*).
3. Examine the **cervical vertebrae** (fig. 6-2, or *Atlas, 368*). Identify the **transverse processes** and the **spinous processes.** Note that the 7th cervical spine is the most prominent of the cervical spines. In the cadaver, run the finger down in the dorsal midline from external occipital protuberance, until it is arrested by the 7th cervical spine.
4. **First thoracic spine** (*Atlas, 458*). Even more prominent than spine of C_7.
5. **Scapula** (*Atlas, 2*). Identify its **spine.** Trace it from the medial border to the **acromion.** Palpate the **superior** and the **inferior angle.** Palpate the **medial or vertebral border** of the scapula.
6. **Iliac crest** (*Atlas, 243*). It terminates posteriorly in the **posterior superior iliac spine** (*Atlas, 271, 273*). Here, the overlying skin often shows a dimple, since there are no fleshy muscle fibers.

With an imaginary line, connect the highest points of the left and right iliac crests. This line crosses the vertebral column at the 4th lumbar spine. The 3rd lumbar interspace is between the 3rd and 4th lumbar spines. A needle is usually introduced into the 3rd lumbar interspace to obtain cerebrospinal fluid (C.S.F.) from the subarachnoid space (spinal tap or lumbar puncture; see page 93).

Plan for Dissection

To save time, skin and superficial fascia of the back will be removed together. The muscles of the superficial and intermediate groups will be reflected. Subsequently, the deep group will be studied. The dorsal aspect of the vertebral column will be exposed. The vertebral canal will be opened, and the spinal cord and its coverings will be studied. Finally, the muscles and nerves of the suboccipital region will be examined.

Skin Incisions

Refer to fig. 6-3. In the midline, make a vertical skin incision from the external occipital protuberance (inion) to the level of the posterior superior iliac spines (*S*). Carry out the following transverse incisions:
1. From *S* to *T* (already done for the dissection of the gluteal region).
2. From *U* to *V*, at the level of the inferior scapular angle.
3. From *R* to *B*, superior to the scapula and to the tip of the acromion, and on to point *F*. Here, make a complete circular skin incision at the root of the arm.
4. From the external occipital protuberance (*X*) laterally to the base of the mastoid process (*M*).

Dissection

Begin dissection with reflection of the skin in the area bounded by points *X*, *M*, and *R* (fig. 6-3). In the underlying subcutaneous tissue, attempt to locate the **greater occipital nerve** and the accompanying **occipital artery** (fig. 6-4 or *Atlas, 477*). The nerve pierces the trapezius muscle about 3 cm inferolateral to the inion. The artery lies lateral to the nerve. The deep

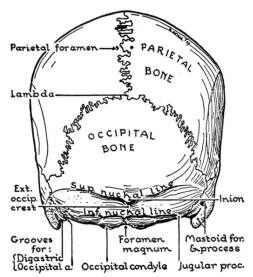

FIG. 6-1. The skull from behind (norma occipitalis). (From *Grant's Method of Anatomy*.)

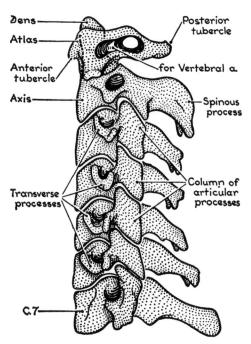

FIG. 6-2. Cervical vertebrae on side view. (From *Grant's Method of Anatomy*.)

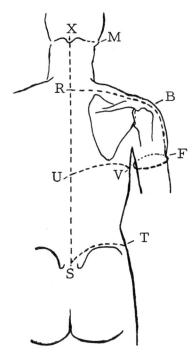

FIG. 6-3. Skin incisions.

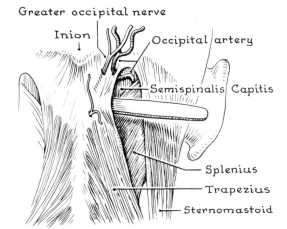

FIG. 6-4. Greater occipital nerve and occipital artery (readily found deep to aponeurosis where there is almost no fat).

fascia in this area is very dense and tough. Therefore, it may be difficult to find the nerve, even though it is large. Using the scissor technique, split the deep fascia parallel to the expected course of the nerve. If you find the occipital artery first, look for the nerve medial to it.

Realize that the greater occipital nerve is the *dorsal ramus* of C₂. Read an account of the **dorsal primary divisions or dorsal rami** of the spinal nerves (fig. 6-5 or *Atlas, 405*). To save time, make no deliberate effort to display other cutaneous branches of the dorsal rami. However, several of these nerves may be seen piercing the trapezius or latissimus dorsi to enter the superficial fascia (*Atlas, 477*).

Reflect skin and superficial fascia of the back together. Be careful **not** to incise the superficial fascia along the anterior border of the trapezius. Here (*Atlas, 472*), the spinal accessory nerve and other structures are in great danger of being cut. The spinal accessory nerve and branches of ventral rami C₂ to C₄ supply the extensive trapezius muscle (*Atlas, 661*).

Clean two extensive muscles of the superficial group: **trapezius** and **latissimus dorsi** (fig. 6-6 or *Atlas, 477*). Notice that they cover almost the entire back. Observe two triangles associated with the latissimus dorsi: triangle of auscultation, and lumbar triangle.

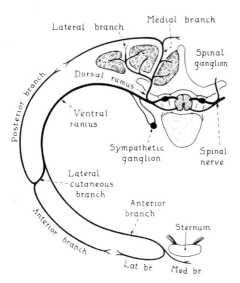

FIG. 6-5. Spinal nerve. Note distribution of dorsal ramus to deep back muscles and to skin of back.

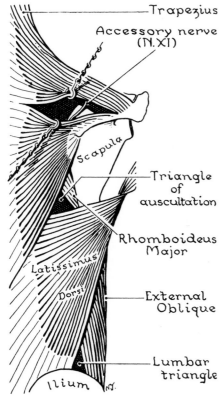

FIG. 6-6. Exposure of dorsal scapular region.

The *triangle of auscultation* (fig. 6-6) is bounded by latissimus dorsi, trapezius, and rhomboid major together with the vertebral border of the scapula. Here, ribs 6 and 7 and intercostal space 6 are free of overlying muscles. Thus, this area is particularly suited for auscultation (listening to sounds produced by thoracic viscera).

The *lumbar triangle* (of Petit) is bounded by latissimus dorsi, obliquus abdominis externus and iliac crest (*Atlas, 477*). Its floor is formed by the obliquus abdominis internus. On rare occasions, this weak triangular space is the site of a 'lumbar hernia.'

Trapezius (*Atlas, 477*). Observe the origin of this triangular muscle from the inion, the ligamentum nuchae, and the spinous processes of C_7 and T_{1-12}. Note that different parts of the muscle take different fiber courses:

1. Fibers of the *superior portion* run inferolaterally and are inserted into the lateral third of the clavicle (*Atlas, 472*).
2. Fibers of the *middle portion* run transversely. These are inserted into the acromion and spine of the scapula (*Atlas, 477*).
3. Fibers of the *inferior portion* run superolaterally. These fibers converge into an aponeurosis near the medial end of the spine of the scapula.

The **trapezius must be reflected** in such a manner as (1) to allow complete access to underlying structures; and (2) to preserve its blood and nerve supply.

1. Ask your partner to push the shoulder backwards. This relaxes the trapezius. Pass your hand under the free lateral and inferior border of the muscle. Feel the loose fat and areolar tissue separating the trapezius from other muscles. Now, detach the muscle from its origin very close to the spinous processes. Start inferiorly. Carefully carry the detachment toward the inion. Frequently, define and loosen the muscle with a finger before you proceed cutting. Then, detach the trapezius from its insertion into the spine and acromion of the scapula. Do this with a scalpel, cutting very close to the bone. Now, the muscle is attached only to the clavicle. Reflect the muscle laterally.
2. Study the deep surface of the trapezius (*Atlas, 477*). In the loose fatty tissue, find blood vessels and nerves. Using the scissor technique, dissect the **spinal accessory nerve** to the upper border of the muscle. Push a probe parallel to the nerve and upwards into the neck. Palpate the probe through the skin. The palpating finger is located over the important *posterior triangle of the neck*. This area will be dissected later with other head and neck structures (p. 134).

Latissimus Dorsi (*Atlas, 477*). Verify the following:

1. Its thin upper border extends laterally from the spinous processes of T_6 and T_7.
2. Its most lateral fibers interdigitate with those of the external oblique below the origin of the serratus anterior (*Atlas, 107*).
3. The muscle arises from the vast thoracolumbar fascia (lumbodorsal fascia) which covers the deep (intrinsic) musculature of the back.
4. Superiorly, the muscle fibers converge (*Atlas, 477*). They form a broad tendon which is inserted into the humerus. Close to the tendon, the muscle receives its nerve supply (*Atlas, 18*). Do not explore either tendinous insertion or nerve supply at this time.

Place your hand deep to the latissimus dorsi and lift it up slightly. With a scalpel, cut through its tendinous origin from the thoracolumbar fascia (*Atlas, 477*). Reflect the muscle laterally.

Next, study the three remaining muscles of the superficial group: **rhomboideus major,** rhomboideus minor, and **levator scapulae.** They are inserted into the medial border of the scapula (*Atlas, 477*). Place your finger deep to the two rhomboids. Then, detach these muscles from the spinous processes. Reflect them laterally. On the deep surface of the muscles, look for nerves and blood vessels. Leave the levator scapulae undisturbed. However, observe 3 or 4 slips arising from the transverse processes of the upper four cervical vertebrae (*Atlas, 478*). Realize that all muscular attachments (with the exception of the levator scapulae) of the shoulder girdle to the vertebral column have been severed. As a result, the shoulder will easily fall forward.

Now, the *intermediate muscle group* is readily accessible. Observe the thin sheets of the *serratus posterior superior* and *serratus posterior inferior*. These muscles are respiratory in action. Note their insertions into the ribs. Cut through the thin aponeuroses of both muscles at their origins from the spinous processes (*Atlas, 478*). Reflect the muscle laterally. Now, only the muscles of the deep group remain (*Atlas, 479*).

The **muscles of the deep group** to be studied at this time include (fig. 6-8; *Atlas, 479*): **splenius capitis et cervicis, semispinalis capitis,** and the enormous musculature collectively called the **erector spinae** and **transversospinalis.** Deep to the semispinalis capitis lie the small muscles of the suboccipital region. The suboocipital region will be studied at the end of this chapter.

Splenius Capitis et Cervicis [Gk., splenion = bandage; L., caput = head; cervix = neck]. Identify the splenius capitis which is inserted into the occipital bone and the mastoid process. The splenius cervicis is inserted into the transverse processes of the upper cervical vertebrae. On one side only, detach the splenius where it arises from the ligamentum nuchae and spinous processes. Reflect the muscle laterally. Now, the semispinalis capitis is fully exposed.

The **semispinalis capitis** (*Atlas, 479, 490*) arises from the transverse processes of the upper thoracic vertebrae. It is inserted into the occipital bone between the nuchal lines. Note, that it is traversed by the greater occipital nerve.

Erector Spinae or Sacrospinalis (fig. 6-7; *Atlas, 479*). Identify *three columns* of the erector spinae: *iliocostalis, longissimus,* and *spinalis*. The iliocostalis is the lateral column. Define its tendinous slips attached to the angles of the ribs. The longissimus is the intermediate column. The spinalis forms the medial column. It is only 2 cm wide and attached to the spinous processes (figs. 6-7, 6-8).

After removal of the spinalis, a number of short

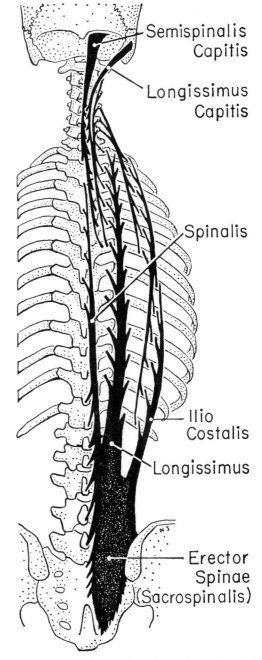

FIG. 6-7. Erector spinae and semispinalis capitis. (After *Cunningham's Anatomy*. From *Grant's Method of Anatomy*.)

muscles (semispinalis, multifidus, rotatores) can be seen filling the groove between transverse and spinous processes of the vertebrae (fig. 6-8; *Atlas, 480*). These muscles are collectively called the **transversospinalis.**

Spinal Cord

Exposure of the Spinal Canal. Place a block under the pelvis to reduce the concavity of the lumbar region. Remove all the dorsal musculature from T₆ to

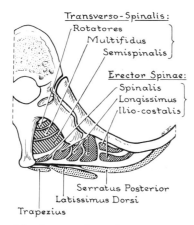

FIG. 6-8. Muscles of the back. Schematic cross section.

L_5. Scoop out the muscles that fill the groove between transverse and spinous processes (fig. 6-8 or *Atlas, 480.1*). In the lower thoracic (T_6) region or in the lumbar (L_1) region, remove several spinous processes with bone pliers. Note that the spines are attached to each other by *supraspinous* and *intraspinous ligaments* (*Atlas, 386*). After removing the spinous processes, observe the strong and elastic *ligamenta flava* (*Atlas, 386, 389*). These ligaments connect the laminae of adjacent vertebrae. They extend laterally to the intervertebral foramina and bound them posteriorly.

Remove the laminae (laminectomy) of several vertebrae. Do this about 1 cm from the midline, using a saw inclined to enter the vertebral canal. Remove individual pieces of bone with bone pliers. Protect your eyes from flying chips of bone.

Identify the *epidural or extradural space*. Remove the fatty tissue and venous plexus from it (*Atlas, 390*). Expose the **dura mater** of the spinal cord. Next, carefully incise the dura mater in the dorsal midline. Try to do this without incising the **arachnoid mater;** i.e. without opening the subarachnoid space (*Atlas, 484*). The subarachnoid space contains the cerebrospinal fluid, the C.S.F. (*Atlas, 484.1*). After identifying the arachnoid, open the subarachnoid space. Note the following:

1. **Spinal cord.** It is completely surrounded with delicate pia mater.
2. On each side of the cord, the pia mater forms strong pointed prolongations. These are the **denticulate ligaments.** They secure the spinal cord to the dura mater (*Atlas, 482*). Usually, there are 21 points of attachment on each side.
3. **Ventral and dorsal roots** (*Atlas, 484*). Using a probe, follow a ventral and a dorsal root to the point where they pierce the dura and enter the intervertebral foramen.
4. In the thoracic region, place a probe into the **intervertebral foramen** to protect the nerve within it. Using bone pliers, remove the articular processes lying posterior to this foramen (*Atlas, 387*). Expose the **spinal ganglion** or dorsal root

ganglion (*Atlas, 483*). If you are careful enough, you can see the spinal nerve dividing into ventral and dorsal rami (*Atlas, 483*).

It will be unnecessary to expose the entire spinal cord if demonstration or museum specimens are available. In these specimens study the following:

1. **Cervical enlargement of spinal cord** from C_3 to T_2, corresponding to the large nerve supply of the upper extremity.
2. **Lumbar enlargement** of spinal cord from T_4 to T_{12}, corresponding to the large nerve supply of the lower extremity. (Realize that these levels T_4 to T_{12} are vertebral levels. They do not correspond to spinal segmental levels.)
3. **Conus medullaris,** the end of the spinal cord, between L_1 and L_2 (fig. 6-9; *Atlas, 484*). Of pediatric importance: At birth, the conus medullaris lies at the level of L_3.
4. **Filum terminale** (fig. 6-9; *Atlas, 484, 484.1*). A delicate filament continuous with the pia mater. Its intradural portion ends at S_2 where it is attached to the end of the dural sac. Its extradural prolongation ends at the coccyx.
5. Cauda equina [L., tail of horse]. Collection of ventral and dorsal roots caudal to the termination of the spinal cord (*Atlas, 484*).
6. Realize that there are 31 pairs of spinal nerves (8 cervical; 12 thoracic; 5 lumbar; 5 sacral; 1 coccygeal).
7. Understand that the cerebrospinal fluid (C.S.F.) can be obtained from the subarachnoid space below the conus medullaris. At this level, there is no danger of penetrating the central nervous system with the puncture needle. However, the needle may injure the nerve fibers in the cauda

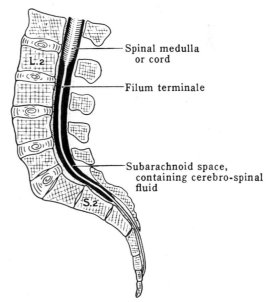

Spinal medulla or cord

Filum terminale

Subarachnoid space, containing cerebro-spinal fluid

FIG. 6-9. Diagram of lower portion of spinal cord. (From *Grant's Atlas of Anatomy.*)

equina. Great care must be taken to avoid infection of the subarachnoid space.

Review the distribution of a spinal nerve (fig. 6-5; *Atlas, 405*). Review also the sympathetic chain and its connections to spinal nerves, the white and gray rami communicates (chap. 2, *Thorax*, fig. 2-18).

Suboccipital Region

Bony Landmarks

Refer to a skull and a vertebral column. Identify the following pertinent landmarks:
1. On the occipital bone: The two **nuchal lines** and the area between them (fig. 6-1 or *Atlas, 485*). **Foramen magnum** (*Atlas, 570*).
2. On the first cervical vertebra or **atlas** (*Atlas, 367, 368*): **Posterior arch** with **posterior tubercle; transverse process; foramen transversarium** for the transmission of the vertebral artery; **groove for the vertebral artery.**
3. On the second cervical vertebra or **axis** (*Atlas, 367, 368*): **Spinous process;** transverse process; foramen transversarium.

Dissection

Once again, identify the **semispinalis capitis** (*Atlas, 490*). If not already done, detach the semispinalis capitis bilaterally close to its attachment to the occipital bone. Carefully reflect the muscle downward. Be cautious not to tear the **greater occipital nerve.** Follow this nerve through the muscle. Deep to the muscle, follow the nerve, as a guiding structure, to

the lower border of the inferior oblique (fig. 6-10 or *Atlas, 490.1*).

The *obliquus capitis inferior* (inferior oblique) forms the lower limit of the suboccipital region. Verify that this muscles extends from the spinous process of the axis (C_2) to the transverse process of the atlas (C_1).

Suboccipital Triangle (fig. 6-10; *Atlas, 490.1–492*). Identify and clean the three muscles bounding the triangle:
1. *Obliquus capitis inferior* (inferior oblique). It bounds the triangle inferiorly.
2. *Rectus capitis posterior major* (rectus major). It bounds the suboccipital triangle medially. Follow it from the spinous process of the axis superolaterally to the inferior nuchal line. (The rectus minor lies medial to the rectus major. It originates from the posterior tubercle of the atlas.)
3. *Obliquus capitis superior* (superior oblique). It bounds the triangle laterally. It lies deep. Follow it from the transverse process of the atlas to the occipital bone.

With the suboccipital triangle well defined, identify the nerves of the region (fig. 6-10). The **greater occipital nerve** (dorsal ramus of C_2; cutaneous) has already been identified. Note that it emerges between vertebrae C_1 and C_2. Find the **suboccipital nerve** (dorsal ramus of C_1) within the suboccipital triangle. Note that the nerve emerges between the occipital bone and vertebra C_1. The suboccipital nerve is motor to the muscles of the suboccipital region.

Next, find the **vertebral artery** (fig. 6-10). On one side of the body, cut all dorsal musculature away from the transverse processes of C_1 and C_2. Identify the vertebral artery as it passes through the **foramina**

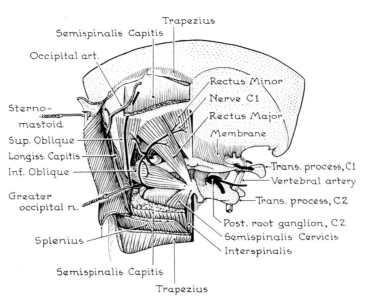

FIG. 6-10. Diagram of suboccipital region.

transversaria of axis and atlas. On the same side, scrape clean the **posterior arch of the atlas.** Note the thin **posterior atlanto-occipital membrane** which stretches from this arch to the posterior margin of the foramen magnum. Observe that the vertebral artery curves around the superior articular process of the atlas. Follow it in its groove on the arch of the atlas. Finally, the artery passes through a hiatus in the posterior atlanto-occipital membrane. (Later, after removal of the membrane and a wedge of occipital bone, the artery will be followed in its course through the foramen magnum into the cranial cavity; p. 121.)

CHAPTER 7

UPPER EXTREMITY

Scapular and Deltoid Regions
General Remarks

The pectoral muscles act on the upper extremity. The pectoralis major and minor were reflected during the dissection of the anterior chest wall. Review these two muscles and their nerve supply (p. 8).

Several muscles acting on the upper extremity were already seen and dissected during exploration of the superficial group of the back muscles (p. 91–92). Once again, identify and review these muscles: Trapezius, latissimus dorsi, rhomboids, and levator scapulae. The latissimus dorsi acts directly on the arm, since it is inserted into the humerus. Trapezius, rhomboids, and levator scapulae act primarily on the scapula. Positional changes of the scapula are transferred to the humerus (since scapula and humerus articulate with each other; *Atlas, 1, 2*).

Four muscles (supraspinatus, infraspinatus, teres major, teres minor) arise from the dorsal surface of the scapula and insert into the upper portion of the humerus. In order to have complete access to these muscles, the deltoid muscle must be detached from its scapular origin.

Bony Landmarks

Refer to a skeleton and study the following bony landmarks:
1. **Scapula** (*Atlas, 2*). The **spine** separates the dorsal surface of the scapula into **supraspinous fossa** and **infraspinous fossa.** At the lateral scapular border, the two spinous fossae are connected by the **great scapular notch.** Observe the **glenoid cavity** for the articulation with the head of the humerus. Above the glenoid cavity, the **supraglenoid tubercle;** below it, the **infraglenoid tubercle. Coracoid process** (*Atlas, 1*). **Suprascapular notch** incising the superior scapular border at the base of the coracoid process.
2. **Humerus** (*Atlas, 1, 2*). **Head** articulating with glenoid cavity. **Greater tubercle** located laterally. **Lesser tubercle** located anteriorly. **Intertubercular sulcus or bicipital groove** between the two turbercles. **Deltoid tuberosity** for insertion of deltoid muscle.

Plan for Dissection

The deltoid muscle will be detached from its scapular origin, and the course of its nerve and artery will be studied. Subsequently, the four muscles arising from the dorsal surface of the scapula (supraspinatus, infraspinatus, teres major, teres minor) will be dissected, and their nerve and blood supplies will be demonstrated.

Dissection

Dissection will be easier if (1) the arm is abducted about 45°; (2) the shoulder is allowed to fall forward. Use a wooden block if necessary.

Define the borders of the **deltoid muscle.** Verify its origin from the lateral third of the clavicle (*Atlas, 14*), spine and acromion of scapula (*Atlas, 24, 25, 30*). With a scalpel, carefully detach the deltoid from spine and acromion of the scapula (*Atlas, 30*). Leave the muscle attached to the clavicle. Reflect the deltoid forward. Observe the **axillary nerve** and **posterior humeral circumflex artery** entering its deep surface (*Atlas, 32*). Using the scissor technique, dissect nerve and vessels. Note the following:
1. The axillary nerve also supplies the teres minor (*Atlas, 10, 32*).
2. The axillary nerve is a branch of the posterior cord of the brachial plexus (*Atlas, 10*).
3. The posterior humeral circumflex artery is a branch of the axillary artery (*Atlas, 3*).

Push your fingers parallel to the axillary nerve and posterior humeral circumflex vessels into a space. This space is the **quadrangular space** (fig. 7-1; *Atlas, 32*). Define the borders of the quadrangular space:
1. Cranially, the capsule of the shoulder joint.
2. Laterally, the surgical neck of the humerus.
3. Medially, the long head of the triceps brachii.
4. Caudally, the upper border of the teres major.

Note the **long head of the triceps brachii** (*Atlas, 32*). Verify that it passes between teres minor and teres major and attaches to the infraglenoid tubercle. With your fingers, separate **long and lateral heads of triceps.** Define the interval between the two heads of the muscle inferior to the teres major. With a probe, explore the floor of the triangular interval. Here you will find the humerus. The **radial nerve** and the

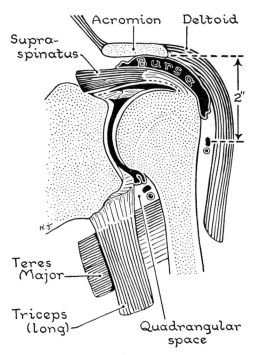

FIG. 7-1. Shoulder region, on coronal section. Quadrangular space.

profunda brachii artery should be seen lying within a broad groove directly on the humerus (*Atlas, 32*). Get into the habit of learning where vessels and nerves originate from and travel to. In this case, the profunda brachii artery is schematized in *Atlas, 3*. A scheme of the radial nerve with its origin and distribution is shown in *Atlas, 10*.

Next, the **supraspinatus** and **infraspinatus muscles** must be explored: To clear the area, reflect the trapezius forward. If dissection of the superficial back muscles has been done properly, the trapezius will remain attached only to the clavicle. Its nerve and blood supply should still be intact. Remove deep fascia from the supraspinatus and infraspinatus. Push your finger into the space bounded by the levator scapulae, superior border of the scapula, and anterior margin of reflected trapezius. Since this space is filled with loose fat, use the scissor technqiue and forceps to remove it. Run your finger along the superior border of the scapula. Feel the ligament that bridges the suprascapular notch medial to the base of the coracoid process (*Atlas, 25, 25.1*). This is the **suprascapular ligament.**

The next objective is to demonstrate the nerve and blood supply to the muscles occupying the supraspinous and infraspinous fossae. Vertically cut across the supraspinatus muscle at the following location (fig. 7-2 or *Atlas, 25.1*): About 5 cm lateral to the superior angle of the scapula; that is, medial to the suprascapular notch and ligament. With the handle of the scalpel, free the lateral portion of the supraspinatus from its fossa. Reflect it laterally. Now, observe and clean the **suprascapular nerve and artery** (fig. 7-2 or

Atlas, 25.1). The nerve passes underneath the suprascapular ligament, while the artery passes above it. Realize that the nerve is derived from cervical segments (*Atlas, 10*). The artery usually originates from the thyrocervical trunk (*Atlas, 25.1, 531*).

Now, about 5 cm from the vertebral scapular border, cut vertically across the **infraspinatus muscle.** Peel the lateral portion of the muscle loose. Reflect it laterally. Note the **suprascapular artery and nerve** reaching the muscle via the greater scapular notch (fig. 7-2 or *Atlas, 25.1*).

Follow the **suprascapular artery** and **nerve** into the fossa bounded by levator scapulae, superior border of scapula, and trapezius (*Atlas, 25*). Both nerve and artery are lateral to a small 'rounded' muscle, the posterior belly of the omohyoid which arises medial to the suprascapular notch. Deep within the fossa, find the **transverse cervical artery** (fig. 7-3, *Atlas, 25*). The transverse cervical artery divides into a superficial and a deep branch at the lateral border of the levator scapulae. The superficial branch follows the accessory nerve to the trapezius. The deep branch (dorsal scapular artery) runs deep to the levator scapulae and the rhomboids along the medial margin of the scapula (*Atlas, 25.1, 25.2*).

The scapular region has an extensive collateral circulation. Its surgical importance becomes apparent during ligation of an injured axillary or subclavian artery. Using the diagrams in figure 7-4 and *Atlas, 3*, realize that the axillary artery may be ligatured between

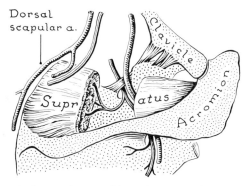

FIG. 7-2. Supraspinatus, with section removed.

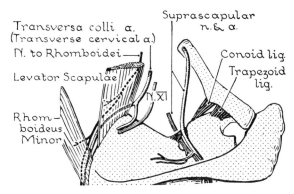

FIG. 7-3. Supraspinous region: Nerves and vessels.

the thyrocervical trunk and the subscapular artery. In this case, the direction of the blood flow in the subscapular artery becomes reversed (*arrows* in fig. 7-4), and arterial blood reaches the distal portion of the axillary artery. Note that the subscapular artery receives its blood via several anastomoses with the suprascapular artery, transverse cervical artery, and some intercostal arteries. Understand the logical approach to placing ligatures. Ligation of the axillary artery distal to the subscapular artery is intolerable.

Finally, study the insertion of the four muscles arising from the dorsal surface of the scapula (fig. 7-5). Verify that the tendons of **supraspinatus, infraspinatus,** and **teres minor** fuse with the capsule of the shoulder joint. These tendons insert into the **greater tubercle** of the humerus. Sometimes, the tendons of infraspinatus and teres minor are inseparable. The teres major inserts into the crest of the **lesser tubercle.** Understand the principal actions of these four muscles (fig. 7-5): The supraspinatus abducts the arm, infraspinatus and teres minor rotate the arm laterally, and the teres major rotates the arm medially.

Attrition of the supraspinatus tendon (*Atlas, 42*) is a common finding among middle aged persons. As the supraspinatus tendon degenerates and wears away, the underlying joint capsule is opened (fig. 7-1 or *Atlas, 38.1*). Between deltoid and acromion superiorly, and the supraspinatus tendon inferiorly, lies a bursa. This bursa (synovial sac) is the subacromial bursa. Attrition of the supraspinatus tendon ultimately leads to wide-open communication be-

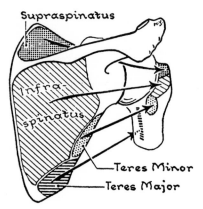

FIG. 7-5. Attachments of the 2 spinati and the 2 teretes muscles. (From *Grant's Method of Anatomy*.)

tween shoulder joint and subacromial bursa. The result is a 'painful shoulder' (rupture of rotator cuff; limitation of rotation).

Superficial Vessels and Cutaneous Nerves

General Remarks

In the living, the superficial veins are conspicuous through the skin. They are most frequently used for drawing blood and injecting medications. In the cadaver, the superficial veins are empty and are not conspicuous through the skin. However, they can be easily demonstrated in the superficial fascia (*Atlas, 4–6*).

The brachial plexus supplies the upper limb with many cutaneous nerves. At various levels, these cutaneous nerves pierce the deep fascia and reach the superficial fascia and skin (*Atlas, 7 and 8*). Although these nerves can be seen in the superficial fascia, it is often easier to identify them as they branch off major nerves. Then, you can quickly follow the cutaneous nerves distally into the subcutaneous tissue.

Plan for Dissection

After removing the skin of the arm and forearm, the more important superficial veins will be identified and followed proximally to the axillary vein. Subsequently, all veins will be removed. Then, it will be easier to demonstrate clearly arteries and nerves.

Skin Incisions

Turn the cadaver into the supine position (face up). Make skin incisions according to figure 7-6. Make additional incisions if convenient.
1. If not already done, make a complete circular incision at the root of the arm from *E* to *I*.
2. At the level of the wrist, make another circular incision from *G* to *H*. Do not injure any structures in the superficial fascia.

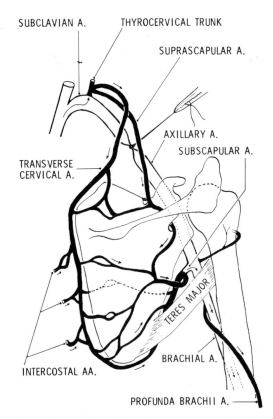

FIG. 7-4. Collateral circulation to arm after ligation of axillary artery. *Arrows* indicate direction of blood flow. Posterior view.

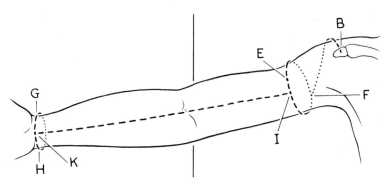

Fig. 7-6. Skin incisions.

3. Join the two circular incisions with a longitudinal one on the anterior aspect of the limb from *I* to *K*.
4. Reflect the skin medially and laterally. Remove it completely. Do not damage the superficial veins and cutaneous nerves in the superficial fascia.

Dissection

Realize that the superficial veins of the upper extremity begin in a **dorsal venous arch** on the back of the hand (*Atlas, 6*). From the medial side of the arch, the **basilic vein** reaches the anterior aspect of the forearm (*Atlas, 4*). From the lateral side of the arch, the cephalic vein reaches the anterior aspect of the forearm (*Atlas, 4, 6*). Identify and dissect the basilic and cephalic veins. Note the **median cubital vein** which joins the basilic and cephalic veins (*Atlas, 4, 44*).

Follow the **cephalic vein** through the deltopectoral triangle (already seen) to the **axillary vein** (*Atlas, 4, 21*). Reflect the pectoralis major and minor upward, and expose the axillary vein. The vein lies within the delicate **axillary sheath.** This sheath not only envelops the vein, but also the axillary artery and parts of the brachial nerve plexus (*Atlas, 15, 16.1*). Carefully incise the axillary sheath to expose the axillary vein.

Follow the **basilic vein** proximally. During its course, it picks up a number of tributaries (venae comitantes of brachial artery; *Atlas, 21*). Finally, at the lower border of the latissimus dorsi, it becomes the **axillary vein** (*Atlas, 21*).

Cut the axillary vein about 2 cm lateral to the first rib. Remove the distal portion of the axillary vein and all its tributaries. This procedure facilitates subsequent dissections in the area.

The **superficial ulnar artery** (*Atlas, 48.1*), present in about 3% of all cases, is of clinical importance. The artery may be mistaken for a superficial vein. If certain drugs are injected into this vessel, the results may be disastrous: Gangrene with subsequent partial or total loss of the hand.

Cutaneous Nerves. Using the scissor technique or a probe, attempt to find the following cutaneous nerves in the superficial fascia (*Atlas, 7, 8*).

1. **Medial cutaneous nerve of forearm.** Large nerve originating from the *medial cord*. Pierces the deep fascia with the basilic vein, medial to the biceps near the midlength of the arm (*Atlas, 7, 44*).
2. **Lateral cutaneous nerve of forearm** (i.e. cutaneous branch of musculocutaneous nerve). Oringates from *lateral cord*. Pierces the deep fascia at the level of the elbow joint, lateral to the biceps and its tendon (*Atlas, 7, 44, 45*).
3. **Posterior cutaneous nerve of forearm.** Branch of radial nerve (i.e. indirectly derived from the *posterior cord*). Look for it along the lateral side of the arm and forearm.
4. **Superficial branch of radial nerve.** Becomes cutaneous about 5 to 8 cm above the wrist joint. Look for it along the lateral aspect (side of thumb) of the lower forearm region (*Atlas, 7, 8, 73*).
5. **Dorsal** (cutaneous) **branch of ulnar nerve.** Becomes cutaneous about 2 to 4 cm above the medial aspect of the hand (*Atlas, 7, 8, 80*).

Axilla

General Remarks

The axilla is the region between the arm or brachium and the chest. Palpate your own axillary fossa and verify that it is a pyramidal space. The axillary fossa possesses an apex, a base, and four walls. The apex is bounded by the clavicle ventrally, the upper border of the scapula dorsally, and the first rib medially. The base of the pyramidal space is the skin and fascia of the arm pit. The four walls of the axilla are (fig. 7-7 or *Atlas, 15.1*):

1. Anterior wall; muscular anterior axillary fold.
2. Posterior wall; consists of muscles clothing the front of the scapula.
3. Medial wall; consists of upper portion of thorax with overlying serratus anterior muscle.

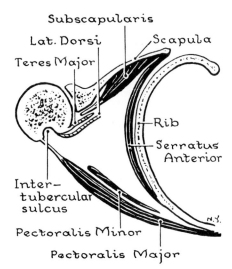

FIG. 7-7. Walls of axilla, on cross section.

4. Lateral wall; the narrow vertical groove of humerus intervening between the converging anterior and posterior walls, i.e. intertubercular sulcus.

The contents of the axilla are: Axillary vessels and lymphatics, brachial plexus, and muscles (*Atlas, 16.1*).

Plan for Dissection

The anterior axillary fold consists mainly of two muscles: Pectoralis major and minor. These muscles were previously dissected. Upward reflection of the pectoral muscles allows convenient access to the other walls and to the contents of the axilla. The axillary vein and its tributaries have already been removed. Therefore, the arteries and nerves of the axilla can be demonstrated with clarity.

Walls of Axilla

Anterior Wall of Axilla. Review the **pectoralis major** and **pectoralis minor** (*Atlas, 13, 14, 16*). These muscles were discussed in detail with the dissection of the pectoral region (p. 8). Reflect the pectoralis minor upward. Reflect the pectoralis major toward the arm. Abduct the arm to a right angle. Have your partner hold the limb in this position with the elbow raised off the table. This procedure relaxes the structures within the axilla.

Posterior Wall of Axilla (fig. 7-7; *Atlas 15–18*). Identify and palpate the three muscles which form the posterior wall of the axilla: **Latissimus dorsi** (responsible for producing the posterior axillary fold), **teres major,** and **subscapularis.** Do *not* clean these muscles at this time. This will be done after tracing nerves and blood vessel from the axillary contents (p. 101).

Medial Wall of Axilla (fig. 7-7; *Atlas, 17*). It is formed by the expansive and flat **serratus anterior**

which covers the ribs and intercostal muscles. Identify the serratus. With your finger tips follow it dorsally toward the medial margin of the scapula. Do *not* clean the muscle at this time so that its nerve and blood supply remain undisturbed.

Lateral Wall of Axilla (fig. 7-7). This narrow wall is the **intertubercular sulcus** of the humerus. The sulcus is also called the **bicipital groove** since the tendon of the long head of biceps brachii lodges in it (*Atlas, 16.1*).

Contents of Axilla

Muscles (*Atlas, 16. 16.1*):
1. Tendinous **long head of biceps brachii.** It lies within the intertubercular sulcus. It arises from the supraglenoid tubercle of the scapula.
2. **Short head of biceps,** lying medial to tendon of long head.
3. **Coracobrachialis,** the most medial of the muscles. Observe that the coracobrachialis and short head of biceps are attached to the coracoid process of the scapula (*Atlas, 16*).

Axillary Sheath (*Atlas, 15*). This sheath envelops the remaining contents of the axilla; i.e. axillary artery, vein, and cords of brachial plexus (*Atlas, 16.1*). If the axillary vein and its tributaries have already been removed (p. 99), the axillary sheath must have been opened.

Axillary Artery and Its Branches (fig. 7-8; *Atlas, 3, 16, 17*). The axillary artery is surrounded by the cords and branches of the brachial plexus (*Atlas, 16, 16.1*). These nerves must *not* be destroyed. They should be retracted (compare *Atlas, 17*) during dissec-

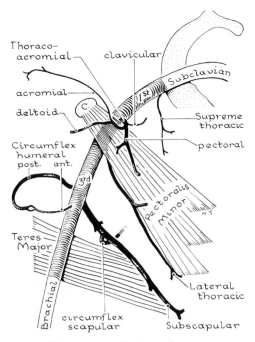

FIG. 7-8. Axillary artery and its branches.

tion of the axillary artery and its branches. Using the scissor technique, clean the following structures:

1. **Axillary artery,** beginning at the caudal border of the teres major. Follow it proximally to the caudal border of the first rib where the name of the vessel changes to subclavian artery (fig. 7-8).

2. **Thoracoacromial artery** (fig. 7-8). Medial to pectoralis minor. This vessel was studied in detail during dissection of the pectoral region (p. 8).

3. **Lateral** (or long) **thoracic artery** (fig. 7-8; *Atlas, 16*). Lateral to pectoralis minor. Follow this vessel to the side of the chest wall, mainly to the serratus anterior.

4. The largest branch of the axillary artery is the **subscapular artery** (fig. 7-8; *Atlas, 17*). Identify one of its branches, the **circumflex scapular artery** as it passes through the triangular space bounded by scapula, teres major, and long head of triceps (fig. 7-9; *Atlas, 18, 32*). This vessel provides collateral circulation of clinical importance (fig. 7-4). Follow other branches of the subscapular artery to the following muscles (*Atlas, 17*): Subscapularis, latissimus dorsi, and serratus anterior.

5. **Posterior humeral circumflex artery** (fig. 7-8; *Atlas, 3*). This large vessel was studied earlier as it passed through the quadrangular space to the deltoid region (compare dorsal aspect, p. 96; *Atlas, 32*). With one finger, approach the quadrangular space from the axilla (fig. 7-9; *Atlas, 17, 18*): Its borders are formed by the tendons of latissimus dorsi and teres major, subscapularis, humerus, and long head of triceps. Identify the posterior humeral circumflex artery as it passes through the quadrangular space. The artery is accompanied by the **axillary nerve** which will be studied later (p. 102).

6. The anterior humeral circumflex artery (fig. 7-8; *Atlas, 3, 17*) is small.

Brachial Plexus (fig. 7-10; *Atlas, 16, 16.1, 19*). The axillary artery is surrounded by the **three cords** of the brachial plexus: Lateral, medial, and posterior. First, identify the **lateral and medial cords** and their branches. Proceed in the following manner (fig. 7-10):

1. Identify the **musculocutaneous nerve.** It is the most lateral nerve of the plexus and enters the substance of coracobrachialis (*Atlas, 16*).

2. Trace the musculocutaneous nerve proximally to the **lateral cord.**

3. Identify the other terminal branch of the lateral cord: this is the lateral root of the median nerve. Follow it distally and identify the **median nerve.**

4. Trace the medial root of the median nerve proximally to the **medial cord** (fig. 7-10).

5. Identify the other terminal branches of the medial cord, the **ulnar nerve.**

Note that the three nerves—musculocutaneous, median, and ulnar—describe the letter *M* in front of

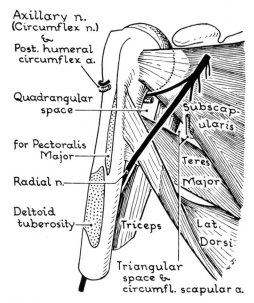

FIG. 7-9. Posterior wall of axilla.

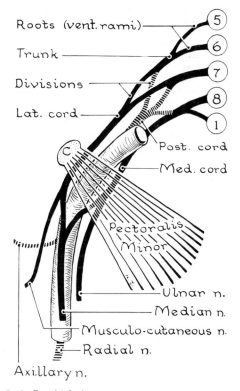

FIG. 7-10. Brachial plexus.

the axillary artery (fig. 7-10). The medial cord has a large collateral branch: The **medial cutaneous nerve of the forearm** (*Atlas, 16, 17*). Trace the pectoral nerves of the reflected pectoral muscles to their origins from lateral and medial cords (or divisions; *Atlas, 9*).

With some tape or a string, retract the axillary vessels and the M-shaped anterior nerves (*Atlas, 17*). This procedure exposes the **posterior cord** of the brachial plexus. Clean the posterior cord and dissect its branches (fig. 7-9; *Atlas, 18*):

1. The **axillary nerve,** passing through the quadrangular space with the posterior humeral circumflex artery.
2. **Subscapular nerves** to subscapularis muscle. Some nerve fibers continue distally to supply the teres major.
3. The **nerve to latissimus dorsi** and the **nerve to subscapularis** run in the loose areolar or fatty tissue ventral to the subscapularis muscle. Use the scissor technique to clean these nerves.

On the lateral axillary and thoracic wall, free the **nerve to the serratus anterior** (*Atlas, 17, 18, 23*). Follow it proximally to the apex of the axilla. This nerve originates separately from lower cervical segments (*Atlas, 10*).

Now, the contents of the axilla have been identified and dissected. Proceed by cleaning the surfaces of all muscles forming the walls of the axilla.

Examine the **contents of the axilla** with special reference to an important bony landmark: The **tip of the coracoid process.** Palpate this landmark. Verify (*Atlas, 16*):

1. The axillary sheath passes about 2 cm medial to it.
2. All structures within the axillary sheath (artery; several nerves) may be easily severed here (stab wounds; piece of shrapnel).

Study the attachments of the **serratus anterior** (fig. 7-7; *Atlas, 23*). It is the essential protractor of the scapula (as when pushing). The muscle also abducts the arm above the horizontal line. Paralysis of the serratus anterior will result in 'winging' of the scapula and in inability to elevate the arm above the horizontal line. The **subscapularis** fills the subscapular fossa (ventral aspect of scapula) and is inserted into the lesser tubercle of the humerus (fig. 7-11; *Atlas, 26*).

The tendons of subscapularis, supraspinatus, infraspinatus, and the teres minor blend to form a continuous musculotendinous sheath. This sheath, which is intimately adherent to the underlying shoulder joint capsule, is called the **rotator cuff** (*Atlas, 39*). Infraspinatus and teres minor *rotate* the arm laterally (fig. 7-5), the

subscapularis *rotates* medially (fig. 7-11), and the supraspinatus abducts (fig. 7-5). Attrition of the rotator cuff may produce a 'painful shoulder' (*Atlas, 42*).

Review the essential anatomical features of the axilla. Study additional cadavers in order to appreciate variations in the distribution of arteries and nerves.

Brachial and Anterior Cubital Regions

General Remarks

The muscles of the arm or brachium are contained in two fascial compartments (fig. 7-12). The anterior compartment houses three muscles, their nerves, and vessels. The posterior compartment houses one extensor muscle, the triceps brachii, and its nerves and vessels (*Atlas, 18*).

Plan for Dissection

Within the cubital fossa, the positions of the brachial artery, median and radial nerve will be investigated. Subsequently, the continuity of median, ulnar, and musculocutaneous nerves will be established. The brachial artery and its important collateral vessels will be demonstrated. Finally, the muscles in the two brachial compartments will be studied.

Dissection

Identify and clean the **biceps brachii** (*Atlas, 45*). In the cubital fossa, note the strong tendon of the biceps. From its medial side, the tendon gives off a strong triangular aponeurosis, the **bicipital aponeurosis** (lacertus fibrosis). It passes obliquely into the deep fascia covering the flexor muscles of the forearm. Note that the bicipital aponeurosis bridges and protects the **median nerve** and the **brachial artery.** Cut across the aponeurosis. Note the relative positions of bicipital tendon, brachial artery, and median nerve

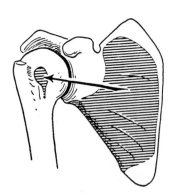

FIG. 7-11. Attachments of subscapularis muscle. (From *Grant's Method of Anatomy*.)

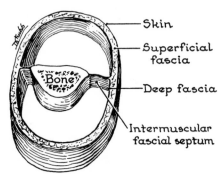

FIG. 7-12. The two compartments of the arm. (From *Grant's Method of Anatomy*.)

(*Atlas, 45*). Do not destroy the **lateral cutaneous nerve of the forearm** (the cutaneous branch of the musculocutaneous nerve). This structure runs between biceps and brachialis, and reaches the cubital fossa lateral to the biceps tendon (*Atlas, 45*).

On the lateral aspect (side of thumb) of the forearm, identify the **brachioradialis muscle** (*Atlas, 45*). With your finger tips, explore the interval between brachioradialis, biceps, and brachialis (*Atlas, 46*). Deep in this interval, find the **radial nerve.**

Follow the **radial nerve** proximally. The next objective is to expose the nerve where it is covered by the lateral head of the triceps brachii (*Atlas, 33*). Proceed as follows: To have better access to the triceps, rotate the arm medially. Push a probe proximally along the course of the radial nerve. The probe lies between lateral head of triceps and humerus (*Atlas, 33*). Using the probe as a protective device to shield nerve and vessels, sever the lateral head of the triceps obliquely. Now, expose the **radial nerve** and the accompanying **profunda brachii artery.**

Establish the continuity of the radial nerve from the axilla to the elbow region. Observe that the radial nerve is in direct contact with the humerus (*Atlas, 33*). This area of contact is called the **sulcus for the radial nerve** or the spiral groove (*Atlas, 2*). Here, with a fracture of the humerus, the radial nerve can be easily injured.

Realize that the **triceps brachii** lodges in the posterior compartment of the arm. Identify the **three heads** of the triceps: **Long, lateral,** and **medial.** Look for muscular branches of the radial nerve to the triceps. There is only one branch to the long head of the triceps (*Atlas, 18*). The other heads receive several branches. Observe that the triceps tendon inserts into the olecranon process of the ulna (*Atlas, 33, 2*).

Identify the three muscles in the anterior compartment of the arm: **Coracobrachialis, brachialis,** and **biceps brachii** (*Atlas, 18, 45, 46*). Observe the tendon of the long head of biceps in the intertubercular sulcus (bicipital groove). Follow the tendon proximally, under the bridge of the transverse humeral ligament, and so to the interior of the fibrous capsule of the shoulder joint (*Atlas, 36*).

Trace the **musculocutaneous nerve** distally through the coracobrachialis (*Atlas, 18*) and between biceps and brachialis (*Atlas, 46*). Sever the biceps about 5 cm proximal to the cubital region. Reflect the severed portions of the biceps. Now, the musculocutaneous nerve can be conveniently traced. Note its motor branches to the three muscles of the anterior brachial compartment (*Atlas, 9, 18*). Follow the nerve distally where it becomes the **lateral cutaneous nerve of the forearm** (*Atlas, 7, 44*).

Trace the **median nerve** from axilla to cubital fossa. Note the communicating branch between the musculocutaneous and the median nerve (*Atlas, 9*). Follow the **ulnar nerve** from the medial cord to the **medial epicondyle** of the humerus. Note that the nerve is applied to the posterior aspect of the medial epicondyle. There, palpate the nerve (*Atlas, 33, 56, 57*). Verify that the median and ulnar nerves do not supply any muscles in the arm (*Atlas, 9*).

The **brachial artery** is the continuation of the axillary artery. It begins at the inferior border of the teres major. It ends at its bifurcation into the ulnar and radial artery (fig. 7-13; *Atlas, 3, 45.1*). Verify that the brachial artery is palpable throughout the arm. It runs with the median nerve which is the only important structure to cross it (*Atlas, 20*). Identify (fig. 7-13 or *Atlas, 45.1*):

1. **Profunda brachii artery.** It is highest in origin. Review its course. Its terminal portion runs with the radial nerve (radial collateral artery; *Atlas, 33*).
2. Several unnamed **muscular branches** (*Atlas, 18, 20*).
3. **Superior** and **inferior ulnar collateral arteries.**

Understand the surgically important collateral circulation around the elbow joint (fig. 7-13; *Atlas, 3, 45.1*). The brachial artery may be tied off distal to the inferior ulnar collateral artery. Under these circumstances, sufficient blood reaches the ulnar and radial arteries via the existing anastomoses. Look for the superior ulnar collateral artery. This artery runs with the ulnar nerve posterior to the medial epicondyle (*Atlas, 45.1, 46*).

Always keep in mind that the brachial artery lies medial to the biceps and its tendon (*Atlas, 45*). At this location, palpate the arterial pulse in yourself and in your partner. Where should you place the stethoscope when taking blood pressure and listening to the pulsations of the brachial artery?

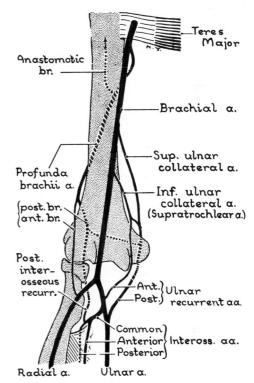

FIG. 7-13. Anastomoses around the elbow.

Flexor Region of Forearm

General Remarks

The flexor muscles of the forearm can be divided into a superficial and deep group. Study a cross section through the middle of the forearm (*Atlas, 63*). Realize that ulnar artery, ulnar nerve, and median nerve are located in an areolar septum. This septum separates the deep from the superficial flexors.

The superficial flexor muscles arise mainly on the medial side of the elbow from the medial epicondyle and its supracondylar ridge (*Atlas, 58*). The deep flexor muscles arise from radius and ulna. Their origin extends to the posterior border of the ulna. Thus, the posterior border of the ulna separates flexor region from extensor region (*Atlas, 63*).

In the living subject, verify the following:

1. Palpate the posterior border of the ulna throughout the forearm region. It lies subcutaneous and is not crossed by muscles or a motor nerve. Therefore, the posterior border of the ulna indicates a convenient 'internervous line,' where the surgeon may incise in order to reach deeper parts of the forearm.

2. Flex your fingers (make a fist). Palpate the contraction of superficial and deep flexors. Note, that the active muscle group originates from the medial region of the elbow and around the medial aspect of the forearm as far as the posterior border of the ulna.

Bony Landmarks

Refer to a skeleton and study the following bony landmarks:

1. **Humerus** (*Atlas, 51*): **Medial epicondyle** and its medial supracondylar ridge give origin to the superficial flexor group (*Atlas, 29*). **Lateral epicondyle** and its lateral supracondylar ridge give origin to extensor muscles (*Atlas, 29*). **Capitulum** for articulation with the radius. **Trochlea** for articulation with the ulna. **Olecranon fossa.**

2. **Radius** (*Atlas, 51*). **Head** for articulation with humerus. **Neck. Tuberosity** for biceps tendon. **Anterior oblique line** for origin of flexor digitorum superficialis. **Styloid process** (*Atlas, 52*). **Interosseous border** for attachment of the important interosseous membrane between radius and ulna (*Atlas, 52, 63*).

3. **Ulna** (*Atlas, 51*). **Olecranon**; observe that it fits into the olecranon fossa of the humerus and thus limits hyperextension of the forearm. Joint surface for articulation with trochlea of humerus. **Head** at the distal extremity of the ulna (*Atlas, 52*). **Interosseous border** for attachment of interosseous membrane.

4. It is essential to understand how the three bones, —humerus, radius, ulna—articulate with each other. On the skeleton, examine the following:
   a. Joint between capitulum of humerus and head of radius (*Atlas, 1*).
   b. Joint between ulna and trochlea of humerus (*Atlas, 1*).
   c. Proximal radio-ulnar joint, between head of radius and a corresponding notch on the proximal end of the ulna (fig. 7-14; *Atlas, 1*).
   d. Distal radio-ulnar joint, between head of ulna and a corresponding notch on the lower end of the radius (fig. 7-14; *Atlas, 1*).
   e. Observe the characteristic movements performed in the proximal and distal radio-ulnar joints. In the position of supination (anatomical position), radius and ulna are parallel. In the position of pronation, the two bones cross each other (fig. 7-14).

5. On the palmar surface of the articulated hand, identify the pisiform bone (*Atlas, 62*).

Plan for Dissection

At the level of the wrist, the relative positions of tendons, vessels and nerves will be identified. After reflecting the superficial flexor group, the deep flexor group will be studied. The student should understand the relations of vessels, nerves, and muscles on cross section (*Atlas, 63*).

Dissection

Remove the superficial and deep fasciae from the front of the forearm as far around as the posterior border of the ulna. Expose the superficial flexor muscles. Follow them distally to the wrist (*Atlas, 59*). Be careful. Do *not* destroy arteries and nerves. From the lateral to medial side, identify the following structures (*Atlas, 59, 66*): **Radial artery,** tendon of **flexor carpi radialis, median nerve,** tendon of **palmaris longus** (absent in 10%), the four tendons of the **flexor digitorum superficialis** (sublimis), **ulnar artery, ulnar nerve,** and the tendon of **flexor carpi ulnaris.**

Palpate these structures in your own wrist (*Atlas, 66*). Do you have a palmaris longus? Feel the pulse in the radial artery. Point to the side of the median nerve. Realize that this important nerve can be easily injured in the wrist region. Palpate the insertion of the flexor carpi ulnaris tendon into the pisiform bone, and through it to the pisohamate and pisocarpal ligaments (*Atlas, 72*). In reference to the pisiform bone, where do you expect to find the ulnar nerve and artery? (*Atlas, 66.1*).

Identify the **brachioradialis.** This muscle is a flexor of the elbow joint. Open the furrow medial to the brachioradialis. There, identify the **superficial**

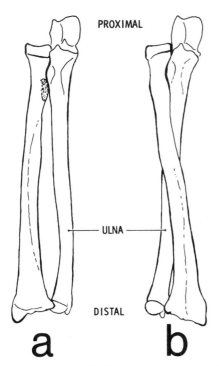

Fig. 7-14. Anterior view of right ulna and radius; *a*, in supination; *b*, in pronation. Note proximal and distal radio-ulnar joints.

superficialis (sublimis) is fully exposed (*Atlas, 60*). Pull on its four tendons and observe that the middle phalanges of fingers 2 to 5 are flexed. Realize that the flexor digitorum superficialis is attached to the common flexor origin and to the anterior oblique line of the radius (*Atlas, 58, 60*). With scissors, carefully detach the superficialis from the radius. Reflect the muscle medially. Identify the **pronator teres.** Understand why it can pronate (*Atlas, 58, 59*). Divide the muscle close to its insertion into the radius. Observe the **median nerve** clinging to the deep surface of the flexor digitorum superficialis. Free the nerve completely, and identify its motor branches.

branch of the radial nerve (fig. 7-15; *Atlas, 46*). Follow the nerve proximally to the point where it arises from the **radial nerve.** Note that the radial nerve divides into its two end branches: Superficial branch, and **deep branch (posterior interosseous nerve).** The deep branch and its relations will be examined later (p. 110).

Pick up the **brachial artery.** Trace it to its subdivision into **ulnar** and **radial arteries** (*Atlas, 60*). Close to the origin of the radial artery, look for the radial recurrent artery. It is part of the anastomotic network around the elbow (*Atlas, 3* anterior view). Quickly, follow the radial artery down to the wrist. Look for muscular branches (*Atlas, 60*). Note: No motor nerve crosses the radial artery. Therefore, the course of the artery indicates a convenient 'internervous line,' where surgeons may incise to reach deeper parts of the forearm.

Pick up the **median nerve.** It is motor to most muscles of the flexor region of the forearm (*Atlas, 9*). Observe that these motor branches arise from the medial side of the median nerve (fig. 7-16; *Atlas, 60, 61*). Study a cross section through the forearm (*Atlas, 63*). Understand that the median nerve runs in the plane between deep and superficial flexors. Therefore, in order to expose the median nerve, the superficial flexor muscles must be reflected. This is the next objective.

Cut the tendon of **palmaris longus** about 3 cm proximal to the wrist. Sever the **flexor carpi radialis** tendon about 5 cm proximal to the wrist. Reflect the muscles and tendons. Now, the **flexor digitorum**

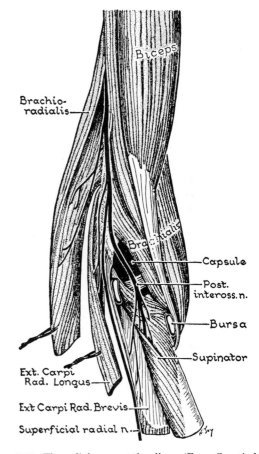

Fig. 7-15. The radial nerve at the elbow. (From *Grant's Method of Anatomy.*)

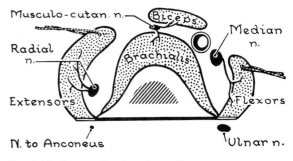

Fig. 7-16. Cross section just above elbow.

With the superficialis reflected, study the **ulnar artery** and its main branches (*Atlas, 60, 61*). First, establish the continuity of the ulnar artery from cubital fossa to wrist. Note that the vessel passes deep to the flexor digitorum superficialis to reach the ulnar (medial) side of the forearm. Refer to a diagram (*Atlas, 3* anterior view). Study the distribution of the **common interosseous artery.** Identify this vessel in the cadaver (*Atlas, 61*). The **anterior interosseous artery** descends on the anterior surface of the interosseous membrane (*Atlas, 63*). It gives off branches to the deep flexors and nutrient branches to the bones. Arterial twigs pierce the interosseous membrane to supply extensors (*Atlas, 52*). The **posterior interosseous artery** reaches the posterior aspect of the forearm and the extensor muscles (*Atlas, 63*). Identify the interosseous arteries (*Atlas, 61*).

Occasionally, the ulnar artery arises high up from the brachial artery. When it does so, it runs almost invariably superficial to the flexor muscles (*Atlas, 48.1*). The artery may be mistaken for a vein. If certain drugs are injected into this vessel, the result may be disastrous: Gangrene with subsequent partial or total loss of the hand.

The ulnar artery is joined by the **ulnar nerve** (*Atlas, 56, 57, 60, 61*). Identify the nerve. Follow it proximally. Observe that the ulnar nerve passes deep to the junction of the 2 heads of the flexor carpi ulnaris. Verify that the nerve lies in a groove between olecranon and medial epicondyle. Here, the nerve is covered only by skin and fascia. In yourself, palpate the nerve. Understand the meaning of the popular term 'funny bone.'

Identify the **supinator** (it belongs to the extensor group). The muscle arises mainly from the radial collateral ligament. It is inserted into the lateral aspect of the radius (*Atlas, 58*). Verify that the **posterior interosseous nerve** (deep branch of radial nerve) pierces the supinator (*Atlas, 46, 60*). Subsequently, the nerve reaches the posterior aspect of the forearm to supply extensor muscles (*Atlas, 63, 79*).

Study the three **deep flexor muscles** of the forearm: **Flexor digitorum profundus, flexor pollicis longus,** and **pronator quadratus** (*Atlas, 61, 62.1*). Pull on the tendon of the profundus, and observe the resulting flexion of the distal phalanges of digits 2 to 5. Pull on the tendon of the flexor pollicis longus; observe the resulting flexion of the distal phalanx of the first digit (thumb). The pronator quadratus runs transversely from ulna to radius in the lower quarter of the forearm (*Atlas, 72*).

Review the major arteries in the anterior forearm (*Atlas, 3* anterior view). Review the nerve supply to the flexor muscles (*Atlas, 9*). Note that the flexor digitorum profundus receives a dual supply: From both the median and the ulnar nerve.

The next objective is to follow tendons, nerves, and arteries from the forearm into the palm of the hand.

Palm of the Hand

General Remarks

There are two superficial muscle masses in the hand: The **thenar group** forming the ball of the thumb, and the **hypothenar musculature** forming the ball of the little (5th) finger. In the middle of the palm is a thick fibrous sheet, the palmar aponeurosis (*Atlas, 59*). Deep to the palmar aponeurosis are the tendons of deep and superficial digital flexors. These tendons reach the palm through the carpal tunnel. Deep in the palm is a series of small muscles.

The palm is supplied with blood by two arterial arches: The superficial arch is mainly derived from the ulnar artery, and the deep arch from the radial artery (*Atlas, 3, 71.1*). The nerve supply of the palmar (or volar) aspect of the hand is derived from the median and ulnar nerves.

Important Landmarks

Refer to an articulated skeleton of the hand. As a group, identify the 8 **carpal bones** (*Atlas, 1*). Distal to the **carpus** [Gk., karpos = wrist] are the 5 **metacarpal bones.** Distal to the metacarpals are the **phalanges.** The thumb (digit 1) has only two phalanges: A proximal one and a distal one. Fingers 2 through 5 have three phalanges: Proximal, middle, and distal (*Atlas, 1, 62, 86*).

Be able to identify the 8 **carpal bones** in the articulated skeleton (*Atlas, 62*). Identify the **pisiform bone** and the hook of the **hamate** on the medial side of the carpus. On the lateral side of the carpus, identify the tubercle of the **scaphoid** and the tubercele of the **trapezium.** These bony landmarks on both sides of the carpus are bridged by a thick fibrous band, the **flexor retinaculum (transverse carpal ligament).** Understand that the wrist is transversely arched and that this arched condition is maintained by the flexor retinaculum. Between carpal bones and flexor retinaculum is an important space, the **carpal tunnel** (*Atlas, 90.1*).

Realize that the **scaphoid** and **lunate** are supported by the radius (*Atlas, 95*). Any transmission of force from hand to forearm or vice versa must pass through these two carpal bones (*Atlas, 95.1*).

Plan for Dissection

After removal of the skin, the palmar aponeurosis and the flexor retinaculum will be examined. The ulnar nerve and artery will be traced into the palm. The carpal tunnel will be opened. Its contents, the median nerve and the long flexor tendons, will be followed into the palm and on to the digits. Subsequently, the long flexor muscles will be served and reflected distally. This procedure will allow convenient access to the deep structures of the palm (muscles, deep palmar arch, and deep branch of ulnar nerve).

Skin Incisions

If the hand is tightly clenched, let your partner hold it open. Make skin incisions as indicated in figure 7-17. Make additional incisions if necessary or convenient:

1. Down the middle of the palm to *M*;
2. Across the palm from *N* to *O*;
3. Down the middle of all fingers (*P*).

Remove the skin from the front and back of the hand and fingers. Note the thinness of the subcutaneous fat at the creases of the fingers. In peeling off the skin flaps from the fingers, proceed with intelligence and caution. Realize that there are digital nerves, vessels, and fibrous sheaths (*Atlas, 70, 70.1*). These structures must not be destroyed.

Dissection

Clean the palmar aponeurosis (*Atlas, 59*). Note that the palmaris longus tendon continues into the palmar aponeurosis. Observe four longitudinal bands of aponeurosis, one to each finger.

Nodular and fibrotic changes of the palmar aponeurosis may lead to a pulling down of one or more fingers via the longitudinal bands of the aponeurosis. This condition is known as Dupuytren's contracture.

Lateral to the palmar aponeurosis observe the thenar fascia enveloping the **thenar muscles.** The **palmaris brevis** muscle arises from the medial aspect of the aponeurosis (*Atlas, 59*). Identify it.

Carefully remove the palmar aponeurosis. Do not damage nerves and blood vessels deep to it (*Atlas, 67*). Detach the palmaris brevis from the palmar aponeurosis and reflect it medially. Now, the ulnar artery and nerve can be freely followed into the palm.

Study the **superficial palmar arch** (*Atlas, 3*). Identify the pisiform bone and verify that the ulnar artery and nerve lie lateral to it (anatomical position). Follow the **ulnar artery** into the palm (*Atlas, 67*). Using the scissor technique, dissect the **superficial palmar arch** and the **digital arteries** springing from it. Subsequently, dissect the **ulnar nerve.** Clean its **superficial branch** which supplies the 5th and the medial part of the 4th finger (*Atlas, 68, 68.1*). The **deep branch of the ulnar nerve** disappears under cover of two of the hypothenar muscles (*Atlas, 68*). Identify its initial portion. Realize that it passes deep into the hand (*Atlas, 72*). Do not trace it at this time.

Review the flexor retinaculum and its role in the formation of the carpal tunnel. Identify the **flexor retinaculum** (*Atlas, 68*). Push a probe deep to the retinaculum through the **carpal tunnel.** With a scalpel, cut through the retinaculum down onto the probe. This procedure will prevent injury to the contents of the carpal tunnel. Examine the contents of the carpal tunnel. It consists of several digital flexor tendons and the median nerve.

Carefully dissect the **median nerve** and its branches. Trace the small but important **recurrent branch** of the median nerve to the **thenar muscles** (*Atlas, 68, 68.1*). The only two other muscles supplied by the median nerve in the hand are the 1st and 2nd lumbricals. Attempt to locate these two small motor branches. Subsequently, follow the **digital branches** of the median nerve to the first 3½ digits (fig. 7-18;

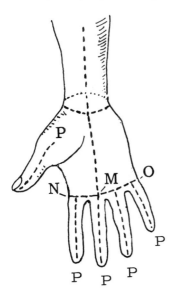

FIG. 7-17. Skin incisions.

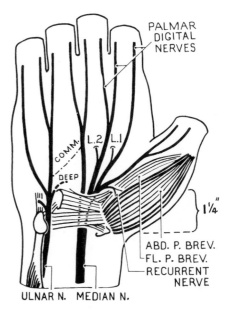

FIG. 7-18. The essential nerves of the hand: Median and ulnar nerves (*L.1* and *L. 2*, lumbrical branches of median nerve).

Atlas, 68). Study the cutaneous nerve supply of hand and fingers. Consult a useful diagram (*Atlas, 83, 84*).

The recurrent branch of the median nerve lies superficial (*Atlas, 66*). Therefore, it can be easily severed during 'minor' cuts. If the nerve is injured, the thenar muscles are paralyzed, and the thumb loses much of its usefulness. In the emergency room, never belittle superficial cuts over the thenar region. Always test the thenar muscles to make sure the important recurrent branch of the median nerve is intact.

Thenar Muscles [Gk., thenar = hand]. Examine the three thenar muscles (*Atlas, 67, 68*):
1. **Abductor pollicis brevis** [L., pollex = thumb; genitive: pollicis]. Raise this superficial muscle. Sever it in the middle (*Atlas, 68*).
2. **Opponens pollicis.** Deep to the severed abductor.
3. **Flexor pollicis brevis.** Note the recurrent branch of the median nerve crossing over it.

Hypothenar Muscles (*Atlas, 67, 68*). Identify:
1. **Abductor digiti quinti,** arising from the pisiform bone.
2. **Opponens digiti quinti.**
3. **Flexor digiti quinti,** sometimes absent.

Clean the **fibrous digital sheaths** of the tendons (fig. 7-19; *Atlas, 72*). Understand that the fibrous digital sheath and the phalangeal bones together form an 'osseofibrous digital tunnel.' In this tunnel, the long flexor tendons are housed (figs. 7-19, 7-20; *Atlas, 70, 72*).

Turn your attention to the long flexor tendons

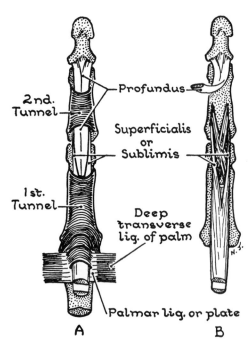

FIG. 7-19. Long flexor tendons and their fibrous sheaths. *A,* a fibrous digital flexor sheath showing the two osseofibrous tunnels. *B,* mode of insertion of the long digital flexors. (From *Grant's Method of Anatomy.*)

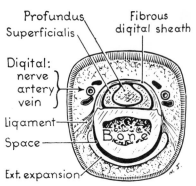

FIG. 7-20. Cross section of a finger. Note osseofibrous digital tunnel with tendons in it. The digital nerve and vessels lie lateral to the tunnel.

which traverse the carpal tunnel. Realize that these tendons are surrounded by synovial sheaths (*Atlas, 69*). These sheaths are lubricating devices. There are two sets of synovial sheaths:
1. **Common synovial sheath** (sac) of the palm. Within the carpal tunnel, and extending proximally and distally to it.
2. **Digital synovial sheaths.** Within the osseofibrous digital tunnels. In most cases, the digital sheath of the little finger and thumb are connected to the common synovial sheath of the palm (*Atlas, 69*).

Frequently, bacterial infection involves the synovial sheaths (bacterial tenosynovitis). The constant movements of the tendons within the synovial sheaths further enhance the spread of infection. Understand that a minor infection of the 5th finger may spread along the flexor tendon sheath, involve the common synovial sheath in the palm, and finally reach the thumb. If time permits, inject some fluid into the common synovial sheath and explore its distribution.

A swelling of the common synovial sheath (as in nonbacterial tenosynovitis) may encroach on the available space in the carpal tunnel. As a result, movements of the flexor tendons are interfered with, and the median nerve may be compressed (carpal tunnel syndrome; pain and paresthesia of thumb, index finger, and middle finger; weakness of thenar muscles).

With your fingers, separate the **flexor digitorum superficialis** from the **profundus.** Cut across the fleshy part of the superficialis. Reflect the tendons distally. During this procedure, the common synovial sheath will be destroyed. In order to reflect the tendons even further, slit open the 1st osseofibrous tunnels (fig. 7-19) of digits 2 through 5.

Now, the **flexor digitorum profundus** is exposed. Identify the four small **lumbrical muscles** originating from the profundus tendons (*Atlas, 68, 69*). Note that these muscles lie on the *radial* side of the corresponding digit. They insert into the dorsal or **extensor expansion** of the digits (*Atlas, 88*). Thus, they flex the metacarpophalangeal joints and extend the interphalangeal joints. Know the nerve supply of the lumbricals (*Atlas, 9*).

On the middle digit, open the fibrous digital sheath.

Study the interactions of the tendons of flexor digitorum superficialis and profundus (fig. 7-19; *Atlas, 72*). Note that the profundus tendon pierces the superficialis tendon. Verify that the superficialis tendon acts on the middle phalanx, whereas the profundus tendon acts on the distal phalanx of fingers 2 through 5. Now, identify the **flexor pollicis longus** (*Atlas, 69, 71*). Leave it intact.

Cut across the fleshy fibers of the **flexor digitorum profundus.** Reflect its tendons and the associated lumbricals as far distally as possible. Now, the **pronator quadratus** is in full view, and the deep palmar space is exposed. This space is of surgical importance. Frequently, it is the site of infections that require surgical drainage.

Deep Structures in the Palm (*Atlas, 71, 72*). The first objective is to follow the deep branches of the ulnar nerve and artery deep into the palm: Detach the flexor digiti quinti from the flexor retinaculum (*Atlas, 68*). Push a probe parallel to the ulnar nerve and accompanying ulnar artery as they pierce the opponens digiti quinti. Carefully remove the muscle tissue in front of the nerve. Now, follow the **deep branch of the ulnar nerve** across the deep structures of the palm (*Atlas, 72*). Identify and clean the triangular **adductor pollicis** (*Atlas, 71, 74*). This muscle draws the thumb toward the palm. This of course, is an important movement. Demonstrate the **deep palmar arch** (*Atlas, 3, 71*).

If time permits, identify the *three palmar interossei* originating from the metacarpal bones of digits 2, 4, and 5. Note that the palmar interossei are inserted into the bases of the proximal phalanges and into the dorsal expansions (*Atlas, 88*). From the diagram in figure 7-21, understand the actions of these muscles. They are adductors. They adduct the finger toward an imaginary line drawn through the long axis of the middle finger. From the dissection, it is obvious that they are supplied by the ulnar nerve (*compare, Atlas, 9*).

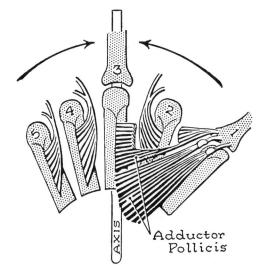

Fig. 7-21. Three palmar interossei and adductor pollicis. (From *Grant's Method of Anatomy*.)

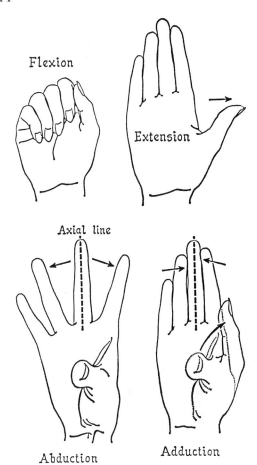

Fig. 7-22. Movements of fingers and thumb. (From *Grant's Method of Anatomy*.)

Review the movements of fingers and thumb. Define: Flexion, extension, abduction, and adduction (fig. 7-22). Which muscles are responsible for flexion? Which muscles are responsible for adduction of the fingers?. Can you name the nerves that innervate the respective muscles? Review the motor branches of the median and ulnar nerves (*Atlas, 9, 68.1*).

Extensor Region of Forearm and Dorsum of Hand

General Remarks

The extensor muscles of the forearm can be divided into a superficial and deep group. The **superficial extensors** arise mainly on the lateral side of the elbow: From the lateral epicondyle, supracondylar ridge, and posterior border of the ulna. The tendons of these muscles reach across the wrist from side to side. They extend the carpus and the phalanges (*Atlas, 77*).

The **deep extensors** arise mainly from the ulna and the posterior aspect of the interosseous membrane. This deep layer is chiefly concerned with supination of the radius and reposition of the thumb into the anatomical position.

The extensors are supplied by the deep branch of the radial nerve (*Atlas, 10, 79*). Nerve and vessels of the extensor compartment run in the plane dividing the superficial from the deep group (*Atlas, 63*).

On the back of the hand, the bones are almost superficial. There are no fleshy extensor fibers here; accordingly, no motor nerve supply is required. The cutaneous nerve supply to the back of the hand is shared by the radial, ulnar, and median nerves. Variation in the pattern of the cutaneous nerve supply are common (*Atlas, 84, 85*).

Dissection

Anatomical 'Snuff Box' (*Atlas, 73, 74*). The **abductor pollicis longus** and **extensor pollicis brevis** bound the 'snuff box' anteriorly. The **extensor pollicis longus** bounds it posteriorly. Identify the 'snuff box' on yourself. Place the tip of the fingers into it, and feel your pulse. In the cadaver, identify and clean the three tendons bounding the 'snuff box.' Deep within the 'snuff box,' find the **radial artery.** Trace it distally to where it disappears between the two heads of the **first dorsal interosseous muscle** (*Atlas, 74*).

The deep fascia at the back of the wrist is thickened to form the **extensor retinaculum** (*Atlas, 78*). All tendons at the back of the wrist are enveloped in synovial sheaths; these extend distally and proximally to the extensor retinaculum (*Atlas, 86.1*).

Trace the three tendons bounding the 'snuff box' proximally into the forearm. The fleshy bellies of the corresponding muscles crop out along a furrow that divides the extensors into a lateral and a medial group. Open this furrow as far as the lateral epicondyle (fig. 7-23; *Atlas. 79*). In doing this, it is necessary to split the intermuscular septum between **extensor carpi radialis brevis** and **extensor digitorum.**

Identify the **supinator** which is wrapped around the upper third of the radius (fig. 7-23; *Atlas, 79*). Once again, verify that the **posterior interosseous nerve** (deep branch of radial nerve) traverses the supinator and sends motor branches to the extensor muscles. Establish the continuity of the posterior interosseous nerve with the radial nerve in front of the elbow joint (*Atlas, 61*).

Muscles (fig. 7-23; *Atlas, 79*). Identify, clean, and study the superficial group of muscles in the following order:

1. Lateral to the outcropping of muscles of the 'snuff box' find the: **Brachioradialis, extensor carpi radialis longus,** and **extensor carpi radialis brevis.**

2. Medial to the outcropping muscles of the 'snuff box' find the: **Extensor digitorum, extensor digiti minimi,** and **extensor carpi ulnaris.**

Follow the flattened tendon of the **extensor digitorum** right to their insertions. Note their cross connections on the back of the hand (*Atlas, 86.1, 87*). Free the extensor digitorum from the extensor retinaculum. Retract it medially. Now, the five muscles of the

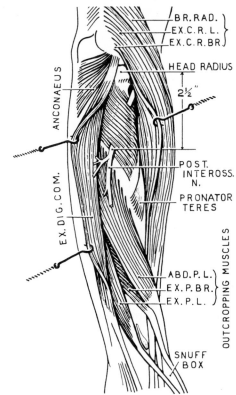

FIG. 7-23. Extensor muscles of forearm.

deep extensor group can be studied in their entirety. These are: The three muscles bounding the 'snuff box,' the **supinator,** and the **extensor indicis** (*Atlas, 79*).

Note that the tendons of the extensor muscles are contained in special tunnels between the bones of the forearm and the extensor retinaculum (*Atlas, 86.1, 86.2*).

Remove the fascia covering the *dorsal interossei muscles.* Note that these muscles occupy the intervals between the metacarpal bones (fig. 7-24; *Atlas, 78*). Follow their tendons into the extensor expansion (*Atlas, 88*). From the diagram in figure 7-25 understand the action of the muscles. They abduct the fingers from an imaginary line drawn through the axis of the middle finger. The dorsal interossei are supplied by the ulnar nerve (*Atlas, 9, 72*).

The 4 dorsal interossei abduct (fig. 7-25). The 3 palmar interossei adduct (fig. 7-21). All 7 interossei are supplied by the ulnar nerve (*Atlas, 9*). That means: If the ulnar nerve is paralyzed, abduction and adduction of the fingers is impossible.

Note that the *radial artery* disappears between the two heads of the first dorsal interosseus (fig. 7-24; *Atlas, 78*). Realize that small arteries exist on the dorsum of the hand; but do not dissect them.

Review the insertion of flexor and extensor tendons into metacarpal bones and phalanges (fig. 7-26). Note that the strongest extensor tendons (extensor carpi radialis longus; extensor carpi radialis brevis; extensor carpi ulnaris) are inserted into the metacarpals. These three extensors of the wrist are the strongest because they work synergistically with the flexors of the digits. Understand and test on yourself: The firmly grasping hand requires an extended wrist (*Atlas, 86.3*). Read an account of the extensor (dorsal) expansion of a finger (*Atlas, 88*).

Joints of the Upper Extremity

General Remarks

It is advantageous to dissect the joints only in one upper extremity. Keep the soft structures of the other limb intact for review purposes.

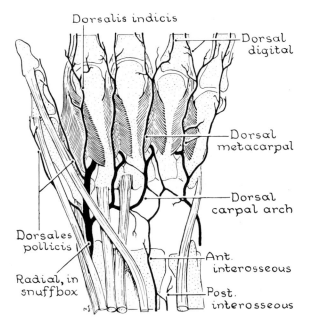

FIG. 7-24. Dorsal interossei. Branches of radial artery on dorsum of hand.

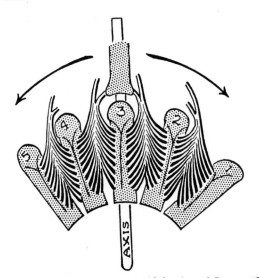

FIG. 7-25. Four dorsal interossei. Abduction of fingers. (From *Grant's Method of Anatomy.*)

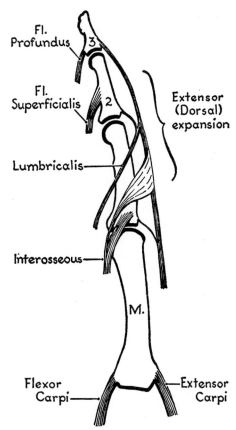

FIG. 7-26. Insertions of tendons of a finger (lateral view). (From *Grant's Method of Anatomy.*)

Refer to the articulated bones of the upper extremity. Identify the following joints (*Atlas, 1, 2*):
1. Sternoclavicular joint.
2. **Shoulder joint.**
3. **Elbow joint.**
4. Radio-ulnar joints (proximal, intermediate, distal).
5. **Wrist joint** (radiocarpal joint).
6. Joints of the digits.

If time permits, refer to the appendix for a detailed text on the dissection of all joints. If time is limited, dissect at least the following joints: Shoulder joint, elbow joint, and wrist joint.

The joints may be dissected in any order. Since the memory of the anatomical details in the forearm is fresh, the wrist joint will be discussed first.

Wrist Joint

By definition, the **wrist joint or radiocarpal joint** is concerned with the movements between **radius** and **carpus.** Review the carpal bones (*Atlas, 62, 86*). Note that the distal end of the radius has two joint surfaces for two carpal bones. In the articulated skeleton, observe that the radius articulates with the **scaphoid** and **lunate** (*Atlas, 95, 95.1*).

Turn to the cadaver. Remove all soft structures

crossing the wrist. On the anterior (palmar) aspect, observe a number of **radiocarpal ligaments** that hold radius and carpus together (*Atlas, 90*).

Force the hand backward (extend). Cut through the ligaments, and open the radiocarpal joint transversely (*Atlas, 91*). Leave the hand attached to the forearm by the dorsal part of the joint capsule.

Identify the smooth proximal surfaces of the **scaphoid, lunate,** and **triquetrum** (*Atlas, 91*). Study the corresponding articular surfaces of the radius and the articular' disc. Verify that the **articular disc** holds the distal ends of radius and ulna firmly together. Understand that the articular disc forms part of the wrist joint. Note that it articulates with the triquetrum, when adducted.

Perform the **principal movements** possible at the wrist joint: *Flexion, adduction, extension,* and *abduction.* Carry out a *circumduction* by combining these movements in a consecutive fashion. Observe the articular surfaces during these movements.

Elbow Joint

Review the bony features of the elbow region (*Atlas, 51*). In the articulated skeleton, verify that the joint consists of three different portions:
1. Portion between trochlea of humerus and trochlear notch of ulna. It is a simple hinge joint (flexion and extension).
2. Portion between capitulum of humerus and head of radius. It is a gliding joint.
3. Portion between circumference of head of radius and radial notch of ulna. Rotation of the radius takes place here.

Turn to the cadaver. Remove the soft structures crossing the elbow joint. Dissect the brachialis off the capsule. Remove the triceps from the back of the thin capsule. Detach the tricipital aponeurosis from the olecranon. Remove the superficial flexor muscles of the forearm from the medial epicondyle.

On the medial side of the elbow joint, free the **ulnar collateral ligament** (*Atlas, 49*). Observe that it consists of a strong anterior cord and a weaker posterior fan-like portion. Define the attachments of the ligament to humerus and ulna.

On the lateral side, detach the extensor muscles from their common tendon of origin. Remove the supinator. Expose the **radial collateral ligament** (*Atlas, 50*). It fans out from the lateral epicondyle to the anular ligament of the radius.

The **anular ligament** encircles the head of the radius. It is in circumferential continuity with the radial notch of the ulna (*Atlas, 53*). Note that the radius can freely rotate in the anular ligament. Place the hand in the pronated position (radius and ulna crossed). Now, pull on the remains of the biceps tendon which is attached to the radial tuberosity. Note the strong supinating action of the biceps brachii.

Open the joint capsule anteriorly by making a transverse cut through the capsule between ulnar and radial collateral ligaments. With a probe, explore the extent of the **synovial capsule** (*Atlas, 54*). Pass the probe (within the capsule) between head of radius and anular ligament. Observe the smooth articular surfaces of the humerus, ulna, and radius (*Atlas, 55*). Notice the thin synovial fold and fat pads intervening between head of radius and capitulum of humerus.

Shoulder Joint

Review the bony features pertinent to the **shoulder joint** (*Atlas, 1, 2*). Remove coracobrachialis, short head of biceps brachii, and long head of triceps. Clean the insertion of the subscapularis. Once again, observe that the tendons of supraspinatus, infraspinatus, and teres minor blend with the joint capsule. Cut these muscles.

The **fibrous capsule** is now completely exposed, except in front where the subscapularis remains intact. Verify that the capsule is attached just proximal to the glenoid cavity. On the humerus, it is attached to the surgical neck (*Atlas, 32, 37, 38.1*).

Remove the posterior portion of the joint capsule. With a probe, explore the extent of the **synovial cavity** (Atlas, 36). With a hammer and chisel, remove the head of the humerus. Now, identify the following structures (*Atlas, 37, 38*):
1. **Glenoid cavity.** Around its margin note a fibrocartilaginous rim, the **glenoid labrum.**
2. Three bands enforcing the front of the joint capsule, the **glenohumeral ligaments.** They converge on the supraglenoid tubercle.
3. **Tendon of long head of biceps.**

Define and clean the strong **coraco-acromial ligament** from coracoid process to acromion (*Atlas, 36*). This ligament, together with acromion and coracoid process, forms a continuous ligamentous and bony protection: The **coraco-acromial arch.** It prevents upward displacement of the head of the humerus.

CHAPTER 8

HEAD AND NECK

Front of Skull and Face

General Remarks

Developmentally, the facial muscles of expression and the muscles of the scalp originate from the right and left *second* branchial arches. The nerve associated with the second arch is the **facial nerve or cranial nerve VII.** This nerve innervates all muscles derived from the second arch including: facial muscles of expression; muscles of scalp and external ear; platysma. The facial muscles are subcutaneous. Most of their fibers are inserted into the skin. They not only express a variety of emotions, but also act as sphincters and dilators for orifices (mouth, nostrils, orbits).

The nerve of the *first* branchial arch is the **trigeminal nerve or cranial nerve V.** It supplies the muscles of mastication which are derived from the first arch. However, the main part of the trigeminal nerve is sensory. Each of the **three divisions** of the trigeminal nerve (V^1, V^2, V^3) supplies an area of skin in the facial region (fig. 8-1 or *Atlas, 470.1*). In general, these areas of skin may be mapped out by drawing two lines: (1) From the nose across the lateral angle of the eye; and (2) from the corner of the mouth to a point about midway between eye and ear. The central V-shaped region (forehead, eyes, nose) is supplied by the **first or ophthalmic division** of the trigeminal nerve (V^1). The intermediate area (cheek) is that of the **second or maxillary division** (V^2). The lower part of the face (mandibular region) is supplied with sensory fibers by the **third or mandibular division** (V^3).

Bony Landmarks

Warning: Handle the skull with great care. Never hold a skull by placing your fingers into the orbital cavities. Their medial walls are paper thin. They are very easily broken.

Orientation: Anatomists have agreed to examine skulls in the following position: The lower margins of the orbital apertures and the upper margins of the external acoustic (auditory) canals lie on a horizontal plane. This position approximates very closely the anatomical position.

Skull on Front View (Norma Frontalis). Examine the front of a skull. Identify the following landmarks (fig. 8-2; *Atlas, 459, 460*):
1. **Frontal bone.**
2. **Maxilla.** It has a *frontal process* which joins the frontal bone.
3. **Zygomatic bone.**
4. **Mandible.**
5. **Anterior nasal aperture** (piriform aperture). Define its borders: Two *nasal bones* superiorly; *two maxillae* laterally and inferiorly; *anterior nasal spine* of maxilla positioned inferiorly in the median plane.
6. **Nasion,** the depression at the root of the nose.
7. **Superciliary arch** (ridge).
8. **Glabella,** the smooth eminence above the nasion and between the superciliary arches.
9. **Entrance to orbit.** Each of three bones—frontal, maxillary, zygomatic—forms approximately one-third of the orbital margin.
10. **Lacrimal bone,** positioned at the anterior part of the medial orbital wall. Together with the frontal process of the maxilla, it forms the **lacrimal fossa** (*Atlas, 518*). The lacrimal fossa is continuous inferiorly with the **nasolacrimal canal.** Gently push a flexible wire through the canal into the nasal cavity.
11. **Teeth.** If fully developed, the adult has 32 teeth, 16 in the upper jaw (maxilla), and 16 in the lower jaw (mandible). The roots of the teeth are embedded in the **alveolar processes.**

If time permits, briefly familiarize yourself with the primary or deciduous teeth (temporary; milk teeth). At the end of the second year, there are normally 20 teeth, 10 in each jaw (*Atlas, 602.1–603*).

Lateral Aspect of Skull (Norma Lateralis). Examine the lateral aspect of the skull. The following bony landmarks are of immediate interest (*Atlas, 461, 462*):
1. **Mandible.** Identify its **body, ramus, angle,** and **posterior border.** The **condylar process** consists of the constricted **neck** and the **articular condyle or head.**
2. **Temporomandibular joint** (T.M. joint), be-

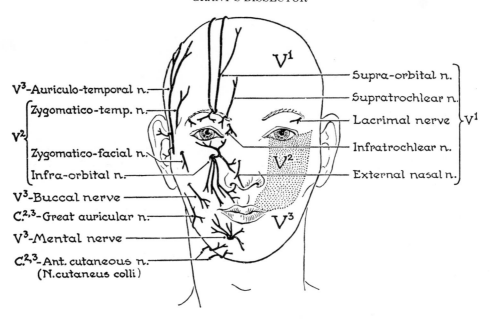

FIG. 8-1. The sensory nerves of the face and front of the scalp. (From *Grant's Method of Anatomy*.)

tween head of mandible and a fossa on the **temporal bone.**
3. **External auditory meatus** (canal), which is part of the temporal bone.
4. **Zygomatic arch.** It is formed by two bony processes: The zygoma of the temporal bone, and the temporal process of the zygomatic bone. Note the suture line in the anterior third of the arch.
5. **Coronal suture.** It separates the frontal from the parietal bones.

Plan for Dissection

After reflection of the skin, the muscles of the face will be exposed. Branches of the facial nerve, which are motor to these muscles, will be identified as they emerge from the substance of the parotid gland. Two important sphincter muscles will receive particular attention: The orbicularis oris (mouth), and the orbicularis oculi (eye). The essential nerves responsible for the sensory supply of the facial skin will be exposed. Finally, the lacrimal apparatus will be explored.

Skin Incisions

Make the following skin incisions (fig. 8-3):
1. In the midline, from vertex to chin (*A* to *B*). Encircle the mouth at the margin of the lips.
2. Start at the nasion (*C*), widely encircle the orbital margins, and return to the nasion.
3. From the vertex, in front of the ear, down to a point just behind the angle of the mandible (*A* to *D*).

First, reflect the skin between eyebrows and vertex. Notice that the skin is closely adherent to the thick and tough subcutaneous fascia. Leave this fascia intact; nerves and vessels run in it. Do not reflect the **frontalis muscle** (*Atlas*, 466). *If the skin is raised without difficulty*, you are probably in the areolar space deep to the frontalis and its aponeurosis.

The skin of the face is thin. There may be a considerable amount of subcutaneous fat. Reflect the skin carefully. Do not damage the underlying pale and inconspicuous facial muscles.

Observe the thin and loose skin of the eyelids. Remove the skin at the margins of the eyelids.

Reflect the skin of the face downward below and parallel to the inferior border of the mandible.

Facial Nerve, Vessels, and Related Structures

The **platysma** (*Atlas*, 526) reaches as far inferiorly as the second rib. This muscle was seen earlier during dissection of the thoracic wall (pp. 7–8). Demonstrate the superior attachment of the muscle sheet to the lower border of the mandible. Subsequently, cut the posterior part of the platysma along the lower border of the mandible, and reflect it toward the angle of the mouth.

Identify the rhomboid **masseter muscle** which extends from the zygomatic arch to the ramus of the mandible (*Atlas*, 465). About 2 to 2.5 cm inferior to the zygomatic arch, the **parotid duct** crosses the lateral aspect of the masseter muscle (fig. 8-4; *Atlas*, 466, 467). Identify the duct. It is empty, collapsed, and flattened like a piece of narrow white tape. Follow the parotid duct to the anterior border of the masseter. Here, the duct makes a right angle turn to pierce

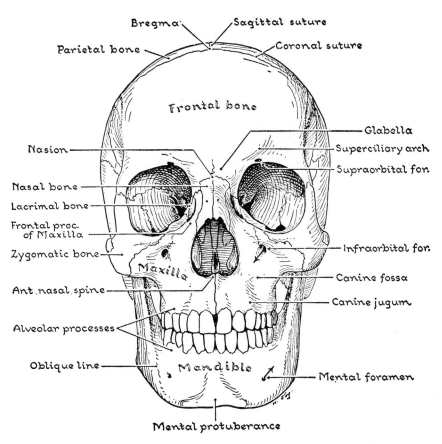

FIG. 8-2. Skull on front view (Norma frontalis). (From *Grant's Method of Anatomy*.)

the buccinator, the muscle of the cheek. Superior to the duct, run the **transverse facial artery** and the *zygomatic branch* of the **facial nerve** (*Atlas, 467*). Preserve the nerve. The artery, unless injected, is often difficult to trace.

The **parotid duct** opens into the oral cavity opposite the upper second molar tooth. Usually, the opening is marked by a slight elevation of buccal mucosa, the **parotid papilla**. Palpate your own right or left parotid papilla with your tongue or your finger. Inspect the papilla in a fellow student. Realize that the parotid duct and the papilla transmit the saliva secreted by the parotid gland.

Facial Nerve (fig. 8-4; *Atlas, 467*). After its emergence at the base of the skull, the facial nerve turns anteriorly and traverses the substance of the parotid gland. Within the gland, the nerve divides into various branches which radiate to the facial muscles of expression. To find these nerve branches, proceed as follows: Follow the parotid duct posteriorly to the point where it emerges from the **parotid gland.** This point is about 5 to 7 mm in front of the posterior border of the mandible. Raise the anterior border of the gland from the masseteric fascia. Find the white, flattened branches of the facial nerve issuing from the substance of the gland. Note that they run deep. They are separated from the masseter only by its fascia.

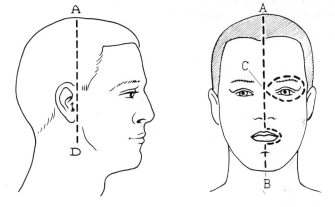

FIG. 8-3. Skin incisions.

Trace the nerve branches to the muscles they supply. The highest of these radiating branches, the *temporal branch*, crosses the zygomatic bone. The lowest branch, the *cervical branch*, runs below the angle of the mandible. This branch sends twigs to the platysma.

Define the free, anterior border of the **masseter** in its entire length. Anterior to the masseter is the extensive **buccal fat pad** (*Atlas, 470*). This buccal fat pad must be removed in order to expose the underly-

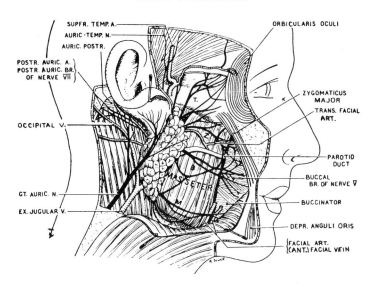

FIG. 8-4. Dissection of side of face.

ing **buccinator muscle** (*Atlas*, *467*). Once again, verify that the **parotid duct** pierces the buccinator. Notice that two different nerves enter the substance of the buccinator:

1. The *buccal branch* of the **facial nerve.** It runs *lateral* to the masseter to supply the buccinator with motor fibers.
2. The **buccal branch of the trigeminal nerve** (**V³**). It runs *medial* to the masseter. Observe its twigs (*Atlas*, *467*, *470*). The nerve does *not* supply the buccinator muscle. It merely pierces the muscle to send sensory fibers to the buccal mucosa of the vestibule of the mouth. (The buccal nerve also sends a small branch to the skin of the cheek (*Atlas*, *470.1*). This branch was destroyed during the dissection.)

Facial Artery and Vein (*Atlas*, *466*). On yourself, palpate the pulse of the **facial artery.** This vessel crosses the mandible at the anterior border of the masseter. The accompanying **facial vein** lies posterior to the artery. Find these vessels in the cadaver. Trace the facial artery to the medial angle of the eye. In its course, the artery crosses successively the mandible, buccinator, and maxilla. Follow the vein to the medial angle of the eye.

Muscles of the Mouth

There are numerous muscles which alter the shape of the mouth and lips. Briefly, define the more important muscles (fig. 8-5; *Atlas*, *470*):

1. **Depressor anguli oris** (depresses corner of mouth; aided by the posterior fibers of the platysma).
2. **Zygomaticus major,** descending from zygomatic bone to corner of mouth (draws angle of mouth upward and backward).

3. **Levator labii superioris,** descending from infraorbital margin to upper lip (elevates upper lip).
4. **Orbicularis oris,** the important sphincter muscle of the mouth. Demonstrate the circular arrangement of its muscle fibers. Realize that the orbicularis oris intimately blends with the fibers of the other muscles (1.–4.).

Clean the surface of the **buccinator** (*Atlas*, *465*). Define its superior and inferior attachments to the outer surfaces of the alveolar processes of maxilla and mandible (*Atlas*, *465.1*, *574*). Note that the buccinator fibers blend with the orbicularis oris.

With a probe, loosen the tissues deep to the levator labii superioris. Carefully cut horizontally through the muscle close to the infraorbital margin. Reflect the muscle downward, and thus expose the **infraorbital nerve** (*Atlas*, *470*). Trace some of its branches to the lower eyelid, side of the nose, and upper lip.

Study the infraorbital foramen and canal in the skull. Pass a wire through the foramen into the canal. For purposes of local anesthesia, the infraorbital nerve is often infiltrated at the level of the foramen or in the canal. In the cadaver, palpate the foramen and push a probe through it.

Lower Lip, External Nose, and External Ear

Lower Lip. Make a midline incision through the entire thickness of the lower lip. Parallel to this incision, make a second vertical incision downward from the angle of the mouth (do this on one side of the body only). Turn down the quadrangular piece of lip. Cut through the mucous membrane along the line of its reflection from lips to gums. Dissect the mucous membrane from the underlying muscle fibers up to the red line of the lip.

Observe the small **labial glands** immediately deep to the mucous membrane. At the red line of the lip, see the **inferior labial artery** (the cut end of the artery may, of course, be seen in the cut edge of the flap). This artery is a branch of the facial artery. The nerve fibers which ascend on the flap, are branches of the **mental nerve.** Now, strip the flap from the bone and locate the **mental foramen.** It is located approximately 3 cm from the median plane. Observe that the mental nerve traverses the foramen (*Atlas, 470*).

The mental nerve is a branch of the inferior alveolar nerve (*Atlas, 654, 656A*). The inferior alveolar nerve runs within the substance of the mandible. Dentists frequently anesthetize the inferior alveolar nerve and, therefore, also the mental nerve. The resulting local anesthesia of the mental nerve involves the region of the chin and the lower lip on the concerned side.

External Nose. The nose is held in shape by the **nasal cartilages** which consist of hyaline cartilage (fig. 8-6; *Atlas, 468*). Palpate the inferior borders of the two nasal bones. Adjacent to these bony borders, identify the paired **lateral nasal cartilages.** They are not independent structures, but merely triangular expansions of the large septal cartilage. This median, unpaired **septal cartilage** extends between the right and left nasal cavities. It forms the anterior part of the nasal septum (*Atlas, 605*).

On each side of the septal cartilage is an **alar cartilage** (fig. 8-6; *Atlas, 468*). These U-shaped cartilages are responsible for the formation of the nares (nostrils). Make a small midline incision at the tip of the nose. Separate the two alar cartilages from the septal cartilage. Follow the free lower edge of the septal cartilage to the anterior nasal spine (*Atlas, 605*).

External Ear (*Atlas, 469*). The external ear consists of the **auricle** and the **external acoustic meatus** (external ear canal). Examine the **auricle** and identify the following parts: *Helix,* the prominent rim. *Antihelix,* the curved prominence anterior to the helix. *Tragus,* usually showing hairs on its medial surface. *Lobule.* The characteristic shape of the auricle is maintained by a single piece of elastic cartilage. There is no cartilage in the lobule.

Time does not permit a detailed dissection of the auricle, its cartilage, and its six tiny intrinsic muscles. Palpate the auricular cartilage on yourself. By palpation, verify that the cartilage is continuous with the cartilage of the external acoustic meatus.

Inspection of Eye and Eyelids

Inspect or palpate the living eye. Your own eye can be examined with the aid of a mirrow. Identify the following structures:
1. **Palpebral commisures or canthi,** uniting the eyelids medially and laterally.
2. **Palpebral rima** or **fissure,** the opening between the lids.
3. **Medial** and **lateral angles** of the fissure.
4. **Cornea,** the transparent anterior ⅙ of the outer coat of the eyeball.
5. **Sclera,** the whitish, opaque, posterior ⅚ of the outer coat of the eyeball.
6. **Iris,** the varied colored diaphragm seen through the cornea.
7. **Pupil,** the aperture in the center of the iris.
8. **Conjunctival sac,** the potential space between eyeball and eyelids.
9. **Conjunctiva,** the membrane lining the sac.
10. **Fornices** (one fornix; two fornices), the regions of conjunctival reflection from eyelid to eyeball.
11. **Medial palpebral ligament,** a fibrous band deep to the medial commissure. It becomes

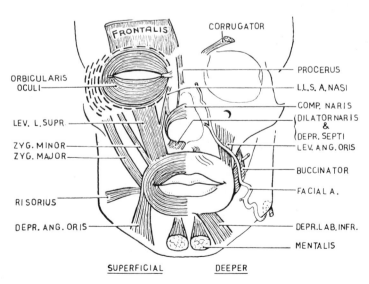

FIG. 8-5. The muscles of the face.

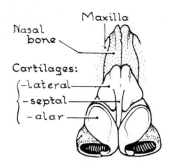

FIG. 8-6. The framework of the external nose (front view).

conspicuous and palpable when the skin at the lateral commissure is pulled laterally (fig. 8-8).

Inspect the **margins of the eyelids** (fig. 8-8; *Atlas, 471*). The margins are flat and thick. They carry double or triple irregular rows of **eyelashes or cilia.** Observe the lack of cilia close to the medial angle of the eye. Posterior to the cilia are the pinpoint orifices of the **tarsal glands.** Examine the inner surfaces of the eyelids. Note yellowish streaks shining through the conjunctiva. These are the tarsal glands.

Inspect the medial palpebral commissure (medial canthus). Here, the upper and lower lids are separated by a triangular space, the **lacus lacrimalis** ('lake of tears'). The lacus contains a small reddish prominence, the **caruncula.** Focus your attention on the area where the base of the triangular lacus lacrimalis meets the eyelids. Here, on both eyelids, find a small elevation, the **lacrimal papilla.** Each papilla has a minute orifice, the **lacrimal punctum.** It is the opening of the **lacrimal canaliculus** which drains lacrimal fluid into the **lacrimal sac** (fig. 8-8; *Atlas, 471.1*).

Dissection of Orbital Region

Dissect the circularly disposed fibers of the **orbicularis oculi** (*Atlas, 466*). Note that this sphincteric muscle consists of two parts: (1) A thick *orbital portion* which surrounds the orbital margin; and (2) a thin, pale *palpebral portion* which is contained in the eyelids. The orbicularis oculi originates from the medial part of the bony orbital margin and from the medial palpebral ligament. Raise the lateral part of the muscle and reflect it medially. Raise the thin palpebral portion off the underlying tarsus, and also turn it medially. Examine the **medial palpebral ligament** (fig. 8-8*B; Atlas, 470*). Its lower border is free. Fibers of the orbicularis oculi arise from its upper border.

The next objective is to reflect part of the frontalis muscle and to expose the supraorbital nerve. Proceed as follows (Fig. 8-7): From the nasion to a point 3 cm above the glabella, make a midline incision through *all* layers of the scalp right down to the bone. Subsequently, make 3 incisions, two parallel and one

horizontal as outlined in fig. 8-7. Turn the quadrangular flap down.

In the flap, identify the following structures (*Atlas, 470*):
1. **Frontalis muscle,** interlacing with the orbicularis oculi.
2. **Supraorbital nerve (V¹) and vessels.** These emerge from the **supraorbital foramen** (or notch).

Turn the flap downward as far as the supraorbital margin and the medial palpebral ligament. Then, remove the flap entirely.

Now, examine the **orbital septum** (palpebral fascia). It is an oval membranous sheet which is attached to the margin of the orbit (fig. 8-8, *A* and *B; Atlas, 470, 471.2*). It is continuous with the periorbita (the endosteum of the orbital cavity). Examine the tarsi. Each *tarsus* is a condensed thickening of the orbital septum, designed to stiffen the eyelid. Evert the larger upper lid and study its free margin. Note the cilia. With the handle of the scalpel, stroke the posterior surface of the upper lid firmly toward its margin. This action will extrude secretions from the **tarsal glands** (compare *Atlas, 471*).

There are about 20 to 30 **tarsal or Meibomian glands** in each tarsus. These are sebaceous glands which secrete an oily substance onto the free margin of the eyelids. This lipid prevents an overflow of lacrimal fluid under normal conditions.

If the duct of a tarsal gland becomes obstructed, a cyst will develop. This is a **chalazion.** Understand that a chalazion will be located between tarsal plate and conjunctiva (*Atlas, 471*).

The chalazion must be distinguished from a **hordeolum** (sty), which involves an inflammation of a small sebaceous gland around the follicle of a cilium.

Cut through the orbital septum in its upper lateral quadrant close to the orbital margin. Pass a probe through the incision. Keep the probe close to the bony orbital roof, and free the **lacrimal gland** (*Atlas, 470*). Attempt to find some of the 6 to 10 ducts which connect the gland to the fornix of the upper part of the conjunctival sac.

The next objective is to study the structures which collect and drain the lacrimal fluid. Once again, refer

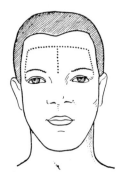

FIG. 8-7. Muscle flap to be turned down.

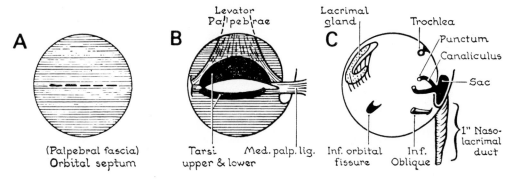

FIG. 8-8. A, the orbital septum. B, the tarsi, ligaments, and levator palpebrae. C, the four corners of the orbital margin, and the lacrimal apparatus (schematic). (From *Grant's Method of Anatomy*.)

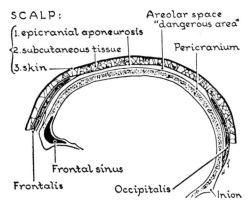

FIG. 8-9. Sagittal section of skull cap and overlying tissues. (From *Grant's Method of Anatomy*.)

to the bony skull, and identify the **lacrimal fossa** for the **lacrimal sac.** Observe the *anterior crest* of the fossa. Understand that the **medial palpebral ligament** is attached to this crest. Consequently, the lacrimal sac lies just posterior to the ligament (*Atlas, 470, 471.1, Horizontal Section*). Turn to the cadaver. With a probe, puncture the lacrimal sac just below and posterior to the medial palpebral ligament. Explore the extent of the sac (*Atlas, 519*). Use a stiff wire or a thin probe and push the instrument downward within the sac. The instrument will traverse the **nasolacrimal duct** and enter the inferior meatus of the nose.

Understand that the normal flow of lacrimal fluid is obliquely across the eye, from the lateral portion of the superior fornix to the medial canthus (fig. 8-8C).

Sensory Nerves of the Face

Review the sensory nerves of the face which are derived from the three divisions of the trigeminal nerve (fig. 8-1; *Atlas, 470, 470.1*):

1. **Supraorbital nerve** (a branch of the ophthalmic division, V^1).
2. **Infraorbital nerve** (a branch of the maxillary division, V^2).

3. **Mental nerve** (a branch of the mandibular division, V^3).

Note that the skin of the nose is supplied by the **external nasal nerve,** a branch of V^1. There are several smaller branches of the trigeminal nerve (*lacrimal, infratrochlear, zygomaticofacial, zygomaticotemporal n.*). Do not dissect these twigs. The auriculotemporal nerve (V^3) will be dissected later (p. 143).

Scalp

General Remarks

The scalp is the covering of the cranial vault. It consists of three layers which are firmly bound together (fig. 8-9):

1. **Skin,** usually covered with hair.
2. **Superficial fascia** (subcutaneous tissue), which is exceedingly tough and dense. Vessels and nerves run in it.
3. **Muscular layer,** consisting of the **frontalis** in front and the **occipitalis** behind. The two muscles are united by a broad aponeurosis, the **galea aponeurotica or epicranial aponeurosis.**

The bones of the cranial vault are intimately covered with **pericranium** or periosteum. The pericranium is separated from the three layers of the scalp by a very **loose areolar tissue.** This loose areolar layer permits the frontalis and occipitalis muscles to produce a limited amount of movement.

Blood vessels and sensory nerves reach the scalp from all around its periphery. These structures are contained in the exceedingly tough superficial fascia. Time does not permit dissection of nerves and vessels in the scalp region. However, be aware of the fact that a rich nerve and blood supply exists (fig. 8-10 or *Atlas, 500*).

The loose areolar layer between scalp and pericranium is of clinical importance. Once an infection has reached the loose layer,

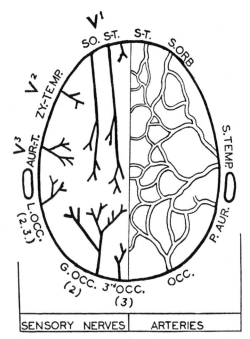

Fig. 8-10. Sensory nerves and arteries of the scalp. (From *Grant's Method of Anatomy*.)

it can spread readily in it. Therefore, this layer has been called the 'dangerous area' (fig. 8-9; *Atlas, 458*). From the 'dangerous area,' the infection is easily carried along veins that traverse the bony vault. As a result, the infection may spread to the substance of the bones, to venous channels within the cranial cavity or to the brain. The physician must be aware of this fact and its anatomical basis.

Bony Landmarks

Refer to a skull and identify the following pertinent landmarks (*Atlas, 459–462*):
1. **Nasion,** the depression at the root of the nose.
2. **Frontal bone.**
3. **Vertex,** the highest point on the **calvaria** or skull cap.
4. **Parietal bones.**
5. **Occipital bone.** Note the **external occipital protuberance or inion.**
6. **Temporal bone** with **mastoid process.**
7. **Zygomatic arch,** jointly formed by processes of the temporal and zygomatic bones.

Skin Incisions and Dissection

Make the following skin incisions (fig. 8-11):
1. In the midline, from nasion (*A*) to vertex (*B*), and on to the external occipital protuberance (*C*).
2. On the right and left sides, from vertex to a point just above and in front of the ear (*B* to *D*).
3. On the right and left sides, from external occipital protuberance transversely to the mastoid process (*C* to *E*).

Reflect the four flaps of scalp downward. Do this by working in the loose areolar space ('dangerous area') with your fingers or the handle of the scalpel. On the side of the skull, reflect the scalp from the underlying **temporalis fascia** (which covers the temporalis muscle; *Atlas, 465*). At the level of the zygomatic arch and at the superior nuchal line, the loose areolar layer is closely adherent to bone (that means, infections of the scalp would not readily spread beyond these areas).

Realize that nerves and vessels are contained within the flaps of scalp. The *occipitalis muscle* is contained in the posterior flap. The anterior flap contains the *frontalis*. Examine the *galea aponeurotica* which unites these two muscles (fig. 8-9).

Next, observe the **pericranium** which intimately covers the skull cap. With a sharp instrument, scrape off the pericranium, but do not remove the temporalis fascia. Now, the **suture lines** separating the individual bones can be seen. In the cadaver and the bony skull identify the following:
1. **Coronal suture,** separating the large unpaired frontal bone from the two parietal bones (*Atlas, 462*).
2. **Lambdoid suture,** separating the unpaired occipital bone from the two parietal bones (*Atlas, 462, 485*).
3. **Sagittal suture,** separating the two parietal bones (*Atlas, 485*).
4. **Lambda,** the point where sagittal and lambdoid sutures meet (*Atlas, 485*).
5. **Bregma,** the point where sagittal and coronal sutures meet (*Atlas, 461*).

In the skull, identify the large unpaired frontal bone. Note the remains of the metopic or frontal suture extending a short distance upward from the nasion (*Atlas, 460*). In about 2% of the population, the frontal bone of the adult is paired, as is normally the case in infants up to 2 years of age (*Atlas, 602 A*). In those cases, the persisting frontal or metopic suture is of radiological importance: it must not be mistaken for a fracture line.

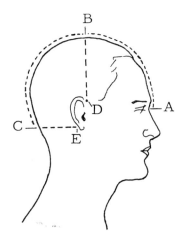

Fig. 8-11. Skin incisions.

Interior of Skull

Removal of Skull Cap [Calvaria]

Refer to the bony skull. Remove the calvaria. Note that the bones of the roof of the skull consist of three parts: A compact *outer lamina*. A compact and very hard *inner lamina*. The *diploe*, a layer of spongy bone which is sandwiched in between the outer and inner laminae. The diploe contains diploic veins (*Atlas, 501*). Observe that there is no diploe in the temporal region where the bones are covered with the thick and fleshy temporalis muscle.

Pull the anterior half of the scalp well down over the face, and the posterior half well down over the nuchal region. With a sharp scalpel, incise the temporalis fascia along the temporal lines (*Atlas, 462*), i.e. incise it in a semicircular fashion along the superior and posterior margins of the temporalis muscle. Now, insert the handle of the scalpel between muscle and bones. Lift off the muscle, and reflect it downward to the level of the zygomatic arch. Scrape the bones clean.

Place an elastic rubber band or a string around the circumference of the skull. Anteriorly, the band must be at least 2 cm above the supraorbital margin. Posteriorly, place the rubber band about 2 cm above the inion (external occipital protuberance). Use the band as a guide, and encircle the calvaria with a pencil line.

With a saw, cut through the external lamina along the pencil line. During the sawing, turn the body alternately on the back or the face. Moist red bone indicates that the saw is well within the diploe. Be particularly careful on the sides, where the bones are thin. If you saw through the inner table, you are liable to damage the underlying dura mater or even the brain. Therefore, break the inner table by repeatedly inserting a chisel into the saw cut, and by striking the chisel gently with a mallet. Continue with this procedure until the calvaria can be pried loose. Remove the calvaria by gently detaching it from the dura mater. Use your fingers, the handle of a scalpel, or a pair of forceps. Do not use more force than necessary. Violent pulling will frequently result in tearing of the dura and in damage to the brain.

In 6% of all female specimens, the frontal bone is of unusual thickness. This condition is known as 'hyperostosis frontalis' (*Atlas, 486*).

Removal of Wedge of Occipital Bone

At this stage, the removal of a large wedge-shaped area of the occipital bone offers many advantages: The brain and its coverings can be more easily examined *in situ*. The superior sagittal and the transverse sinuses can be demonstrated *in situ*. After removal of the cerebellum, the brain stem, its 4th ventricle, and the emerging cranial nerves can be studied *in situ*. Finally, the removal of the brain is greatly facilitated.

Turn to the bony skull. Examine the landmarks pertinent to the removal of the bony wedge:
1. **Mastoid process.**
2. **Foramen magnum.**
3. **External occipital protuberance or inion.**
4. Examine the *internal* surface of the **occipital bone** (*Atlas, 508*): **Groove for superior sagittal sinus. Grooves for right and left transverse sinuses. Two fossae for cerebellum,** inferior to grooves for transverse sinuses. **Two fossae for occipital poles** of cerebral hemispheres, superior to grooves for transverse sinuses.

On the right and left side of the skull, identify (1) the **lateral margin of the foramen magnum**; and (2) the point where the cut edge of the skull intersects with the **lambdoid suture** (suture between occipital and parietal bone). On the right and left sides, connect points (1) and (2) with pencil lines. You have now demarkated the wedge that is to be removed in the cadaver (fig. 8-12).

Turn to the cadaver which must be in the prone position (face down). Briefly review the suboccipital region (chap. 6, p. 94; *Atlas, 490.1*). Detach all muscles from the occipital bone. Clearly identify the interval between **occipital bone** and **atlas** (C₁).

Preserve the **vertebral arteries.** Using fine scissors, carefully incise the **posterior atlanto-occipital membrane** transversely from vertebral artery to vertebral artery.

Scrape the occipital bone clean of muscle remains and pericranium. With pencil lines, mark the bony wedge as explained above (compare 'bony skull'). Cut along these lines with a small saw (Hey's saw). As in the removal of the calvaria, do not cut through the inner compact layer of bone. Loosen the bony wedge with chisel and mallet. Carefully pry it loose from the moistened dura mater. Protect the vertebral arteries.

Examine the inner surface of the removed bony wedge. Verify that the two **cerebellar fossae** (*Atlas, 508*) were in contact with the dura mater overlying the **cerebellum.** Demonstrate that the **grooves for the transverse sinuses** were in contact with these venous channels.

Meninges of Brain

The brain is covered with three membranes, the **meninges** [Gk., meninx = membrane]. These are (fig. 8-14):
1. **Dura mater,** the outer tough membrane.
2. **Arachnoid,** the intermediate membrane with spiderweb-like processes toward the pia mater.

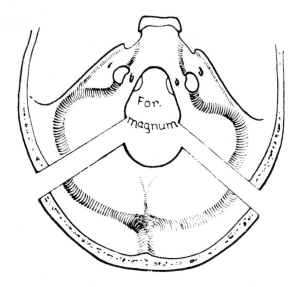

FIG. 8-12. Large wedge removed from occipital bone.

3. **Pia mater,** a soft delicate membrane which is closely applied to the brain tissue.

The *dura mater* [L., dura = hard] is also known as **pachymeninx** [Gk., pachys = thick]. The two soft membranes, *arachnoid* and *pia mater*, are also collectively called **leptomeninx** [Gk., leptos = thin; delicate]. The meninges of the brain are continuous with those covering the spinal cord (chap. 6, p. 93).

Dura Mater (*Atlas*, 502). It consists of two layers:
1. A rough, outer layer. It was adherent to the cranial bones where it formed an endocranium (periosteal covering) for them.
2. A smooth inner layer.

The two dural layers are indistinguishable except where they separate to enclose the venous sinuses.

Examine the rough, outer layer of the dura mater which covers the cerebral and cerebellar hemispheres. In the outer dural layer, observe the branches of the important **middle meningeal artery** (*Atlas*, 502). This vessel supplies the dura mater. The bulk of blood, however, reaches the adjacent cranial bones: Examine the internal surface of the removed calvaria. Note the distinct **grooves** for the branches of the middle meningeal artery. In the immediate vicinity of these grooves, observe numerous, tiny nutrient foramina leading to the substance of the bones.

The **middle meningeal artery** is of great clinical importance. If it is torn in a head injury, blood will quickly accumulate between bony skull and dura mater (epidural hematoma). The expanding hematoma may exert fatal pressure on the brain, unless it is promptly recognized and surgically treated. Surgeons must be aware of the course of the middle meningeal artery and its projection on the surface of the cranium (*Atlas*, 499).

In certain areas the two layers of dura split to enclose the venous sinuses. Identify the **superior sagittal sinus** and the right and left **transverse**

sinuses (fig. 8-13). With scissors, slit these sinuses open. Examine closely the **superior sagittal sinus,** and verify that:
1. It increases in caliber as it passes backward (direction of venous blood flow).
2. It is triangular in cross section (fig. 8-14).
3. It has lateral expansions, the *lacunae laterales* (fig. 8-14).

In relation to the superior sagittal sinus and its lacunae, observe numerous cauliflower-like masses, the **arachnoid granulations** (fig. 8-14).

The **arachnoid granulations** are projections of the subarachnoid space which is filled with cerebrospinal fluid (C.S.F.). The C.S.F. is constantly produced by the choroid plexuses in the ventricular system of the brain. To avoid undue and harmful pressure, any excess of C.S.F. must be removed. This is accomplished by the arachnoid granulations. They empty the C.S.F. into the venous sinuses by a process of osmosis.

The arachnoid granulations are responsible for small shallow depressions on the inner aspect of the calvaria. Examine the removed calvaria. Note these depressions, the *foveolae granulares*, in the vicinity of the sulcus for the superior sagittal sinus.

On both sides, **reflect the dura mater** from the cerebral and cerebellar hemispheres in the following manner:
1. Make an incision through the dura corresponding to the coronal suture. Be very careful not to injure the underlying arachnoid: With a forceps, produce a small fold of dura, nick it, and insert the scissors.
2. Cut the dura parallel to the superior sagittal and transverse sinuses. Stay about 2 cm clear of the venous channels. Now, expose the cerebral hemispheres by reflecting the dural flaps downward. Note the smooth inner surface of the dura.
3. Cut the dura just inferiorly to the transverse sinuses. Then, cut it along the margins of the removed bony wedge. You may enlarge the exposed area by carefully resecting the posterior arch of the atlas. Remove the dura, but leave a small, sickle-shaped dural fold between the two cerebellar hemispheres. This is the *falx cerebelli* (*Atlas*, 458).

Now, with the dura mater reflected, the arachnoid is widely exposed. Realize that there is an extensive potential space between the dura mater and the delicate membrane of the arachnoid.

As a complication of head injury, bleeding into the potential space between dura mater and arachnoid may occur (subdural hematoma). Because the potential space is only limited by the falx cerebri and the tentorium cerebelli, a subdural hemorrhage may spread thinly and widely over a hemisphere. The *subdural hematoma*, which is venous in origin, is a serious and insidious complication of head injuries. It must be distinguished from the *epidural hematoma*.

Arachnoid [Gk., arachne = spider; referring to the

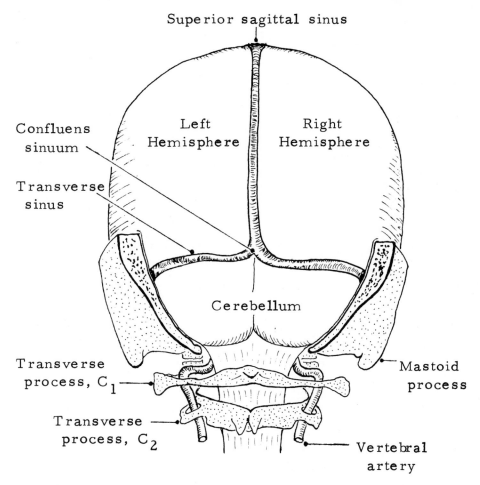

Superior sagittal sinus

Left Hemisphere

Right Hemisphere

Confluens sinuum

Transverse sinus

Cerebellum

Transverse process, C₁

Mastoid process

Transverse process, C₂

Vertebral artery

FIG. 8-13. Calvaria and large wedge of occipital bone removed. Dura mater and venous sinuses in posterior view (schematic).

fine spiderweb-like processes between arachnoid membrane and pia]. The arachnoid is a thin, nonvascular membrane which surrounds the brain loosely. The **subarachnoid space** is a real space which contains cerebrospinal fluid (C.S.F.). In the living, this fluid-filled space acts as an effective shock absorber. In the embalmed cadaver, the C.S.F. is absent. Restore it artificially over a limited area of the cerebral hemisphere: Use a syringe with a fine needle. Puncture the arachnoid membrane obliquely. Inject 5 to 10 cc of fluid (colored or plain water) into the subarachnoid space. An effective fluid cushion is being formed which covers several gyri and sulci. Note that the arachnoid smoothly covers all gaps and fissures of the brain surface.

Substantial intervals between pia and arachnoid are known as cisternae. Find the largest of these, the *cisterna cerebellomedullaris* (cisterna magna). It is the enlarged subarachnoid space between the caudal part of the cerebellar hemispheres and the medulla oblongata. In the patient, the cisterna cerebellomedullaris can be tapped by a needle inserted through the posterior atlanto-occipital membrane.

Pia Mater [L., pius = tender; faithful]. On part of one cerebral hemisphere, remove the arachnoid. Identify the pia. It is a delicate membrane which follows (faithfully) the brain tissue in between all sulci and fissures. The pia carries the blood vessels which supply the brain (fig. 8-14). Observe the **cerebral veins** that empty into the superior sagittal sinus.

Exposure of Brain Stem and Fourth Ventricle

It is desirable to maintain the structural integrity of the brain so that it can be used for future detailed studies (courses in Neuroanatomy or Neurosciences). Therefore, efforts must be made to preserve the brain. Only half of the cerebellum will be sacrificed to expose the brain stem and the 4th ventricle.

The objective is to expose the brain stem and the cranial nerves emerging from it, as depicted in *Atlas, 495*. The cerebellum covers the brain stem posteriorly (fig. 8-15; *Atlas, 458*). Remove the *right half* of the cerebellum in the following manner:

With a scalpel, carefully split the narrow median

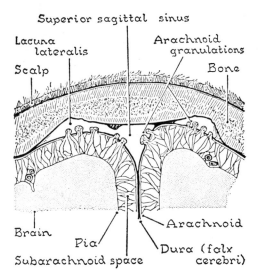

FIG. 8-14. Coronal section through superior sagittal sinus and related structures. (From *Grant's Method of Anatomy*.)

portion (vermis) of the cerebellum in the midsagittal plane. Start just inferior to the confluens of the sinuses (fig. 8-13) and just to the right of the falx cerebelli. Avoid cutting into the medulla. Next, make a parasagittal cut about 5 mm lateral to the midsagittal incision. Remove the narrow slice of cerebellar tissue. Gently force the two cerebellar hemispheres apart to obtain a partial view of the 4th ventricle. Remove several more thin slices of cerebellum. Finally, cut through the attachments of the right cerebellar hemisphere to the brain stem. Remove the remains of the right half of the cerebellum. The right half of the brain stem and of the 4th ventricle is now exposed. On the right side only, identify the following important structures (*Atlas*, 495):

1. **Vertebral artery,** entering the cranial cavity through the foramen magnum.
2. **Trochlear nerve (IV).** It is the most delicate of the cranial nerves. See it just caudal to the colliculi of the midbrain (also compare *Atlas*, 513).
3. **Trigeminal nerve (V).** It is the largest of the cranial nerves emerging from the brain stem (*Atlas*, 495).
4. **Facial nerve (VII)** and **vestibulocochlear nerve (acoustic nerve; VIII),** taking a common course toward the internal acoustic meatus.
5. Three cranial nerves which converge on the jugular foramen: **glossopharyngeal nerve (IX), vagus (X),** and **accessory nerve (XI).**

Folds of Dura Mater

The *inner layer* of dura mater forms **inwardly projecting folds** which serve as incomplete partitions of the cranial cavity. Three of these folds will be

examined now: **tentorium cerebelli, falx cerebelli,** and **falx cerebri** (fig. 8-15; *Atlas*, 503).

Tentorium Cerebelli [L., tentorium = tent]. In the cadaver, examine the inferior surface of the tentorium where the right cerebellar hemisphere was removed. Verify that it separates the cerebellum from the occipital poles of the cerebral hemispheres. In fact, in the anatomical position, the tentorium supports the weight of the occipital poles. Observe in the cadaver: The *posterior convex border* of the tentorium. It encloses the transverse sinuses. Review its attachments to the inner surface of the occipital bone, along the grooves for the transverse sinuses. The *anterior and medial borders* of the tentorium. They are free and concave and form the tentorial notch which surrounds the midbrain (*Atlas*, 514).

Falx Cerebelli [L., falx = sickle]. It is small. Observe its anterior free border which projects between the cerebellar hemispheres in the median plane (fig. 8-15; *Atlas*, 503).

Falx Cerebri. This large, sickle-shaped membrane lies in the midsagittal plane between the two cerebral hemispheres (figs. 8-15, 8-16; *Atlas*, 503). Anteriorly, it is attached to the *crista galli* of the ethmoid bone. Posteriorly, it is fused with the tentorium cerebelli. The superior convex border encloses the **superior sagittal sinus** (figs. 8-14, 8-16). Review its attachments to the inner surface of the calvaria, along the groove for the superior sagittal sinus. On the right and left sides, cut the **cerebral veins** which empty into the superior sagittal sinus. Free the **falx cerebri.** Gently pull the cerebral hemispheres apart, and observe the **free inferior border** of the falx. It lies above the *corpus callosum* of the brain (fig. 8-15).

The inferior concave border of the falx cerebri encloses the **inferior sagittal sinus** (fig. 8-16). This sinus joins the great cerebral vein (of Galen) to form the **straight sinus.** The straight sinus runs obliquely between the falx cerebri and the tentorium cerebelli. Find the straight sinus as it empties into the **confluens of the sinuses** (fig. 8-13). Push a thin probe anterosuperiorly from the confluens sinuum into the straight sinus.

Review the folds of dura mater and obtain a clear concept of their arrangements. These dural folds will be detached during removal of the brain from the cranial cavity.

Removal of Brain

All attachments of the brain to the cranium must be freed. With the cadaver in the prone position (face down), transect the following structures (*Atlas*, 495):

1. The **spinal cord** at the level of the atlas (C_1).
2. Both **vertebral arteries,** anywhere between the foramen magnum and the transverse processes of the atlas.
3. On the right side, where the cerebellum has been

removed, cut with fine scissors the following **cranial nerves** close to the brain stem: **IV, V, and VII through XI.** Reflect nerves X and XI posteriorly, and expose the fiber bundles of the **hypoglossal nerve (XII).** Sever this nerve.

Which structures must still be severed to completely mobilize the brain? Cranial nerves I, II, III, and VI on the right side; all cranial nerves on the left side; blood vessels; attachments of dural folds.

At this stage, it is necessary that you familiarize yourself with **relevant bony landmarks** and certain

soft structures. In the bony skull identify the following (*Atlas*, *508*):

1. **Crista galli.** A triangular plate of the ethmoid bone projecting into the interior of the skull in the median plane.
2. **Cribriform plate** [L., cribrum = sieve]. A plate on either side of the crista galli. Its numerous foramina transmit the filaments of the olfactory nerve. The olfactory bulb rests on the cribriform plate.
3. **Optic foramen** (canal). A round opening traversed by the optic nerve and the ophthalmic

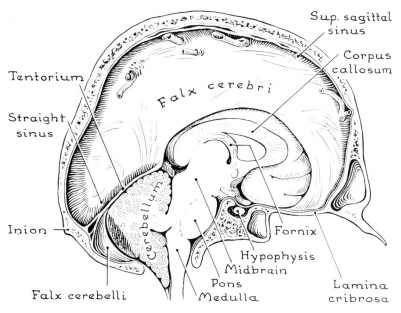

Fig. 8-15. Folds of dura mater and related structures.

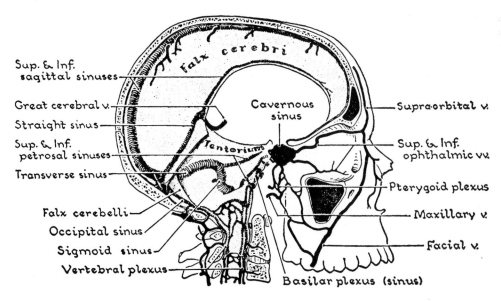

Fig. 8-16. Folds of dura mater and venous sinuses. (From *Grant's Method of Anatomy.*)

artery. View this foramen from the orbital cavity (*Atlas, 518*).

4. **Groove for the internal carotid artery,** just inferior to the optic canal (*Atlas, 508*).

5. **Petrous portion of the temporal bone** (*Atlas, 510*). Note its sharp **superior margin.** The tentorium cerebelli is attached here. The margin also contains a small groove for the superior petrosal sinus (*Atlas, 512*).

Examine the base of a brain (demonstration specimen) and identify the following **pertinent soft structures** (*Atlas, 506*):

1. **Olfactory bulbs and tracts** (cranial 'nerves' I).
2. Right and left **optic nerves** (cranial 'nerves' II). They unite to form the **optic chiasma.**
3. **Infundibulum,** just posterior to the optic chiasma. Essentially, it is the stalk of the hypophysis cerebri (pituitary). The gland must be severed from its stalk during removal of the brain.
4. Right and left **internal carotid arteries,** lying in their grooves just inferior to the optic nerves (*Atlas, 513, 514.1*).
5. **Oculomotor nerve (III),** just cranial to the pons (*Atlas, 506*).
6. **Abducent nerve (VI),** just caudal to the pons.

Procedure. Turn the cadaver into the supine position (face up). Ask your partner to support the brain posteriorly with one or two hands. Gently separate the frontal poles of the cerebral hemispheres. Cut the **falx cerebri** close to the **crista galli** (*Atlas, 503*). Pull the falx upward and backward.

Gently lift up the frontal poles. To both sides of the crista galli, note the **olfactory bulbs and tracts.** Dislodge the bulbs from the cribriform plates. Accomplish this with the aid of forceps and probe. Elevate the brain further until you see the **infundibulum** just posterior to the **optic chiasma.** Cut across the infundibulum. Next, sever the **optic nerves** and the two **internal carotid arteries** close to the optic foramina. Lift up the brain further. Identify the two **oculomotor nerves** and cut them.

With a scalpel, **detach the tentorium cerebelli** on both sides. Start the cut at the free border of the tentorial notch. Carry the cut backward, close to the **superior margin of the petrous bone.** Complete the detachment by cutting all the way to the free margin of the excised occipital wedge. Ask your partner to support the weight of the brain.

Next, identify and cut the two **abducent nerves.** Subsequently, sever the remaining cranial nerves on the *left side* (IV, V, VII through XII). Pull the brain gently backward, and remove it from the cranial cavity.

Gross Examination of the Brain

Examine the cerebral hemispheres and identify the following (fig. 8-17):

1. **Frontal pole**

2. **Temporal pole.**
3. **Occipital pole.**
4. **Lateral sulcus** (lateral cerebral fissure; fissure of Sylvius).
5. **Central sulcus** (fissure of Rolando).
6. **Frontal lobe,** the largest of the lobes. It is bounded posteriorly by the central sulcus, inferiorly by the lateral sulcus.

Refer to a skull, and identify the **three cranial fossae:** *anterior, middle,* and *posterior* (fig. 8-19). By placing the brain back into the cranial cavity, verify the following:

1. The frontal pole is located in the anterior cranial fossa.
2. The temporal pole fits into the middle cranial fossa.
3. The occipital pole is located in the posterior cranial fossa (above the grooves for the transverse sinuses).

Examine the base of the brain. Note that it is covered with arachnoid. Remove the arachnoid. Note the arteries at the base of the brain (fig. 8-18; *Atlas, 505, 505.1*). The two vertebral and the two internal carotid arteries supply the brain. These arteries join to form the **cerebral arterial circle** (of Willis). Verify the following:

1. The right and left **vertebral arteries** join to form the **basilar artery.**
2. The **basilar artery** gives off several branches: Posterior inferior cerebellar; anterior inferior cerebellar; superior cerebellar; posterior cerebral. Note the *oculomotor nerve* (III) emerging between **posterior cerebral artery** and **superior cerebellar artery** (also compare *Atlas, 513*).
3. After giving off the *ophthalmic artery,* each **internal carotid artery** terminates by dividing into: **Middle cerebral artery** and **anterior cerebral artery.**
4. The **arterial circle** is completed by communicating arteries. Anteriorly, the two anterior cerebral arteries are united by the unpaired and very short **anterior communicating artery.** Posteriorly, the **posterior communicating arteries** connect the internal carotid arteries with the posterior cerebral arteries.

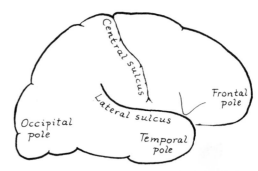

FIG. 8-17. Lateral aspect of right cerebral hemisphere (schematic).

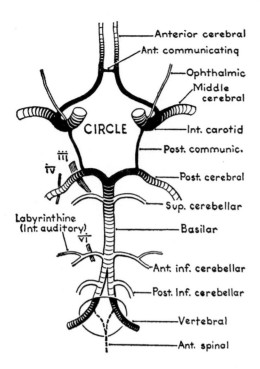

FIG. 8-18. The two vertebral and two internal carotid arteries supply the brain. These arteries join to form an arterial circle. (From *Grant's Method of Anatomy*.)

Note that the flat *medial surfaces* of the cerebral hemispheres are supplied by the anterior and posterior cerebral arteries. Specifically, the *anterior cerebral artery* supplies the anterior and superior aspects of the medial surface. *The posterior cerebral artery* supplies the posterior aspect of the medial surface and the inferior surface of the hemisphere.

Follow the large *middle cerebral artery* through the lateral sulcus. Gently widen the sulcus by retracting the gyri which bound it above and below. This procedure will expose the *insula*. Note that the insula is supplied by branches of the middle cerebral artery. Follow the artery on to the convex aspect of the hemisphere. Note that the superolateral surface of the cerebral hemisphere is predominantly supplied by branches of the middle cerebral artery.

If time permits, examine more closely the middle cerebral artery within the lateral cerebral fissure. Note several small but important branches which supply the corpus striatum and the internal capsule. These branches are also known as 'arteries of cerebral apoplexy' since they are frequently involved in apoplexy (stroke).

At the base of the brain, identify **cranial nerves I through XII** (*Atlas, 506*). After completion of your studies, moisten the brain with embalming fluid, and store it in an air-tight plastic bag. Detailed studies of the brain must be conducted in a separate neuroanatomy course.

Anterior Cranial Fossa

Refer to the bony skull. Note that the interior of the base of the skull is subdivided into three fossae: Anterior, middle, and posterior (fig. 8-19). The **anterior cranial fossa** is sharply marked off from the middle cranial fossa by three concave crests: The sharp posterior borders of the *right and left lesser wings of the sphenoid bone*, and the *anterior margin of the chiasmatic groove* (fig. 8-20).

Identify the three bones which participate in the formation of the anterior cranial fossa: *Sphenoid bone;* crista galli and cribriform plate of *ethomoid bone;* and orbital plates of *frontal bone*, forming the roofs of the orbital cavities.

Recall the topographic relations of soft structures and bony landmarks: The olfactory bulbs rest on the cribriform plates. The falx cerebri is attached to the triangular crista galli. The frontal poles of the cerebral hemispheres rest on the orbital plates of the frontal bone.

Posterior Cranial Fossa

Refer to the bony skull and the cadaver specimen. Realize that the **posterior cranial fossa** is the largest and the deepest of the three fossae (fig. 8-19). It is separated from the middle fossa by the dorsum sellae and the superior borders (margins) of the right and left petrous bones.

The posterior cranial fossa is dominated by the enormous, unpaired and oval **foramen magnum.** At the level of this foramen, the medulla oblongata becomes continuous with the spinal cord. The inclining bony surface anterior to the foramen magnum is the **clivus.** It is topographically related to the pons and the medulla oblongata (*Atlas, 458*). The fossae for the cerebellum and the occipital poles of the cerebral hemispheres were examined earlier (p. 121).

In the bony skull, identify the following openings (*Atlas, 510, 512*):
1. **Hypoglossal canal** for nerve XII.
2. **Jugular foramen,** which transmits nerves IX, X, XI, and the sigmoid sinus.
3. **Internal acoustic meatus** for nerves VII and VIII.

Turn to the cadaver. Identify the **stumps of cranial nerves VII through XII,** and follow them to their respective foramina (fig. 8-21). Note the large **trigeminal nerve (V)** as it curves over the most medial part of the superior margin of the petrous bone. The nerve passes below the attached margin of the tentorium into the middle cranial fossa to enter the trigeminal cave.

Slit open the **transverse sinus.** After leaving the tentorium, it becomes the **sigmoid sinus.** Open the sigmoid sinus. Verify that it leads to the jugular foramen (*Atlas, 643*). Slit open the **superior petrosal**

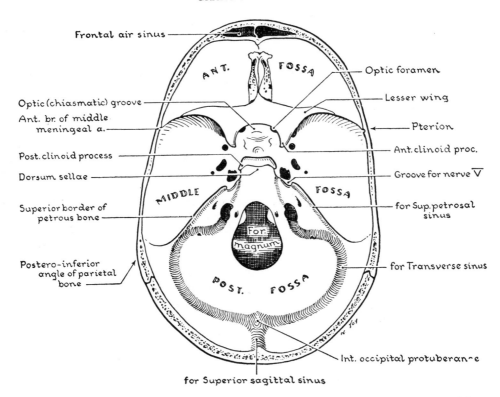

FIG. 8-19. The interior of the base of the skull: The three cranial fossae. (From *Grant's Method of Anatomy*.)

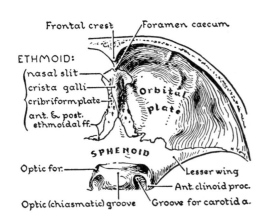

FIG. 8-20. Anterior cranial fossa. (From *Grant's Method of Anatomy*.)

sinus. Note that it runs in the attachment of the tentorium cerebelli to the superior margin of the petrous bone. This small sinus connects the large cavernous sinus with the transverse sinus. Finally, identify the stump of the **abducent nerve (VI).** It pierces the dura within the posterior cranial fossa, in close relationship to the inferior petrosal sinus (*Atlas, 643*).

Middle Cranial Fossa

In the bony skull, identify the **middle cranial fossa** (fig. 8-19). Note that the main part of the fossa is composed of two bones: *Sphenoid bone* and *temporal bone*. On each side, the greater wing of the sphenoid contains a crescent of foramina (*Atlas, 509*). Of these, the following are of particular importance:

1. **Superior orbital fissure,** which transmits cranial nerves III, IV, V¹, VI, sympathetic nerve fibers, and the superior ophthalmic vein.
2. **Foramen rotundum** for nerve V².
3. **Foramen ovale** for nerve V³.
4. **Foramen spinosum** for the middle meningeal vessels. The **groove for the middle meningeal artery** leads from it.

In addition, identify the following pertinent bony landmarks (*Atlas, 507–512*):

5. **Hypophyseal fossa** for the hypophysis cerebri (pituitary gland).
6. **Chiasmatic sulcus,** leading on each side to the optic canal.
7. **Optic canal,** for optic nerve and ophthalmic artery.
8. **Dorsum sellae.**
9. **Foramen lacerum,** situated between hypophyseal fossa and apex of petrous bone.
10. **Carotid groove** for the internal carotid artery.

Recall that the middle cranial fossae are occupied by the temporal poles and lobes of the cerebral hemispheres. Identify the optic nerve which traverses the optic canal. During removal of the brain, the **hypophysis cerebri** (pituitary gland) was severed from its stalk. This small but important master gland lies beneath a circular dural fold which covers the hypophyseal fossa. This fold is the **diaphragma sellae.** With a probe, define the circular aperture of the diaphragma sellae. Enlarge the opening, and scoop out the gland.

Certain soft structures of the middle cranial fossa lie between *two layers* of dura. Therefore, the dura must be split to expose these structures: **Cavernous sinus; internal carotid artery; cranial nerves III, IV, V, and VI.**

If not already done, slit open the **superior petrosal sinus** (*Atlas*, *643*). Carry the cut anteromedially into the **cavernous sinus.** The sinus is large and important. Study a coronal section through the cavernous sinus (*Atlas*, *515*). Realize that the sinus is actually traversed by the internal carotid artery and by cranial nerves.

These relations (*Atlas*, *515*) are of clinical significance. In fractures of the base of the skull, the internal carotid artery may rupture within the cavernous sinus. As a result, an arteriovenous fistula (shunt) occurs. There is an abnormal reflux of blood from the cavernous sinus into the ophthalmic veins, which normally drain the contents of the orbital cavity. As a result, the eye is protruded, engorged, and is pulsating in synchrony with the radial pulse (pulsating exophthalmos).

During injuries or infections of the cavernous sinus, the cranial nerves in it may also be affected.

Pick up the **abducent nerve (VI)** in the posterior cranial fossa. Slit open the dura. Follow the nerve into the **cavernous sinus** (*Atlas*, *643*). Trace the **oculomotor nerve (III)** forward by slitting the dura. Iden-

tify a portion of the **internal carotid artery** within the cavernous sinus.

Pick up the **trigeminal nerve (V)** where it crosses the superior border of the petrous bone (*Atlas*, *643*). Here, the nerve lies in a 1 cm long cave which is lined with arachnoid. Slit open the roof of the cave. In doing so, you will necessarily cut across the superior petrosal sinus. Remove the dura from the greater wing of the sphenoid to expose the **trigeminal ganglion** and the **three trigeminal divisions** (*Atlas*, *513*). Trace the **mandibular division (V³)** to the foramen ovale. Follow the **maxillary division (V²)** to the foramen rotundum. Trace the small **ophthalmic division (V¹)** toward the superior orbital fissure.

Clean the **internal carotid artery** and demonstrate its sinuous course. Note its close relations to cranial nerves III, IV, and VI (fig. 8-22 or *Atlas*, *514.1*, *Atlas*, *513*).

The **middle meningeal vessels** are embedded in the *outer layer* of the dura mater. Follow these vessels to the foramen spinosum.

If time permits, find a very small branch of the facial nerve, the *greater petrosal nerve*. It carries important parasympathetic fibers to the pterygopalatine ganglion (*Atlas*, *513.1*). The nerve lies extradurally. Therefore, remove the moistened dura in the vicinity of the foramen lacerum. Be sure the dura is moist. If it is dry it will break. The fine nerve may be seen running from the facial hiatus of the petrous bone to the foramen lacerum (*Atlas*, *513*, *514*). After traversing this foramen, the nerve enters the pterygoid canal.

The tiny *lesser petrosal nerve* carries parasympathetic fibers to the otic ganglion (*Atlas*, *513.2*). The nerve runs lateral to the greater petrosal nerve to the foramen ovale or to a tiny foramen just posterior to the foramen ovale (*Atlas*, *513*).

Read an account of the dural sinuses, and review them in the cadaver (fig. 8-16 or *Atlas*, *504*).

Orbit and Contents

General Remarks

The two orbits are deep bony sockets for the eyeballs and their related structures (muscles, nerves, vessels). Certain vessels and nerves traverse the orbit in close contact with its roof or floor, to reach the scalp or face.

Each orbit is pyramidal in shape (fig. 8-23). It has four walls. The orbital margin is at the base. The apex is at the optic canal. The medial walls are parallel, and about 25 mm apart. The lateral walls are at right angles to each other.

The eyeball is about 25 mm long; i.e. it is half as long as the orbit. It occupies the anterior half of the orbit (fig. 8-23). The posterior half of the orbit is largely filled with muscles and loose fatty tissue.

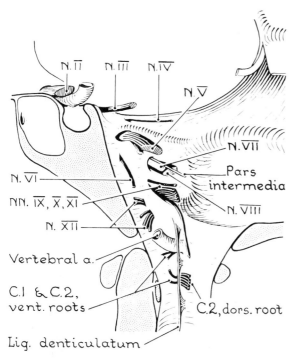

Fig. 8-21. The stumps of the cranial nerves.

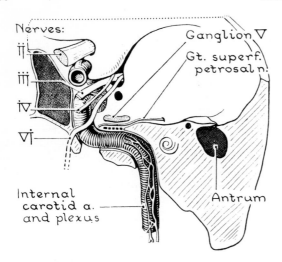

FIG. 8-22. Internal carotid artery and its relations.

Bony Landmarks

Refer to a skull and verify that a number of different bones participate in the formation of the **orbital cavity** (fig. 8-24 or *Atlas, 518*):

1. **Maxillary bone.**
2. **Zygomatic bone.**
3. **Frontal bone.**
4. **Lacrimal bone.**
5. **Ethmoid bone.**
6. **Sphenoid bone.**

In addition, observe the following details:

7. **Optic canal,** at the junction of lesser wing and body of the sphenoid (*Atlas, 507.1*).
8. **Superior orbital fissure,** positioned between the greater and the lesser wing of sphenoid.
9. **Inferior orbital fissure,** a gap between maxilla and greater wing of sphenoid.
10. **Infraorbital groove,** continuous with the infraorbital canal, which ends as the infraorbital foramen.
11. An object pushed through the **roof** of the orbit will enter the anterior cranial fossa (fig. 8-25).
12. An object pushed through the **floor** of the orbit will enter the large maxillary air sinus (fig. 8-25).
13. An object pushed through the **paper-thin medial wall** of the cavity, the **lamina papyracea** of the ethmoid bone, will enter the ethmoidal sinuses of the nasal cavity.
14. **Anterior and posterior ethmoidal foramina,** on the medial wall of the cavity, leading between the ethmoidal air sinuses to the anterior cranial fossa (*Atlas, 520, 521*).
15. The **lateral wall** of the orbit is stout and strong.
16. Explore this realistic possibility: A sharp object (pencil, nail) or a bullet entering the orbit in an anteroposterior direction will traverse the supe-

rior orbital fissure and enter the middle cranial fossa. The physician will be confronted with such penetrating injuries; and he must understand which anatomical substrates have been injured.

The bones of the orbital cavity are lined with periosteum called **periorbita.** At the optic canal and the superior orbital fissure, the periorbita is continuous with the dura mater of the cranial cavity.

Plan for Dissection

It is recommended that the right orbital cavity be approached from above through its roof. In contrast, the left orbital cavity should be dissected from in front.

Right Orbit from Above. The orbital plate of the frontal bone must be removed. This procedure will reveal nerves, vessels, and muscles which are in contact with the roof of the orbit. The extraocular muscles will be studied. Two muscles will be divided and reflected to expose various important nerves and vessels located in the posterior half of the cavity. It will be seen that the optic canal transmits the optic nerve and the ophthalmic artery. The ophthalmic vein and nerves III, IV, V^1, and VI will be followed through the superior orbital fissure.

Left Orbit from in Front (Surgical Approach). General knowledge of the topographic anatomy in the orbit is a prerequisite for this most useful exercise. Eventually, the dissection is concluded with the enucleation of the right eyeball. Subsequently, the interior of the removed eye may be dissected.

Special Technique. In most cases, the eyeball is partially collapsed. Distend it by injecting preservative fluid or glycerin into it with a fine needle attached to a syringe. Insert the needle very obliquely through the transparent cornea in front of the pupil.

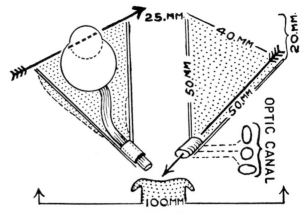

FIG. 8-23. The orbital cavities on horizontal section, and their dimensions. (From *Grant's Method of Anatomy.*)

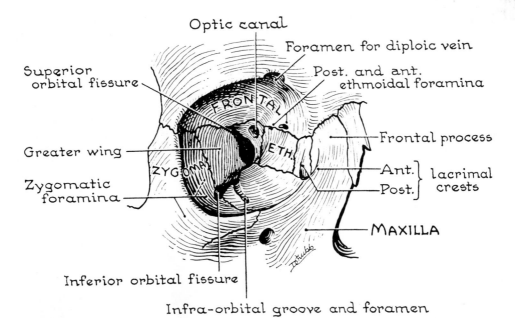

FIG. 8-24. The bony walls of the orbital cavity. (From *Grant's Method of Anatomy*.)

Right Orbit from Above

In the cranial cavity, incise the moistened dura mater along the posterior sharp margin of the lesser wing of the sphenoid and along the lateral margin of the cribriform plate. Now, strip the dura from the anterior cranial fossa (roof of the orbital cavity).

With a chisel or another suitable metal instrument, break the center of the roof of the orbit. With bone forceps, nibble away the whole roof piece by piece:

Anteriorly, the bone is hollow. The exposed spaces belong to the **frontal air sinus** (*Atlas, 520*). Note its mucosal lining. Remove the roof as far anteriorly as possible, but leave the superior orbital margin intact.

Medially, the roof may also be hollow. Here, the **anterior and posterior ethmoidal air cells** will be exposed. Understand that the ethmoidal air cells have a tendency to invade the adjacent frontal bone (*Atlas, 614*). Observe the mucosal lining of the air cells (*Atlas, 520*). At this stage, identify the tough membrane just inferior to the removed roof of the orbit. This is the **periorbita** which envelops the contents of the orbital cavity.

Posteriorly and *laterally*, the lesser wing of the sphenoid must be removed. This procedure will expose the superior orbital fissure and the optic canal. Push a probe between bony roof and periorbita posteriorly through the **superior orbital fissure.** With the probe still in a guiding position, remove the lesser wing of the sphenoid which forms the upper margin of the superior orbital fissure. Next, with the aid of a probe, carefully break away the roof and lateral wall of the **optic canal.** Finally, remove the anterior clinoid process. Shell it out of the investing dura with a pair of forceps.

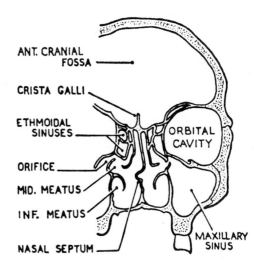

FIG. 8-25. The skull, on coronal section. (From *Grant's Method of Anatomy*.)

Next, incise the **periorbita** transversely near the anterior margin of the orbit. Make a second incision in an anteroposterior direction, but only as far posteriorly as the periorbita is free. Reflect or remove the flaps. Now, the most superior orbital contents are exposed (*Atlas, 520, 523.6*).

Locate the intracranial stump of the delicate **trochlear nerve** (*Atlas, 513*). Using the scissor technique, carefully follow it anteriorly. Observe the nerve along the lateral wall of the cavernous sinus and lateral to the internal carotid artery. In the superior orbital fissure, nerve IV is in intimate contact with the **frontal nerve.** Separate the nerves with fine sharp-sharp scissors ('scissor technique'). Follow the trochlear nerve to the upper border of the **superior oblique** muscle in the orbit (*Atlas, 513, 520*).

Trace the **frontal nerve** from the first trigeminal division through the superior orbital fissure (*Atlas, 513*). In the orbit (*Atlas, 520*), trace the nerve forward to its division into the small supratrochlear nerve and the large **supraorbital nerve.** Push a probe through the supraorbital notch or foramen, and establish the continuity of the supraorbital nerve onto the forehead and scalp region (*Atlas, 470, 470.1*). At this stage, you may extend the dissection field. If you wish to do so, carefully remove the part of the frontal bone which forms the superior orbital margin. This procedure completely exposes the upper eyelid and the *levator palpebrae superioris.*

The delicate **lacrimal nerve** (*Atlas, 513*) enters the superior orbital fissure lateral to the frontal nerve. In the orbit (*Atlas, 520*), trace the nerve forward to the **lacrimal gland.** Arteries accompany the frontal and lacrimal nerves. With forceps, pick out fine lobules of loose fatty tissue, and expose the surface of the most superiorly positioned muscle, the levator palpebrae superioris.

Examine the **levator palpebrae superioris.** Gently pull on the muscle. Verify that it raises the upper eyelid. Understand that various layers of the muscle are inserted into different parts of the lid (*Atlas, 471.2*). Cut the muscle as far anteriorly as possible, and reflect it backward. Now, the underlying **superior rectus** lies exposed. Clean it. Note that the muscle is attached to the eyeball by a tendinous expansion. Cut the superior rectus close to the eyeball, and reflect it backward. Note that a branch of the **oculomotor nerve (III)** reaches its deep surface (fig. 8-26; *Atlas, 520*). Examine the **superior oblique** and trace it forward to its pulley, the **trochlea.** Note that the tendon of the muscle bends at an acute angle and passes to its insertion into the lateral and posterior portion of the eyeball.

At this stage, the origin of the four recti muscles must be considered. They arise from a tough tendinous ring or cuff, the **anulus tendineus** (fig. 8-27 or *Atlas, 525*). This fibrous ring surrounds the optic canal and its contents. In addition, the ring partially includes the superior orbital fissure. The two heads of the **lateral rectus** are attached to the ring. The narrow interval over the superior orbital fissure, encircled by the fibrous ring and bounded by the heads of the lateral rectus, is of strategic importance. Several structures pass through this gap: *Nasociliary nerve; abducent nerve; oculomotor nerve;* and *ophthalmic vein.* Identify the **lateral rectus** and its superior head. Gently push a probe through the interval between the two heads of the muscle. Carefully sever the superior head and the anulus tendineus. Now, all structures passing through the narrow interval can be studied:

Nasociliary Nerve (fig. 8-26; *Atlas, 520, 521*). It is

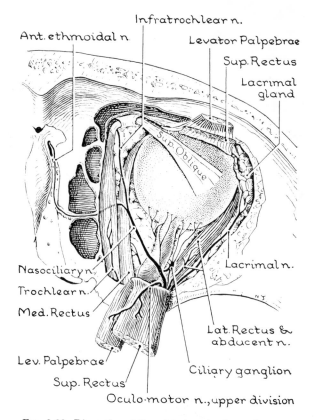

FIG. 8-26. Dissection of the orbital cavity from above.

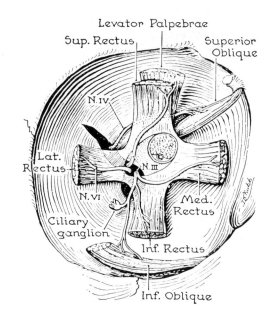

FIG. 8-27. Anulus tendineus. Distribution of nerves III, IV, and VI. (From *Grant's Method of Anatomy.*)

a branch of the first trigeminal division (V^1). Follow it into the orbit. As the nerve crosses the optic nerve, it gives off two or three delicate **long ciliary nerves** to the posterior part of the eyeball. Subsequently, the nasociliary nerve runs obliquely toward the medial wall of the orbit, at the level between the **superior oblique** and the **medial rectus.** To clarify the dissection field, pick out the numerous tiny lobules of loose fatty tissue which fill the interval between muscles, nerves, and vessels.

A small branch of the nasociliary nerve, the *anterior ethmoidal nerve*, passes through the anterior ethmoidal foramen (fig. 8-26). The nerve enters the cranial cavity, runs lateral to the cribriform plate, and enters the ethmoid bone to reach the nasal cavity. It supplies part of the mucous membrane in the nasal cavity. Finally, it terminates as the sensory *external nasal nerve (Atlas, 470.1).*

Abducent Nerve (VI). Once again, follow it through the cavernous sinus and lateral to the internal carotid artery to the superior orbital fissure (*Atlas, 513, 514*). In the orbital cavity (fig. 8-26; *Atlas, 520*), find the nerve applied to the medial surface of the lateral rectus.

Oculomotor Nerve (III). In the cranial cavity, identify the nerve where it pierces the dura between the anterior and posterior clinoid processes (*Atlas, 514*). Follow it to the superior orbital fissure. Here it divides into two divisions. Identify the *upper division* which supplies the reflected levator palpebrae superioris and the superior rectus (fig. 8-26). The *lower division* supplies the **medial rectus, inferior rectus,** and **inferior oblique** (fig. 8-27 or *Atlas, 525; Atlas, 521*). Identify the **ciliary ganglion** which receives parasympathetic fibers from the lower division of nerve III. This parasympathetic ganglion is only 1 to 2 mm in diameter. Find it lateral to the optic nerve, about 1 cm anterior to the apex of the orbit (*Atlas, 523.6*). Delicate short ciliary nerves connect the ganglion to the posterior portion of the eyeball. Understand the functional importance of the ciliary ganglion and the ciliary nerves (*Atlas, 653*).

Look for the **superior ophthalmic vein** (fig. 8-16 or *Atlas, 504*). At the medial angle of the eye, this vein anastomoses with tributaries of the facial vein. In the orbit, the superior ophthalmic vein and its tributaries accompany the ophthalmic artery. Identify the vein on the basis of two facts: (1) It passes through the **superior orbital fissure;** and (2) it drains into the cavernous sinus.

The anastomoses between facial vein and ophthalmic veins (*Atlas, 504*) are of clinical importance. Infections (boils) of the nasal cavity, upper lip, cheeks, and forehead region may spread along venous channels into the ophthalmic veins and on into the cavernous sinus. The resulting *cavernous sinus thrombosis* is a most dangerous complication.

Optic Nerve (*Atlas, 521*). If not already done, open the roof of the optic canal. The optic 'nerve' is actually a brain tract. Therefore, it is surrounded with the three meningeal layers: Dura, arachnoid, and pia (*Atlas, 523.1*). Pass a thin probe below the external (dural) sheath and slit it open. Cut across the optic nerve inside the sheath. Lift up the nerve. Examine the cut surface of the nerve, and identify a dark spot at the center. This is the sectioned **central artery of the retina.**

Ophthalmic Artery (*Atlas, 524*). Identify the artery where it arises from the internal carotid artery. In the optic canal, the vessel lies inferior and lateral to the optic nerve. With the tip of a probe, elevate the optic nerve slightly and observe the ophthalmic artery. Follow the artery into the orbital cavity. Note that it curves over the optic nerve and, subsequently, reaches the medial wall of the orbit. Observe the fine **ciliary arteries** to the eyeball. If time permits, examine other branches of the ophthalmic artery (*Atlas, 524*).

The *central artery of the retina* was already seen on the sectioned surface of the optic nerve (*Atlas, 523.1*). The artery enters the nerve about 13 mm posterior to the eyeball, runs in the center of the nerve, pierces the sclera, and reaches the retina. Its occlusion leads to instant and total blindness of the concerned eye.

Remove the optic nerve and its sheath. Now, the muscles at the floor of the orbital cavity can be observed (*Atlas, 521*). Identify the **inferior rectus.** Raise the posterior pole of the eyeball, and observe the insertion of the **inferior oblique** into the sclera (*Atlas, 522.1*). Study the **medial rectus.** Review the distribution of the lower division of nerve III (*Atlas, 521, 525*).

Review the insertion of the extraocular muscles (*Atlas, 522–523*): The *four recti* muscles are inserted by thin, wide tendons into the scleral coat near the cornea. The *two oblique* muscles are also inserted by thin wide tendons; but they are attached to the sclera of the posterior half of the eyeball.

Students particularly interested in the orbit and its contents should consider an additional or alternative procedure: the *lateral approach.* This useful approach was devised by Professor Laurenson. It allows an excellent exploration of the orbital contents. Refer to *Atlas, 523.6.*

Left Orbit from Facial Aspect (Surgical Approach)

Review the extent of the **conjunctival sac** (*Atlas, 471.2*). Verify that the conjunctiva is firmly adherent to the cornea, but loosely attached to the sclera (*Atlas, 522*). With a sharp scalpel, make a complete circular incision through the conjunctiva, about 6 to 8 mm from the sclerocorneal junction. Push a probe through the incision, and find at least one of the recti muscles.

In order to facilitate the dissection, remove both eyelids and the orbital septum. (Compare your field of dissection with *Atlas, 519*. The *Atlas* depicts the right orbit; you are dissecting the left one).

Examine three corners of the orbit. Notice:
1. Upper lateral: lacrimal gland
2. Upper medial: trochlea for superior oblique
3. Lower medial: lacrimal sac; origin of inferior oblique

Observe the insertion of the **four recti muscles.** Study the insertions of the **superior and inferior obliques.** Notice that the obliques pass *inferior* to the corresponding recti.

Enucleation of Eyeball. With a probe, hook up each rectus tendon and cut across it. Cut all four recti. Adduct the eyeball (turn medially) and pull it forward. Insert a cutting instrument (preferably long curved scissors) into the orbit from the lateral side. Cut the optic nerve. Now, pull the eyeball forward and sever the two oblique muscles. Remove the eyeball. Keep it moist, and store it in a small plastic bag.

Study the socket (fig. 8-27 or *Atlas, 525*). Remove the loose fatty tissue from the posterior portion of the orbital cavity. Pick up the nerve to the inferior oblique and follow it backward as far as possible. Trace the **four recti** to their origin from the **anulus tendineus.** Identify the structures which pass between the two heads of the lateral rectus: **Nerve VI,** lower and upper divisions of **nerve III,** and **nasociliary nerve.**

Dissection of Human Eyeball

In most cases, the removed human eyeball is not well enough preserved to warrant its dissection. If the eye is in acceptable condition, cut it into two halves along a sagittal plane. Use a sharp scalpel (new blade!). Carefully remove the remains of the vitreous body. Gently wash it out, if necessary. Note the following essential features (*Atlas, 523.1*):

1. **External or fibrous coat,** consisting of **sclera** (posterior ⅚) and **cornea** (anterior ⅙). The cornea is more convex than the sclera.
2. **Middle or vascular coat,** consisting of **choroid, ciliary body,** and **iris.** Blood vessels and the ciliary nerves are contained in this coat.
3. **Internal or retinal coat.** In the cadaver, the retina is gray and partially detached (*Atlas, 523.5*). In well preserved specimens, you may find the macula. Identify the region where the optic nerve and retinal vessels enter or leave. This is the **optic papilla or disc.**
4. Two of the **four refractive media** are still present: **cornea** and **lens.** The now empty space between cornea and lens is normally filled with **aqueous humor.** The jelly-like **vitreous body** has been removed earlier.

The gross structures of the eye can be conveniently examined in the large and fresh eye of the bull. If time permits this study, refer to the Appendix, IV.

Posterior Triangle of Neck

General Remarks

The **boundaries** of the posterior triangle of the neck are (fig. 8–29; *Atlas, 540*):
1. Anteriorly, the posterior border of the **sternomastoid** muscle.
2. Posteriorly, the anterior border of the **trapezius.**
3. Inferiorly, the middle third of the **clavicle.**

The posterior triangle has a **fascial roof** of deep fascia which stretches between the two muscles forming its boundaries. This fascia splits to envelop the trapezius and the sternomastoid. Superficial veins lie superficial to the fascial roof. The roof is pierced by cutaneous nerves.

The **floor** of the triangle is formed by a series of muscles which are covered with a thin, firm layer of fascia.

The **contents** of the posterior triangle consist largely of nerves and vessels connecting the neck region with the upper limb.

Plan for Dissection

Following reflection of the skin and a portion of the platysma, the posterior triangle will be fully exposed. First, the accessory nerve, being an important guiding structure, must be identified (fig. 8–29). Subsequently, a number of sensory nerves radiating from the posterior border of the sternomastoid, will be dissected. At the base of the triangle, tributaries of the external jugular vein and branches of the thyrocervical trunk will be observed. Dissection in this area will be greatly facilitated by partial resection of the clavicle.

Finally, the fascia forming the floor of the triangle will be removed and the underlying muscles will be exposed. The important brachial plexus will be followed from the neck into the axilla.

Skin Incisions

If not already done, make an incision along the clavicle from its medial end to a point 3 cm beyond the acrominon (*Thorax*, fig. 2-7).

Make an incision from the base of the mastoid process to the medial end of the clavicle (fig. 8-28, *E* to *F*). Reflect the skin posteriorly. Subsequently, remove the triangular flap along the anterior border of the trapezius. Anteriorly, reflect the skin overlying the sternomastoid muscle.

Superficial Structures and Contents of Triangle

The postero-inferior portion of the **platysma** covers the basal part of the triangle. The platysma passes

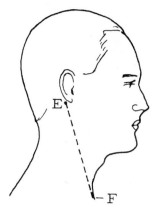

E

F

FIG. 8-28. Skin incisions.

over the whole length of the clavicle (*Atlas, 13*). The **supraclavicular nerves,** which cling to the deep surface of the platysma, also cross the clavicle. Reflect the platysma upward. Do not injure the supraclavicular nerves.

Find the **accessory nerve** (fig. 8–29; or *Atlas, 471.3*). Its approximate course is marked by a line connecting two points: (1) A point slightly above the middle of the posterior border of the sternomastoid; and (2) a point about 5 cm above the clavicle at the anterior border of the trapezius. Incise the roof of the triangle along the course indicated. Using the scissor technique, find the accessory nerve (XI) and free it from its surrounding tissue. Be aware of the function of nerve XI (*Atlas, 661*).

Find the lesser occipital nerve (*Atlas, 472*). It emerges from the posterior border of the sternomastoid in close proximity to nerve XI. Trace the lesser occipital nerve upward, along or near the posterior border of the sternomastoid. The nerve supplies the scalp (*Atlas, 500*). At the apex of the posterior triangle, briefly search for the occipital artery.

In addition to nerve XI and the lesser occipital nerve ($C_{2,3}$), three other nerves radiate from the posterior border of the sternomastoid (*Atlas, 472*):

1. **Great auricular nerve** ($C_{2,3}$). Together with the external jugular vein, it ascends vertically on the surface of the sternomastoid. The nerve supplies the back of the auricle and a cutaneous area extending from the angle of the mandible to the mastoid process.
2. **Transverse cervical nerve** ($C_{2,3}$). Follow it transversely across the middle of the sternomastoid. It supplies the skin of the *anterior triangle* of the neck.
3. **Supraclavicular nerves** ($C_{3,4}$). Note *medial, intermediate,* and *lateral* branches.

External Jugular Vein (*Atlas, 472*). This vein runs superficially from an area posterior to the angle of the mandible to a point about 3 cm above the clavicle. At this point, the vein pierces the roof of the posterior triangle. Clean the vein and follow it through the fascia. Then, remove the remains of the fascial roof.

Resection of Middle Portion of Clavicle. With a small saw, cut through the clavicle at two points (*Atlas, 474, 475*): (1) Laterally, close to the anterior attachments of the trapezius and deltoid muscles; and (2) close to the medial end of the clavicle. Detach the clavicular head of the sternomastoid as far as necessary. Remove the middle portion of the clavicle. Observe the slender **subclavius muscle,** then remove it. Now, the structures at the base of the posterior triangle can be displayed.

Next, the slender **omohyoid muscle** must be examined (*Atlas, 540*). Its inferior (posterior) and superior bellies are separated by an intertendon (*Atlas, 542*). This intertendon is held down to the clavicle by a fibrous expansion. Note this fibrous band (omohyoid fascia) deep to the clavicular attachment of the sternomastoid. Remove the omohyoid fascia, thereby exposing the blood vessels at the base of the posterior triangle.

Blood Vessels (*Atlas, 474, 475*). Follow the **external jugular vein** through the omohyoid fascia to the subclavian vein. Note the **suprascapular vein** which runs posterior to the clavicle. Note the **transverse cervical artery** (transversa colli a.) running about 2 to 3 cm above the clavicle and deep to the omohyoid (*Atlas, 475*). This artery heads toward the levator scapulae. The **suprascapular artery** takes a retroclavicular course to reach the suprascapular notch. Review the origin and destination of the two arteries (*Atlas, 25.1*). Recall their importance in the collateral circulation around the scapula (*Upper Extremity,* fig. 7-4). Note that both arteries pass anterior to the scalenus anterior. Variations in the origin of the transverse cervical and suprascapular arteries are common. In over 50% of the cases, one of the arteries does not arise from the thyrocervical trunk (examples: *Atlas, 532, 536, 567*).

Structures Deep to Floor of Triangle

Now, after securing the contents of the posterior triangle, the **fascial floor** of the triangle (fascial carpet) can be removed (*Atlas, 473, 474*). Expose the underlying muscles: **Splenius capitis, levator scapulae,** and the three scaleni, **scalenus posterior, scalenus medius,** and **scalenus anterior.**

Define the **scalenus anterior** and the **scalenus medius.** Clean the area. Observe the following (*Atlas, 475*):

1. The two muscles are inserted into **rib 1.**
2. An elongated triangular space is formed by the two muscles and rib 1. This is the **interscalene triangle.** Through this interval pass two important structures: **Subclavian artery** and **brachial plexus.**
3. The **subclavian vein** passes in front of the scalenus anterior.
4. The **transverse cervical artery** and **supra-**

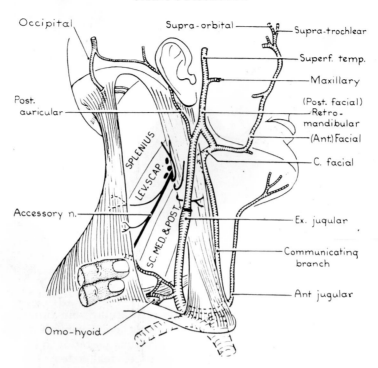

Occipital · Supra-orbital · Supra-trochlear · Superf. temp. · Maxillary · Post. auricular · (Post. facial) Retro-mandibular · (Ant.) Facial · C. facial · Accessory n. · SPLENIUS · LEV. SCAP. · S.C. MED. & POST. · Ex. jugular · Communicating branch · Ant jugular · Omo-hyoid

FIG. 8-29. Posterior triangle of neck. Superficial veins and nerve XI.

scapular artery commonly cross in front of the scalenus anterior.

5. The **phrenic nerve** ($C_{3, 4, 5}$) descends vertically across the surface of the scalenus anterior toward the thorax. The nerve is intimately applied to the muscle; therefore, nerve and muscle are crossed anteriorly by the three vessels: transverse cervical artery, suprascapular artery, and subclavian vein.

6. The scalenus medius is pierced by motor nerves to the rhomboids (C_5) and to the serratus anterior ($C_{5, 6}$).

If not already done, clean the **axillary artery** and the **brachial plexus** at the level of the scaleni. Review the brachial plexus, its rami, trunks, and divisions (*Atlas, 476*).

The **interscalene triangle** becomes of clinical significance when it is too narrow and, therefore, compresses the structures passing through it. Anatomical variations such as additional muscular slips, an accessory cervical rib, or exostosis on the first rib may narrow the available interval. As a result, the subclavian artery and/or the brachial plexus may be compressed. This compression may lead to ischemia and to disturbances in nerve function in the upper extremity.

The supraclavicular nerves and the phrenic nerve have essentially the same segmental origin: $C_{3, 4}$. This fact explains the phenomenon of 'referred pain' in pleurisy. Irritation of the phrenic nerve in the diaphragmatic region may produce pain sensations in the cutaneous area supplied by the supraclavicular nerves (shoulder; clavicular region).

Anterior Triangle of Neck

General Remarks

The **boundaries** of the **anterior triangle** of the neck are (*Atlas, 540*):

1. Anteriorly, the median line of the neck.
2. Posteriorly, the anterior border of the sternomastoid.
3. Superiorly, the lower border of the mandible.

The anterior triangle is further subdivided into smaller triangles: *muscular, carotid, submandibular,* and *submental.*

Study a cross section through the neck (*Atlas, 535*). The anterior part of the neck may be regarded as a **'cervical cavity'** It is bounded by walls:

1. Posteriorly, the cervical vertebrae.
2. Posterolaterally, the scaleni.
3. Laterally, the sternomastoid.
4. Anteriorly, the strap-like infrahyoid muscles.

The 'cervical cavity' houses the **cervical viscera,** which lie in the median plane (*Atlas, 535*):

1. Upper part of digestive tract: **Pharynx** and **esophagus.**
2. Upper part of respiratory tract: **Larynx** and **trachea.**
3. **Thyroid gland,** in front of the tube-like digestive and respiratory tracts.

The big vessels and nerves lie to each side of the cervical viscera. Three major structures, **carotid ar-**

tery, **internal jugular vein, and vagus nerve,** are wrapped together in the fascial **carotid sheath.**

Arterial Supply (*Atlas, 505.2*). The **common carotid** artery bifurcates into the internal and external carotid arteries. The **external carotid artery** supplies almost all structures of the head and neck outside the cranial cavity. The **internal carotid artery** supplies the structures within the cranial and orbital cavities. The **vertebral arteries,** which ascend in the neck through the foramina transversaria, enter the cranial cavity through the foramen magnum to contribute to the cerebral arterial circle. A branch of the subclavian artery, the **thyrocervical trunk,** supplies the lower part of the neck.

Exposure of Anterior Triangle

Make a skin incision in the midline from the tip of the chin to the suprasternal notch. Remove entirely the skin from the front of the neck.

Once again, observe the fibers of the **platysma** (*Atlas, 526*). Reflect and remove it. Review the cutaneous nerve to the region of the anterior triangle, the **transverse cervical nerve** (*Atlas, 472*).

Superficial Veins (fig. 8–29 or *Atlas, 543*). *Expect to find variations* in the venous pattern. Review the course of the **external jugular vein.** Trace the **facial vein** along the lower border of the mandible to a point where it joins the **retromandibular vein.** Retromandibular and facial vein unite to form the **common facial vein.** This vein drains into the internal jugular vein deep to the sternomastoid. Following the common facial vein for a short distance. If present, find the small *anterior jugular vein.* On occasion, this vein is connected to the common facial vein by a *communicating branch.* Clean the deep fascia within the confines of the anterior triangle.

Study bony and cartilaginous **landmarks** which will be used as reference structures (*Atlas, 621–623*):

1. **Hyoid bone,** at the angle between floor of mouth and upper end of neck. Palpate your own hyoid bone. Distinguish *body, greater horn,* and *lesser horn.*
2. **Thyroid cartilage,** the large cartilage of the larynx. In the midline, note and palpate the **laryngeal prominence** (Adam's apple).
3. **Thyrohyoid membrane,** stretching between thyroid cartilage and hyoid bone.
4. **Cricoid cartilage,** inferior to thyroid cartilage and superior to the first tracheal ring. It lies at the level of C_6.
5. **Cricothyroid membrane,** stretching between cricoid and thyroid cartilages. The **cricothyroid muscles** unite the two cartilages more laterally.
6. **Trachea.** Note its upper three rings.

Muscular Triangle

The **muscular triangle** is separated from the carotid triangle by the superior belly of the omohyoid (*Atlas, 540*). On each side of the median line are four ribbon-like muscles which descend from the hyoid bone or the thyroid cartilage. These are the **infrahyoid muscles** (fig. 8–30; *Atlas, 527*). Their names are descriptive of their attachments. In a *superficial plane,* identify the superior belly of the **omohyoid** and the **sternohyoid.** *Deep* to these two muscles are the **sternothyroid** and the short **thyrohyoid.** The muscles are supplied by nerve branches from C_{1-3} via the **ansa cervicalis** (*Atlas, 662*). These nerves to the infrahyoid muscles will be identified later (p. 138).

Widen the gap in the midline between the right and left infrahyoids by gently pulling the muscles laterally. Now, palpate and identify (*Atlas, 528*): **Laryngeal prominence, cricoid cartilage, cricothyroid membrane, first tracheal ring,** and **isthmus of thyroid gland.**

Tracheotomy (tracheostomy), the formation of an opening into the trachea. As an emergency operation, it must be rapidly performed in cases with sudden obstruction of the vital airways (aspiration of foreign body; edema of larynx; paralysis of vocal cords). A superior (high) tracheotomy is performed above the level of the isthmus of the thyroid gland. An inferior (low) tracheotomy is done below the isthmus.

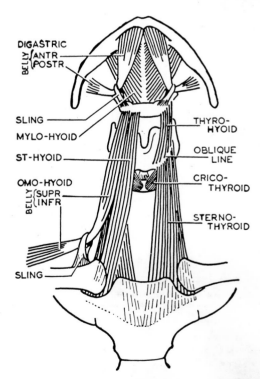

FIG. 8-30. The muscles bounding the median line of the neck. Diagram of infrahyoid muscles. (From *Grant's Method of Anatomy.*)

The simplest and most rapid tracheotomy may be performed by opening the cricothyroid membrane. Perform this important emergency procedure in the cadaver. Palpate the thyroid and cricoid cartilages and the membrane stretching between them. Then, incise the membrane transversely.

Carotid Triangle

The **carotid triangle** is bounded by the superior belly of the omohyoid, the posterior belly of the digastric, and the anterior border of the sternomastoid. The **common carotid artery** ascends through the triangle, and its pulse can be palpated and auscultated within the boundaries of this triangular space.

Nerves in the Carotid Triangle (*Atlas,* *540.2–543.1*). The first objective is to find the **accessory nerve (XI)** as it enters the sternomastoid muscle. Transect the sternomastoid muscle about 5 cm above its insertion into sternum and clavicle. Using the scissor technique, free and clean the upper portion of the sternomastoid from its surrounding fascia. Do not damage the nerves which radiate from the posterior border of the muscle into the posterior triangle. Note the arterial branches which enter the muscle; then cut them. Find the **accessory nerve** where it enters the *deep surface* of the sternomastoid: About 5 cm inferior to the tip of the mastoid process, and about 2 cm behind the anterior border of the muscle (*Atlas,* *542*). Trace the accessory nerve upward as far as possible. The nerve may cross the internal jugular vein anteriorly or posteriorly. Nerve and vein pass through the same opening, the jugular foramen. Review nerve XI (*Atlas,* *661*).

To allow better access to deeper structures, cut the **common facial vein** where it empties into the internal jugular vein.

The **tip of the greater horn of the hyoid bone** is an important reference point for many structures. The greater horn on one side is palpable only when the greater horn of the opposite side is steadied. Palpate the greater horn on the side of the dissection with one index finger, while you press against the greater horn of the opposite side with your other index finger (fig. 8–31).

The next objective is to find the **hypoglossal nerve (XII).** It is the motor nerve to the tongue; therefore, it courses forward. Once again, palpate and locate the **tip of the greater horn** of the hyoid bone. Then, pick up the large, flat hypoglossal nerve just above the tip (fig. 8–32 or *Atlas,* *541.1, 542*). At this point, the nerve gives off the **nerve to the thyrohyoid.** Follow this slender branch across the tip of the greater horn to the lateral border of the thyrohyoid muscle.

Trace the **hypoglossal nerve** forward to where it disappears under the posterior belly of the digastric (fig. 8–33 or *Atlas,* *540.2*). Then, trace the hypoglossal nerve backward to where it appears from under cover of the posterior belly of the digastric. Here, the

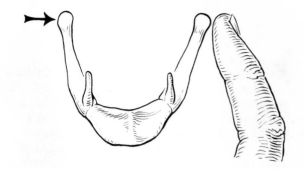

FIG. 8-31. Steady the tip of one horn while palpating the other.

sternomastoid branch of the occipital artery hooks over the nerve. At this point, find the *superior root* of the ansa cervicalis which is closely adherent to nerve XII (fig. 8–32 or *Atlas,* *541.1; Atlas,* *542*). Study the components of the **ansa cervicalis** (*Atlas,* *662*). The superior root (descendens hypoglossi) is composed of fibers from $C_1(+C_2)$. It joins the inferior root of the ansa (descendens cervicalis; $C_{2,3}$) to form the loop or ansa. Dissect the ansa. Trace nerve branches from it to the **infrahyoid muscles** (*Atlas,* *542*).

The next objective is to find the **vagus (X)** and one of its branches. The vagus lies in the carotid sheath, in the posterior angle between internal jugular vein and the great arterial trunk. Pull the internal jugular vein and nerve XI laterally, and pull the carotid arteries and nerve XII medially. This will expose the vagus (fig. 8–33). Using the scissor technique, trace the vagus downward.

Now, find the **superior laryngeal nerve** and its major branch, the **internal laryngeal nerve** (fig. 8–34 or *Atlas,* *543.1*). Proceed as follows: Relax the structures by bending the head forward. With scissors, sever the omohyoid and the sternohyoid close to the hyoid bone. Reflect the muscles downward. Next, carefully sever the exposed thyrohyoid muscle close to the hyoid bone; reflect it downward. Now, the **thyrohyoid membrane** lies exposed. The substantial **internal laryngeal nerve** pierces it to supply the upper portion of the larynx with sensory fibers. Once again, palpate the tip of the greater horn of the hyoid bone. Find the nerve just inferior to it.

If time permits, find the **external laryngeal nerve** which supplies the cricothyroid muscle and the adjacent part of the inferior constrictor (fig. 8–34 or *Atlas,* *543.1*). Proceed as follows: Trace the internal laryngeal nerve proximally to a point where it is crossed by the internal carotid artery. Here, find the external laryngeal nerve. Trace the delicate nerve inferiorly. Carefully sever the sternothyroid muscle from the oblique line of the thyroid cartilage. Raise the muscle. Find the external laryngeal nerve deep to it. Trace the nerve to the cricothyroid muscle.

Arteries in the Carotid Triangle (fig. 8–35 or *Atlas,* *543.2*). The arteries in this triangle are: (1) Parts of the common, internal, and external carotid arteries; and (2) the stems of most of the six collateral

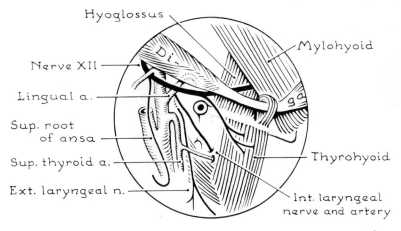

FIG. 8-32. The tip of the greater horn is the reference point for many structures: nerves, arteries, and muscles.

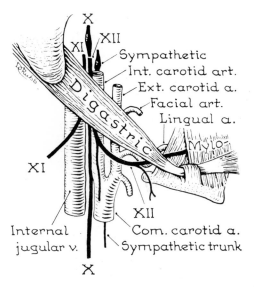

FIG. 8-33. Posterior belly of digastric, and the structures deep to it.

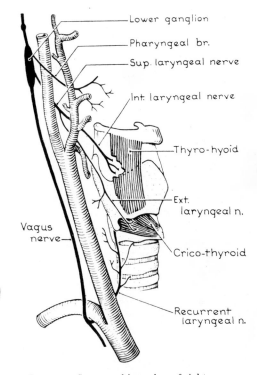

FIG. 8-34. Laryngeal branches of right vagus.

branches of the external carotid artery.

Remove the **carotid sheath** as the dissection proceeds. Note: The **common carotid artery** and the **internal carotid artery** lie in medial contact with the internal jugular vein. These arteries have *no collateral branches* in the neck. The **external carotid artery,** which lies anteromedial to the internal carotid artery, gives off several branches before reaching the posterior belly of the digastric. Identify these branches (fig. 8–35):

1. **Superior thyroid artery.** Identify its origin just inferior and posterior to the tip of the greater horn of the hyoid bone (compare fig. 8–32). The artery descends to the upper pole of the thyroid gland. Identify one of its branches, the **superior laryngeal artery.** This artery pierces the thyrohyoid membrane together with the internal laryngeal nerve.

2. **Lingual artery.** Identify its origin just posterior

to the tip of the greater horn of the hyoid bone (compare fig. 8–32).

3. **Facial artery,** arising just superior to the lingual artery. In 20% of all cases, the lingual and facial arteries have a common stem. Expect to find variations (*Atlas, 566.1*).

4. **Occipital artery.** It gives off a muscular branch to the sternomastoid muscle.

5. *Ascending pharyngeal artery.* Usually, it is the first branch to arise from the external carotid artery close to the bifurcation. It is often difficult to find.

Clean the **bifurcation** of the common carotid artery. Notice the dilation of the upper end of the

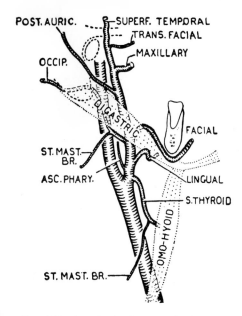

FIG. 8-35. Arteries in the carotid triangle.

common carotid and the beginning of the internal carotid. Here, the walls of the artery are thinner, less muscular, and more elastic. This dilated region is the **carotid sinus.** The wall of this sinus contains pressoreceptors which respond to changes in blood pressure.

If time permits, look for the carotid body (*Atlas, 659.1*). It is a small mass of tissue, darker and more firm than fat, and located on the medial aspect in the crotch of the bifurcation. The carotid body responds to changes in the chemical composition of the blood. Cranial nerves IX and X supply the carotid body and sinus.

Veins in the Anterior Triangle (*Atlas, 543.3*). Briefly identify the following tributaries to the **internal jugular vein: Common facial vein, lingual vein,** and **superior thyroid vein** which accompanies the respective artery. To clarify the dissection field, remove the tributaries of the internal jugular vein.

Submandibular Triangle

The **submandibular or digastric triangle** is bounded by (*Atlas, 540*):
1. Inferior border of mandible.
2. Anterior belly of digastric.
3. Posterior belly of digastric.
In the skull, identify the following relevant **landmarks:**
1. On the temporal bone examine (*Atlas, 461*): **Mastoid process** and **styloid process.** In many skulls, the long and sharp styloid process is broken off.
2. Examine the inner aspect of a **mandible** (Atlas, 553.1) and identify: **Digastric fossa** for the

attachment of the anterior belly of the digastric; **mylohyoid line,** for the attachment of the mylohyoid; **submandibular fossa,** inferior to the mylohyoid line; **mylohyoid groove,** in which the nerves and vessels to the mylohyoid and the anterior belly of the digastric run.

Part of the submandibular salivary gland and some lymph nodes fill the submandibular triangle (*Atlas, 541*). The **submandibular gland** is wrapped around the free posterior border of the mylohyoid like the letter U on its side, thus ⊏ The deep part of the gland and its duct (*Atlas, 597*) must not be disturbed. The superficial part of the gland, lying within the boundaries of the submandibular triangle, may be severed and removed. Proceed as follows: Clamp a hemostat or a forceps to the gland. Pull the gland medially. Using the scissor technique, free the superficial part of the gland from its surrounding fascia. Separate the **facial artery and vein** from the gland. Note blood vessels supplying the glandular tissue. Now, cut through the gland at the posterior border of the mylohyoid, and remove it.

Now, the **anterior and posterior bellies of the digastric** can be well defined. Note that the two bellies are connected to each other by an **intermediate tendon** (fig. 8-36; *Atlas, 541.1, 542*). This tendon is held to the body and the greater horn of the hyoid bone by a fibrous sling. Note that the intermediate tendon perforates a slender, round muscle, the **stylohyoid.** Verify that the posterior belly of the digastric arises from the medial aspect of the mastoid process. The anterior belly arises from the digastric fossa of the mandible.

Trace the **hypoglossal nerve (XII)** into the submandibular triangle (*Atlas, 542, 546*). Observe that the nerve disappears under cover of the mylohyoid muscle.

Pull the anterior belly of the digastric medially to expose the **mylohyoid nerve,** a branch of V³. Observe that the nerve is sheltered by the lower border of the mandible. Its more distal portion is closely applied to

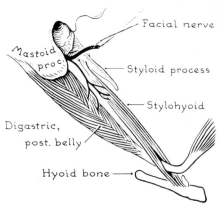

FIG. 8-36. Stylohyoid muscle perforated by intermediate tendon of digastric.

the mylohyoid. A branch reaches the anterior belly of the digastric (the posterior belly of the digastric and the stylohyoid are supplied by a branch of VII; *Atlas, 552, 657*).

Submental Triangle

The boundaries of the submental (suprahyoid) triangle are (fig. 8–30 or *Atlas, 527.1; Atlas, 540*):
1. Inferiorly, the body of the hyoid bone.
2. Laterally, the right and left anterior bellies of the digastric muscles.

The floor of the triangle is formed by the two **mylohyoid muscles.** These muscles arise from the mandible and are inserted into the body of the hyoid bone. The fibers of the right and left muscles meet in a median fibrous raphe (cf. bulbospongiosus, *Atlas, 192*).

If not already done, clean the anterior bellies of the digastrics. Occasionally, these anterior bellies are fused and, therefore, may hide the underlying mylohyoid muscle. If this is the case, separate the digastrics from each other and expose the floor of the submental triangle.

Cervical Viscera

The upper parts of the digestive tract (pharynx and esophagus) and the respiratory tract (larynx and trachea) will be dealt with in special assignments (p. 151; p. 161). The thyroid gland can be conveniently explored at this time.

Thyroid Gland (fig. 8–37 or *Atlas, 529.1*). The infrahyoid muscles and the sternomastoid were reflected earlier. Therefore, the thyroid gland lies exposed. Verify that it extends between the carotid sheaths of the two sides (*Atlas, 530.1*). Identify the **right and left lobes.** The two lobes are connected by the **isthmus,** which usually covers the 2nd to 4th tracheal rings. In 50% of all cases, the gland has a **pyramidal lobe** which ascends from the isthmus upward, sometimes as high as the hyoid bone. Expect to find variations (*Atlas, 539*).

Being an endocrine organ, the thyroid gland has a rich blood supply and drainage. Once again, identify the **superior thyroid artery.** Demonstrate the three veins which drain the thyroid gland: **Superior, middle,** and **inferior thyroid veins** (*Atlas, 529*). To find the **inferior thyroid artery,** on the respective side, pull the lobe of the thyroid gland forward. See the origin of the artery from the thyrocervical trunk (*Atlas, 531, 536*).

Cut the isthmus of the gland, and turn the lobes laterally. Define and then sever the fascial band

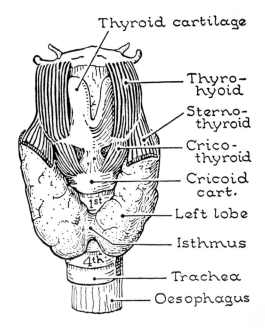

FIG. 8-37. The thyroid gland, front view. (From *Grant's Method of Anatomy.*)

which attaches the capsule of the gland to the first tracheal ring (*Atlas, 530*). With a probe, display the **recurrent laryngeal nerve** which ascends just posterior to the gland on the side of the trachea (*Atlas, 534*).

On the left side only, cut all blood vessels leading to or from the left lobe of the thyroid gland. Then, enucleate this lobe. Cut into the substance of the gland, and observe its characteristic colloid structure. Preserve the posterior aspect of the lobe, where the parathyroid glands may be found.

Parathyroid Glands (*Atlas, 534, 626*). These small but vital glands lie along the posterior border of the thyroid gland between its capsule and its sheath. On the posterior aspect of the removed thyroid lobe, look for small brownish bodies, measuring about 5 mm in diameter. Usually, there are two parathyroid glands on each side. However, the total number may vary from 2 to 6.

Physicians must be fully aware of the close relationship between thyroid gland, parathyroids, and the recurrent laryngeal nerves. If, during thyroidectomy (removal of thyroid gland), one or both recurrent laryngeal nerves are injured, paralysis of the laryngeal muscles will occur. Note how intimately the recurrent laryngeal nerve is related to the thyroid gland (*Atlas, 534, 626*). Understand that a malignant tumor of the thyroid may easily lead to destruction of the recurrent laryngeal nerve or nerves.

The parathyroids play a vital role in the regulation of calcium and phosphorus metabolism. During thyroidectomy, these small endocrine glands are in danger of being damaged or of being removed. Appreciate this fact by studying the close relations between thyroid and parathyroid glands (*Atlas, 626*).

Root of the Neck

The sternomastoid, sternohyoid, sternothyroid, and the superior belly of the omohyoid were reflected earlier. If not already done, remove the fascia (loop) that binds the intermediate tendon of the omohyoid to the clavicle (*Atlas, 527.1*). Now, the root of the neck lies exposed, particularly on the left side, where the left lobe of the thyroid gland was resected (*Atlas, 536*).

To clarify the dissection field, cut the **common carotid artery** and the **internal jugular vein** (but not the vagus) about 2 cm above the clavicular level. Reflect the large vessels upward. Fix them in the reflected position with needles or a hemostat.

The next objective is to find the **thoracic duct.** The duct opens at (or near) the angle between the **left subclavian vein** and the **left internal jugular vein** (*Atlas, 533, 534*). The duct has approximately the same diameter as the superior thyroid vein. Usually, it is pale, collapsed, inconspicuous, and very easily torn.

To find the **thoracic duct,** proceed as follows (fig. 8–38 or *Atlas, 536 B*): Pull the lower portions of the severed common carotid artery and internal jugular vein forward. Now, the duct lies exposed as it arches from the side of the esophagus laterally to the angle between internal jugular and subclavian veins. To clarify the dissection field, remove the vertebral vein. Usually, this vein descends posterior to the thoracic duct to empty dorsally into the brachiocephalic vein (*Atlas, 536*).

Realize that delicate **lymphatic trunks** empty into the *right* subclavian and jugular veins (*Atlas, 453*). You are not required to search for these lymph vessels.

Clean the vagus and the phrenic nerve, and follow

these structures into the thorax. Once again, note that the **phrenic nerve** is intimately applied to the ventral surface of the scalenus anterior. The **transverse cervical and suprascapular arteries** pass directly anterior to the nerve and muscle (*Atlas, 531, 536*). Trace these two arteries back to their origin from the **thyrocervical trunk.** This arterial trunk arises near the medial border of the scalenus anterior. Identify a third branch of the thyrocervical trunk, the **inferior thyroid artery.** It passes posterior to the carotid sheath to enter the inferior pole of the thyroid gland. Expect to find variations: Often, the thyrocervical trunk does not give rise to all three arteries. On occasion, the arteries arise separately from the subclavian artery.

Opposite the thyrocervical trunk notice the origin of the **internal thoracic artery** (fig. 8–39 or *Atlas, 536 A*).

The next objective is to find and partially trace the **vertebral artery.** It is the first and largest branch of the subclavian artery (fig. 8–39 or *Atlas, 536 A*). Identify this deeply running vessel in relation to two muscles: Scalenus anterior and longus colli. These muscles form the two sides of the '*triangle of the vertebral artery.*' The apex of this triangle is the **transverse process of C$_6$.** The anterior tubercle of this transverse process is an important landmark: The common carotid artery passes in front of the tubercle and may be compressed against it ('carotid tubercle'; fig. 8–39). Trace the vertebral artery to the apex of the triangle where it enters the transverse foramen of C$_6$. Review the course of the vertebral artery (*Atlas, 505.2*).

The *sympathetic trunk* and its ganglia may be examined now (*Atlas, 537*). However, these structures can be more conveniently studied in the prevertebral region, after removal of the head (p. 149).

Parotid Region

Bony Landmarks

Refer to a skull and study the following **pertinent landmarks:**

1. On the temporal bone (*Atlas, 461*): **Styloid process, mastoid process, external acoustic meatus,** and **mandibular fossa** for the head of the mandible.
2. On the **mandible** (*Atlas, 461, 462*): **Head, neck,** and posterior border of **ramus.**
3. On the exterior of the base of the skull (*Atlas, 569, 570*): **Stylomastoid foramen,** located between the base of the styloid process and the mastoid process. The important facial nerve (VII) passes through this foramen.

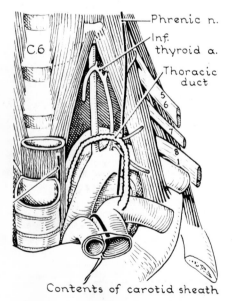

FIG. 8-38. To display the thoracic duct in the neck.

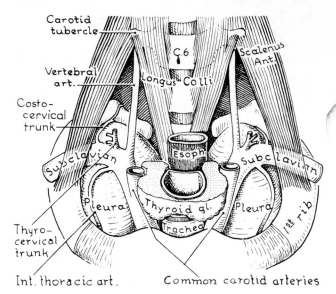

FIG. 8-39. Root of the neck: Triangle of vertebral artery, and branches of the subclavian artery.

General Remarks

The parotid region is a restricted space occupied by the parotid gland and certain soft structures associated with it. Refer to a skull and define the bony space which forms the boundaries for the parotid bed (*Atlas, 461*):

1. Posteriorly, mastoid process.
2. Anteriorly, ramus of mandible.
3. Superiorly, floor of external acoustic meatus.
4. Medially, styloid process.

The posterior wall of the parotid region extends between the mastoid and styloid processes. Therefore, the muscles attached to these processes (sternomastoid; posterior belly of digastric; stylohyoid) are closely related to the gland (fig. 8-40; *Atlas, 550-552*). The anterior wall of the parotid region is formed by the ramus of the mandible and the two muscles (masseter; medial pterygoid) applied to it (fig. 8-40 or *Atlas, 584*).

The parotid gland is traversed by branches of the facial nerve, arteries, and veins. This fact must be appreciated during dissection and during surgery.

Dissection

Observe the superficial extent of the parotid gland and the structures radiating from its margin (*Atlas, 467*): **Parotid duct,** transverse facial artery, and branches of the **facial nerve.** These structures have already been cleaned. Note that the parotid gland is enclosed within fascia, the **parotid sheath.**

The first objective is to find the **stem of the facial nerve** (VII) as it emerges from the stylomastoid foramen (fig. 8-41; *Atlas, 550*). Proceed as follows:

Make sure that the sternomastoid is well cleaned up to the mastoid process. Reflect it. With the handle of the scalpel, ease the parotid sheath and the contained gland forward. Hold it in this position with a hemostat. Again, refer to a skull, and examine how you must aim the handle of the knife in order to reach the stylomastoid foramen. Push the handle upward, anteromedially to the mastoid process, until it catches between mastoid and styloid processes. With a probe, reveal the facial nerve as it leaves the stylomastoid foramen to enter the parotid sheath.

Follow the **temporal branches of the facial nerve** backward. Trace them through the glandular tissue (*Atlas, 550*). You may find two large communications with the **auriculotemporal nerve** (V^3), which carry secretory fibers to the parotid gland. Using blunt dissection, shell the gland out of its fascial bed. Follow facial nerve branches deep through the substance of the gland. Trace the auriculotemporal nerve toward the neck of the mandible. The nerve runs medial and deep to the parotid gland (*Atlas, 552*).

The next objective is to identify the vessels which traverse the tissue of the parotid gland. Using the scissor technique, establish the course of the **retromandibular vein** (fig. 8-41; *Atlas, 550*). Next, trace the **external carotid artery** through the gland. The artery is deeply placed and sheltered by the ramus of the mandible (*Atlas, 552*). Posterior to the neck of the mandible, the external carotid artery divides into its

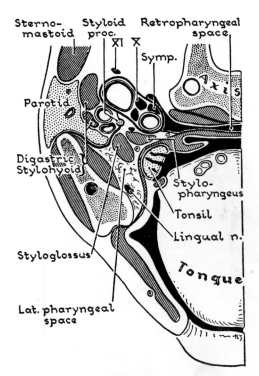

FIG. 8-40. Cross section of the head, at the level of the parotid gland. (From *Grant's Method of Anatomy*.)

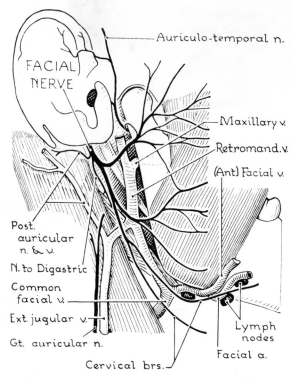

FIG. 8-41. Facial nerve and veins in the parotid bed.

two terminal branches: **Maxillary artery** and **superficial temporal artery** (*Atlas, 543.2, 556*).

Cut the parotid duct close to the gland. Pull the gland backward and downward. Sever the facial nerve about 2 to 3 cm distal to the stylomastoid foramen. Remove the parotid gland.

Now, examine the **parotid bed** (*Atlas, 552*). Identify the **posterior belly of the digastric** and the **stylohyoid.** Palpate the styloid process. Clean the auriculotemporal nerve posterior to the temporomandibular joint. Mark the severed facial nerve by tying a piece of thread to it.

Appreciate the close relationship between external ear canal and parotid gland [Parotid: Gk., para = near; otos = ear]: A painful swelling of the parotid gland (mumps) characteristically pushes the ear lobe upward and outward.

During parotidectomy (surgical excision of parotid gland), the facial nerve is in constant danger. In cases of benign parotid tumors, the stem of the facial nerve may be isolated at the stylomastoid foramen, and the facial nerve branches may remain intact during removal of lobules of parotid tissue. In malignant tumors, the facial nerve must be sacrificed. What will happen if the orbicularis oculi is paralyzed?

Temporal and Masseteric Regions

Bony Landmarks

Refer to a skull and study the following pertinent landmarks (*Atlas, 461, 462*):

1. **Temporal lines,** curving backward from the frontal process of the zygomatic bone, and indicating the margin of origin of the temporalis muscle. The temporal lines surround the **temporal fossa.** Note that this fossa is formed by several bony components: *Parietal* bone, *frontal* bone, squamous part of *temporal* bone, and greater wing of *sphenoid* bone.
2. **Zygomatic arch,** composed of the *zygoma* of the temporal bone and the *zygomatic process* of the zygomatic bone.
3. **Mandible** (*Atlas, 462, 553*). Identify: **Ramus, angle,** and **mandibular notch** which is located between **coronoid process** and head of mandible.

Dissection

Remove the remains of the masseteric fascia and clean the **masseter** (*Atlas, 465*). Detach the posterior third of the muscle from the zygomatic arch. Turn the detached portion of the masseter forward to display the **masseteric nerve and vessels** passing through the mandibular notch.

Next, the masseter must be reflected downward together with its bone of origin. Proceed as follows (fig. 8-42); Pass a probe or closed forceps deep to the zygomatic arch to protect the underlying soft structures. Saw obliquely through the zygomatic bone as far forward as possible. Then, saw through the zygoma as far backward as possible. Turn down the section of the zygomatic arch together with the attached masseter muscle. During this process, the nerve and vessels to the masseter will be torn. With the handle of a scalpel, detach the muscle fibers of the deep portion of the masseter from the superior portion of the ramus and from the lateral surface of the coronoid process. Detach the superficial portion of the muscle from the ramus of the mandible. Leave the masseter attached to the lower margin of the mandible (Atlas, 551).

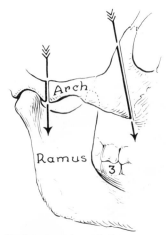

FIG. 8-42. Saw cuts through the zygomatic arch.

Now, the **temporal fascia** is fully exposed. Review its attachment to the temporal line (it cannot be fully traced where the calvaria has been removed). Make a deep vertical cut through the fascia and evert it (*Atlas*, 465). Observe:

1. Muscle fibers of the temporalis partly arise from the fascia.
2. The temporalis inserts into the coronoid process of the mandible (*Atlas*, 551).
3. The anterior portion of the temporalis is thick. Its fibers take a vertical direction (jaw closure). The fibers of the smaller posterior portion take a backward sweep from the coronoid process.

The temporal fascia splits to enclose a small fat pad between the temporalis and the lateral wall of the orbit. Notice that this fatty tissue is continuous with the buccal fat pad on the buccinator (*Atlas*, 470). Remove the fat. Realize: In the emaciated person, the loss of the continuous fat pads is responsible for the sunken cheeks and temples.

Infratemporal Region

General Remarks and Bony Landmarks

The infratemporal fossa contains two muscles of mastication, the mandibular nerve (V³), and the maxillary vessels. The fossa lies deep; its lateral wall is the ramus of the mandible. Therefore, access to the infratemporal fossa will necessitate partial removal of the ramus.

Profitable dissection of this region requires a thorough knowledge of the **pertinent bony features.** Refer to a skull and identify:

1. On the inner aspect of the **mandible** (*Atlas*, 553.1):
   a. **Coronoid process.**
   b. **Lingula** for the attachment of the sphenomandibular ligament.
   c. **Mandibular foramen,** for the transmission of the inferior alveolar nerves and vessels.
   d. **Mylohyoid groove,** for the nerve and vessels to the mylohyoid and anterior belly of the digastric.
2. Remove the mandible from the bony skull, thus gaining access to the bony landmarks of the infratemporal fossa. View this area inferolaterally (*Atlas*, 558) or from the base of the skull (*Atlas*, 569). Identify:
   a. **Lateral pterygoid plate** of sphenoid bone
   b. **Infratemporal** (posterior) **surface of maxilla**
   c. **Pterygopalatine fossa,** a wedge-shaped cleft which transmits blood vessels.
   d. **Greater wing of the sphenoid,** with two

important foramina: **Foramen ovale** and **foramen spinosum.**

Now, identify the **walls of the infratemporal fossa** (*Atlas*, 557, 558):

1. *Laterally,* the ramus of the mandible.
2. *Anteriorly,* the posterior aspect of the maxilla. It is limited above by the inferior orbital fissure, medially by the pterygopalatine fossa.
3. The *medial wall* is the lateral plate of the pterygoid process.
4. The *roof* of the infratemporal fossa is flat and formed by the greater wing of the sphenoid. The large foramen ovale transmits nerve V³. The foramen spinosum is traversed by the middle meningeal vessels. The sphenomandibular ligament is attached near the spine of the sphenoid.

Dissection

First Saw Cut (fig. 8-43). To detach the coronoid process, proceed as follows: Pass a probe or the blade of a forceps (*arrow* in fig. 8-43) through the mandibular notch. Push the instrument obliquely downward and forward, in contact with the mandible. Now, the soft structures deep to the coronoid process are protected from the saw blade. Cut obliquely through the **coronoid process.** Reflect it, together with the insertion of the **temporalis muscle.**

Raise the anterior and posterior borders of the temporalis until the nerves to the muscle are seen lying on the bone. These nerves are accompanied by deep temporal arteries (*Atlas*, 559). Now, remove the temporalis muscle entirely and discard it.

Second Saw Cut (fig. 8-43). The objective of this procedure is to remove the superior part of the ramus of the mandible. However, the nerves and vessels just medial to the mandibular ramus must not be damaged. Proceed as follows: With a pencil, mark the approximate position of the **lingula** (center of ramus) on the lateral surface of the ramus. Below this pencil mark, the inferior alveolar nerve and vessels enter the

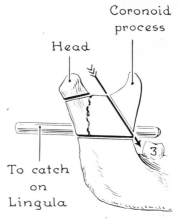

Fig. 8-43. Saw cuts through mandible.

mandible on its medial aspect (*Atlas, 559*). In order *not* to damage the inferior alveolar structures, the saw cut across the mandible must be made *above* the pencil mark. Pass the blade of an open forceps medial to the neck of the mandible. Keep in close contact with the bone. Work the instrument downward until it is arrested by the lingula. Carefully make the prescribed saw cut, but do not cut through the entire thickness of the mandible. With bone pliers, nibble away the remainder of the ramus. Guard your eyes against flying bone fragments.

Third Saw Cut (fig. 8-43). Cut through the neck of the mandible, just inferior to the **temporomandibular joint.** During the sawing procedure, protect the underlying soft structures with a probe or forceps.

Now, the **contents of the infratemporal fossa** lie exposed (*Atlas, 559*). Identify the **inferior alveolar nerve and artery** (the structures may be obscured by mandibular periosteum inadvertently left behind during bone removal). Trace the nerve downward: it enters the mandibular foramen. Trace the nerve upward: it leads to the lower border of the lateral pterygoid.

If time permits, follow the inferior alveolar nerve and vessels into the (bony) mandibular canal. With small bone pliers (or with a dental drill), open the canal. Note branches of the nerve and arteries to the teeth (*Atlas, 654*). Finally, follow the distal portion of the inferior alveolar nerve through the mental foramen into the region of the chin and lower lip.

Mandibular block: Local anesthesia applied to the inferior alveolar nerve at the level of the mandibular foramen. Understand from your dissection that this block will not only anesthetize the mandibular teeth on the corresponding side, but also the lower lip and the chin below it.

Pick up the **lingual nerve** which is closely applied to the ramus of the mandible (*Atlas, 559*). This large nerve runs in front of the inferior alveolar nerve. Trace it to the lower border of the lateral pterygoid, from where it emerges. Posterior to the inferior alveolar nerve is the delicate **mylohyoid nerve.**

Maxillary Artery (fig. 8-44 or *Atlas, 556*). Trace the artery through the infratemporal region. In most cases, it crosses superficial to the lateral pterygoid. However, in approximately one-third of all cases, it passes deep to the muscle (*Atlas, 559, 560*).

To obtain a complete and extensive view of the infratemporal region, the **lateral pterygoid muscle** must be removed. Notice that the muscle has two heads: One arises from the roof of the fossa; the other from the lateral pterygoid plate. With the handle of the scalpel, free the upper border of the lateral pterygoid from the roof. Next, define the lower border of the muscle by inserting the handle into the interval between lateral and medial pterygoids. This interval is marked by the lingual and inferior alveolar nerves. Work the handle anteriorly and upward, and free the muscle from the lateral pterygoid plate. Finally, sever

the muscle close to its pointed insertion into the neck of the mandible and into the articular disc (*Atlas, 555*). Remove the muscle completely. Do so in a piecemeal fashion to preserve superficially positioned nerves and vessels.

Now, the nerves and vessels in the infratemporal fossa can be examined in detail (*Atlas, 560*):
1. Identify the delicate **chorda tympani.** It joins the lingual nerve from behind.
2. Follow the **inferior alveolar and lingual nerves** to the foramen ovale in the roof of the fossa.
3. Push a thin probe through the **foramen ovale.** Locate the tip of the probe in the middle cranial fossa.
4. Identify and clean the **buccal nerve.** Its branches pierce the buccinator to supply the buccal mucosa with sensory fibers.
5. Once again, identify the **auriculotemporal nerve.** Follow it to the foramen ovale.
6. Clean the **maxillary artery.** Identify two branches which pass through bony foramina: **Inferior alveolar artery,** and **middle meningeal artery** traversing the foramen spinosum. Stick a needle through the **foramen spinosum.** Find the needle tip in the middle cranial fossa.
7. Notice **muscular branches** to the muscles of mastication. Most of these branches are torn or cut by now.
8. Within the pterygopalatine fossa, the maxillary artery gives off several branches (*Atlas, 559, 560*). Identify the **posterior superior alveolar artery** (fig. 8-44). The *infraorbital artery* and the *greater palatine artery* will be seen later (p. 157).

Review the distribution of the mandibular division of the trigeminal nerve (*Atlas, 654, 655*). Understand the importance of the delicate chorda tympani (*Atlas, 657*).

Temporomandibular Joint

Refer to a skull and examine the following bony landmarks (*Atlas, 555, 569*): **Mandibular fossa, articular tubercle,** and **articular condyle** on the **head** of the mandible.

Although the superior portion of the mandibular ramus has been removed, the head and neck of the mandible are still intact. The capsule of the temporomandibular joint is lax. It is thickened laterally to form the **temporomandibular ligament** (*Atlas, 551*).

Enter the point of the scalpel into the mandibular fossa close to the bone. Open freely the upper cavity of the joint (*Atlas, 555*). *Remove the articular disc* together with the head of the mandible.

In the isolated specimen (head and neck of mandible with articular disc) study the following:
1. The insertion of the severed lateral pterygoid.

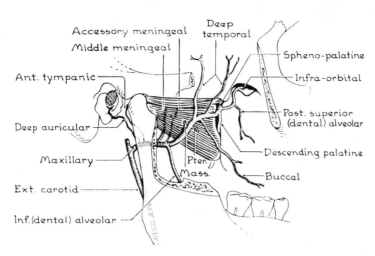

Accessory meningeal
Middle meningeal
Deep temporal
Ant. tympanic
Spheno-palatine
Infra-orbital
Deep auricular
Post. superior (dental) alveolar
Maxillary
Pter. Mass.
Descending palatine
Ext. carotid
Buccal
Inf. (dental) alveolar

Fig. 8-44. Maxillary artery and its branches.

The remains of the muscle are attached to the neck and articular disc.

2. Cut the disc anteroposteriorly, and so open the lower cavity of the joint. Observe the shape and varying thickness of the disc (*Atlas, 555*).

AXIOM: In man, an articular disc implies two types of movements, one on each side of the disc. In the lower cavity, simple hinge movements between head and disc occur. In the upper cavity, the disc and head together glide on the articular tubercle during protraction of the mandible.

Place the little finger in the cartilaginous portion of your own external ear canal. Perform simple hinge movements of the mandible. Then, protract and retract your lower jaw. By finger palpation, study the movements of the head of your mandible.

Craniovertebral Joints and Removal of Head

General Remarks and Orientation

The objective of the next dissection procedure is: The head with the cervical viscera and the major nerves and vessels must be detached from the vertebral column and its associated musculature. This procedure will allow a posterior approach to the cervical viscera. Study a midsagittal section of the head and neck region (*Atlas, 458*) and understand:

1. The logical plane for separation is the **retropharyngeal (retrovisceral) space** which extends from the base of the skull into the upper part of the thorax.

2. The joints between cranium and vertebrae (craniovertebral joints) are the logical site for separation between head and vertebral column. All ligaments holding these joints together must be severed in order to achieve separation.

3. In addition, the muscles connecting the verte-

brae with the base of the skull must be severed (fig. 8-47 or *Atlas, 561*). These muscles are the *rectus capitis lateralis* and *anterior* and the uppermost portion of the *longus capitis.*

Study a cross section of the neck (fig. 8-45; *Atlas, 584*). Identify the **retropharyngeal (retrovisceral) space.** Now, turn to the cadaver. Reflect the two sternomastoids. On both sides at once, insert the fingers of your right and left hands behind the carotid sheaths. Push your fingers medially until they meet posterior to the cervical viscera. Your fingers are now in the retrovisceral space. Work your fingers upward as high as the base of the skull; here is the superior limit of the retropharyngeal space. Work your fingers downward toward the thorax; here, the space ends at the level of T₃ where part of the prevertebral fascia fuses with the buccopharyngeal (visceral) fascia.

Before the head together with the cervical visera can be removed, the craniovertebral joints must be studied and, subsequently, disarticulated. Knowledge of pertinent bony reference points is essential.

Bony Landmarks

Refer to a skeleton (or skull and cervical vertebral column) and identify the following pertinent bony landmarks:

1. **Axis,** C₂ (*Atlas, 367, 368*). Note its **dens or odontoid process** which is in apposition with the anterior arch of the atlas.

2. **Atlas** (*Atlas, 563*). Identify: **Posterior arch; anterior arch** with facet for dens; **transverse process; superior articular facet.** Understand that the dens of the axis is held tight to the anterior arch by the *transverse ligament,* which is bow-shaped and very strong.

3. On the occipital bone identify (*Atlas, 569*): Anterior and lateral margins of **foramen magnum; occipital condyle.** The joint between the

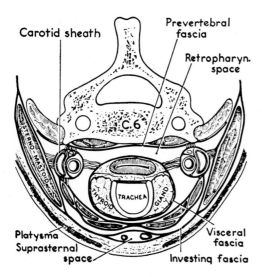

FIG. 8-45. The retropharyngeal (retrovisceral) space. (From *Grant's Method of Anatomy.*)

occipital condyle and the superior articular facet of the atlas is the **atlanto-occipital joint.**

Craniovertebral Joints

Turn the cadaver into the prone position (face down). A large wedge-shaped portion of the occipital bone was removed earlier. If not already done, resect the posterior arch of the atlas. Define the anterior border of the foramen magnum. Note the median knuckle-like eminence produced by the dens of the axis. Palpate the dens while rotating the head to the right and the left.

To expose the underlying ligaments, the dura mater and the membrana tectoria must be reflected (*Atlas, 562*). First, excise the **dura mater** in the following fashion (fig. 8-46; *Atlas, 565*): Make a transverse incision through the dura, about 3 cm inferior to the dorsum sellae. From each end of this incision carry an obliquely vertical cut downward to the point where the vertebral artery pierces the dura. This is just medial to the points of exit of the hypoglossal nerves. With a probe, ease the dura from the underlying membrana tectoria. Turn down the flap of dura as far as possible.

Next, examine the exposed **membrana tectoria.** Cut the membrane transversely above the anterior border of the foramen magnum. With the handle of a scalpel and a probe, raise the membrane and reflect it downward as far as possible. Now, the major ligaments of the craniovertebral region are exposed.

Ligaments of Craniovertebral Region (fig. 8-46; *Atlas, 562, 563, 565*). Identify the **transverse ligament** of the atlas. It holds the dens of the axis firmly to the anterior arch of the atlas. The transverse ligament and the vertically orientated upper and lower bands are collectively known as the *cruciform ligament.*

Next, identify the **alar ligaments or check ligaments.** They extend from the dens to the lateral margins of the foramen magnum. These strong paired ligaments are nearly as thick as a pencil. They *check* the lateral rotation and the side-to-side movements of the head. Observe the extent of rotation possible in the cadaver. Next, cut the alar ligaments close to the dens. Note that the rotation of the head is now very easy and extensive.

Removal of Head

With a scalpel, cut along the anterior border of the foramen magnum, thereby severing a fine median strand extending from the tip of the dens to the anterior border of the foramen. Next, cut close to the lateral margins of the foramen magnum, thereby cutting the attachments of the alar ligaments. Carry cuts close to the medial and posterior aspects of the occipital condyles; this procedure will open the atlanto-occipital joints. Force a chisel into the **atlanto-occipital joints** and disarticulate the joints as much as possible.

Now, it is advantageous to turn the cadaver into the supine position (face up). Once again, place your hands into the already defined **retrovisceral space.** Pull forward the cervical viscera and the big vessels and nerves. Thus, a convenient working space is created in front of the prevertebral region. Now, proceed as follows:

1. Identify the **sympathetic trunk** and the large **superior cervical sympathetic ganglion** (*Atlas, 561*). Sever the sympathetic trunk on one side, thus leaving it attached to the prevertebral

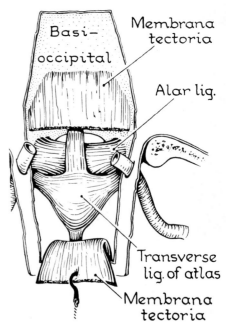

FIG. 8-46. Removal of dura mater and membrana tectoria. Exposure of some ligaments of the craniovertebral region.

region. On the other side, reflect the sympathetic trunk and its superior ganglion together with the cervical viscera.

2. Hold the cervical viscera forward. Pass the knife between the transverse process of the atlas and the occipital bone. This procedure will sever the *rectus capitis lateralis* on each side (fig. 8-47 or *Atlas, 561*).

3. Next, carry the cut more medially. Cut the *rectus capitis anterior* and the thick *longus capitis*.

4. Carry the blade across the median plane just above the anterior arch of the atlas. This procedure will sever the **anterior atlanto-occipital membrane.**

Now, detach the head and the cervical viscera with relative ease. At this point you have *two options:*

1. Reflect the head and the attached cervical viscera downward and forward. This procedure will leave certain cervicothoracic relations intact. At the same time, it permits a posterior approach to the cervical viscera.

2. *Or,* isolate the head and the cervical viscera. In that case, mobilize the trachea and the esophagus. If not already done, cut the esophagus in the thorax. Sever the contents of the carotid sheaths. Remove the head together with the attached cervical viscera.

Keep the cadaver moist at all times to make dissection possible.

Prevertebral and Lateral Vertebral Regions

The head has been detached at the atlanto-occipital joint. During this procedure, the muscles between transverse processes of atlas and occipital bone were cut, and the uppermost portion of the longus capitis was severed.

Examine the deep investing fascia covering the lateral vertebral (scaleni) and prevertebral muscles. The fascia in front of the vertebral column and extending between the transverse processes of the vertebrae is the *prevertebral fascia* (fig. 8-45). It actually consists of two layers which are separated by loose connective tissue. With a forceps, pick up a fine fold of the more anterior layer (alar fascia). Insert a probe into the interval between the two layers of the prevertebral fascia. You are now in a space which has been termed by clinicians the 'danger space,' since it constitutes a passageway for infections from the neck region all the way down into the posterior mediastinum.

On one side of the cadaver, the cervical part of the **sympathetic trunk** was left in place on the prevertebral muscles (*Atlas, 561*). Locate it. Identify the *superior, middle,* and *inferior cervical sympathetic ganglia.* The inferior cervical ganglion is positioned

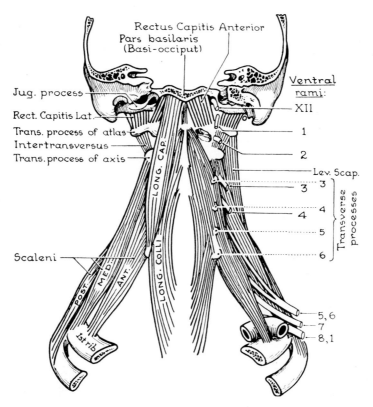

FIG. 8-47. Prevertebral muscles. Ventral roots of cervical spinal nerves.

close to the anterior aspect of the head of rib 1. Frequently, the ganglion is fused with the *first thoracic ganglion* to form the *stellate ganglion* (*Atlas,* 537). Observe *gray rami communicantes* which connect the sympathetic ganglia with the cervical spinal nerves.

Identify the *longus colli, longus capitis* and **scalenus anterior** (fig. 8-47 or *Atlas,* 561). Remove these muscles from the anterior tubercles of the transverse processes of C$_3$ through C$_6$.

Now, the **cervical spinal nerves are exposed.** Trace a ventral ramus to the gutter-like end of the corresponding transverse process on which it rests (*Atlas,* 538.1). Review the contributions of ventral rami C$_{5-8}$ to the brachial plexus (*Atlas,* 476, 561).

Follow the **vertebral artery** to the transverse foramen of C$_6$. Be aware of possible variations (*Atlas,* 567).

Exterior of Base of Skull

Bony Landmarks

Refer to a bony skull and study the following pertinent features:

Anterior Transverse Line (fig. 8-48 or *Atlas,* 571.2). Pass a pencil or the handle of a probe through both mandibular notches across the base of the skull (*Atlas,* 571). The instrument marks a line which passes across the **foramen ovale** on each side.

Posterior Transverse Line (fig. 8-48 or *Atlas,* 571.2). This line stretches across the base of the skull between the mastoid and styloid processes of the two sides. Observe that the line crosses the **stylomastoid foramen, jugular foramen, hypoglossal canal, occipital condyles,** and the **foramen magnum.** Examine the **jugular foramen** more closely, and observe that *three compartments* may be distinguished (*Atlas,* 497):

1. *Anterior compartment.* It transmits the inferior petrosal sinus. In the posterior cranial fossa, note the groove for this sinus running toward the anterior compartment of the jugular foramen. The inferior petrosal sinus joins the internal jugular vein.
2. *Intermediate compartment,* for the transmission of cranial nerves IX, X, and XI.
3. The large *posterior compartment.* It transmits mainly the sigmoid dural sinus, which here becomes the internal jugular vein.

Dissection

Examine the nerves and vessels at the exterior of the base of the skull (*Atlas,* 573, 574). Pick up the cut end of the **common carotid artery.** Trace the **sympathetic trunk** (which lies posterior to the common and internal carotids) up to the carotid canal. Observe the long fusiform ganglion, the **superior cervical sympathetic ganglion.**

The pharynx hangs from the pharyngeal tubercle, well in front of the foramen magnum. The great vessels and nerves lie posterolateral to the posterior wall of the pharynx.

Identify the soft structures which traverse the foramina marked by the 'posterior transverse line':

1. **Facial nerve,** emerging from the stylomastoid foramen.
2. **Internal jugular vein,** beginning at the posterior compartment of the jugular foramen, where it is continuous with the sigmoid sinus and the inferior petrosal sinus.
3. **Nerves IX, X, and XI,** traversing the intermediate compartment of the jugular foramen. If time permits, use bone pliers to remove the bone posterior to the jugular foramen. Now, follow the nerves from the neck into the posterior cranial fossa.
4. **Nerve XII,** emerging from the hypoglossal canal.

The **vagus** (X) belongs to the digestive and respiratory tracts; therefore, it must proceed straight downward. Trace the nerve between internal jugular vein and internal carotid artery. Just below the jugular foramen, observe a 2 cm long swelling, the **jugular ganglion or inferior ganglion of the vagus.** The **superior laryngeal nerve** arises from the vagus about 2.5 cm below the base of the skull. Trace this nerve to the larynx. The **pharyngeal branch** of the vagus arises at a high level. Follow the branch between the internal and external carotid arteries to the pharyngeal wall. Here it joins the pharyngeal plexus. Review the vagus and its essential branches (*Atlas,* 543.1, 660).

The **accessory nerve (XI)** supplies the sternomastoid and the trapezius. At the base of the skull, it lies immediately lateral to the vagus. Follow nerve XI through the interval between internal jugular vein and internal carotid artery toward the substance of the sternomastoid. The accessory nerve crosses anterior to the internal jugular vein in 70%, and posterior to it in about 30% of all cases (*Atlas,* 566.2). Review nerve XI (*Atlas,* 661).

The **hypoglossal nerve** (XII) supplies the muscles of the tongue. The quickest way to positively identify the nerve is to follow it backward from the digastric triangle (*Atlas,* 574). At the base of the skull, the hypoglossal nerve is closely adherent to the inferior ganglion of the vagus. Review nerve XII (*Atlas,* 662).

The **glossopharyngeal nerve** (IX) is destined for the pharynx and the back of the tongue; therefore, it must swing forward (*Atlas,* 573, 574). In doing so, it passes between the internal and external carotid arteries. Separate the two carotid arteries. Observe a lumbrical-like muscle descending from the styloid process between the two arteries. This is the **stylopharyngeus.** The glossopharyngeal nerve is closely

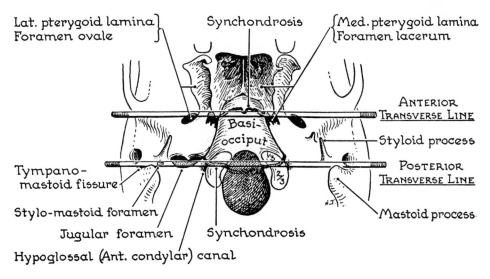

Lat. pterygoid lamina
Foramen ovale
Synchondrosis
Med. pterygoid lamina
Foramen lacerum

Basi-occiput

ANTERIOR TRANSVERSE LINE

Styloid process

POSTERIOR TRANSVERSE LINE

Tympano-mastoid fissure

Stylo-mastoid foramen

Jugular foramen

Synchondrosis

Hypoglossal (Ant. condylar) canal

Mastoid process

FIG. 8-48. 'Anterior transverse line' and 'posterior transverse line' on exterior of base of skull. (From *Grant's Method of Anatomy*.)

applied to its lateral side. Review nerve IX (*Atlas, 659*).

Pharynx

General Remarks

The pharynx is the upper end of the respiratory and digestive tubes. It extends from the base of the skull to the lower border of cricoid cartilage (vertebra C_6).

The **pharyngeal wall** consists of four layers or coats:

1. **Areolar coat or layer.** It is continuous with the areolar layer of the buccinator. Therefore, it is called the **buccopharyngeal fascia.** This layer facilitates movements of the pharynx. It also contains the pharyngeal plexus of veins and nerves.

2. **Muscular layer,** It is composed of (*a*) an *outer circular layer;* and (*b*) an *inner longitudinal layer.*

3. **Fibrous layer or pharyngobasilar fascia.** It corresponds to the tunica submucosa. It is especially strong where it anchors the pharynx to the base of the skull.

4. **Mucous layer.**

The outer circular part of the muscular layer consists of **three constrictors:** *Superior, middle,* and *inferior* (fig. 8-49 or *Atlas, 573.1*). Each constrictor is fan-shaped. The narrow ends of the fans are fixed anteriorly. Posteriorly, the fans of the opposite sides meet in a median raphe. Laterally, there are gaps between the constrictors. Through these spaces pass vessels, nerves, and muscles (Atlas, 574). The constrictors overlap each other to some degree.

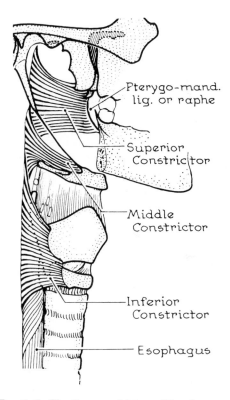

Pterygo-mand. lig. or raphe

Superior Constrictor

Middle Constrictor

Inferior Constrictor

Esophagus

FIG. 8-49. The three constrictors of the pharynx.

External Aspect of Pharynx

Inspect and clean the posterior aspect of the pharyngeal constrictors (*Atlas, 572, 573*). It is easiest to identify the **middle constrictor** first. Its fibers arise from the greater horn of the hyoid bone and from the lower portion of the stylohyoid ligament (figs. 8-49, 8-50). Palpate the greater horn of the hyoid bone. Positively identify the middle constrictor.

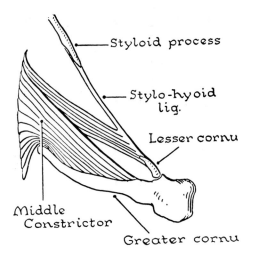

Fig. 8-50. The angular origin of the middle constrictor. (From *Grant's Method of Anatomy.*)

The muscle fibers above the middle constrictor belong to the **superior constrictor.** This muscle arises from the pterygomandibular raphe or ligament and from the bone at either end of it.

The muscle fibers below the middle constrictor belong to the **inferior constrictor.** Observe the continuous origin of this muscle from the **thyroid and cricoid cartilages** (fig. 8-49). Demonstrate that the inferior constrictor overlaps the middle constrictor. Display the interval between the two muscles. Here, the **internal laryngeal nerve** and the superior laryngeal vessels pierce the thyrohyoid membrane (*Atlas, 574*). Examine the free lower border of the inferior constrictor. Here, the **recurrent laryngeal nerve** enters the pharyngeal wall. Note that the most inferior fibers of the inferior constrictor are continuous with the circular fibers of the **esophagus.**

Demonstrate the interval between the middle and superior constrictors (*Atlas, 572–574*). The **stylopharyngeus** and the **glossopharyngeal nerve** (IX) pass through this gap. Verify this fact.

Internal Aspect of Pharynx

Incision. With scissors, slit open the posterior wall of the esophagus and the pharynx. Carry the median section all the way up to the base of the skull (*Atlas, 578*).

The interior of the pharynx communicates anteriorly with three cavities: Nose, mouth, and larynx (fig. 8-51; *Atlas, 578*). Accordingly, the pharynx is divided into three parts: **Nasal pharynx, oral pharynx,** and **laryngeal pharynx.** The soft palate, ending in the uvula, separates the nasopharynx above from the oral pharynx below.

Nasal Pharynx or Nasopharynx. It lies above the soft palate. Verify that it is a backward extension of the nasal cavities. Refer to a skull (*Atlas, 569*), and identify the two posterior nasal apertures or **choanae** which are separated by the bony **nasal septum.** Look through the choanae. Identify scroll-like bones projecting from the lateral wall of each nasal cavity. These are the **middle** and **inferior conchae.** Turn to the cadaver (*Atlas, 578*). Identify the nasal septum, choanae, and conchae.

On each side of the nasopharynx, 1 to 1.5 cm posterior to the inferior concha, is the **pharyngeal orifice of the auditory tube** (*Atlas, 587*). Place a probe into the opening. Posterior to it, identify the **torus tubarius** which is produced by the underlying cartilage of the auditory tube. Behind the torus, explore the **pharyngeal recess** which extends laterally and backward almost to the carotid canal.

The bony curved roof of the nasopharynx is formed by the sphenoid and occipital bones. The mucous membrane on the roof and posterior wall contains a mass of lymphoid tissue, the so-called pharyngeal or **nasopharyngeal tonsil** (*Atlas, 458, 579*). Enlarged nasopharyngeal tonsils are known as 'adenoids.' Understand that large adenoids will obstruct the airpassages from the nose through the nasopharynx, making mouth breathing necessary.

Examine the close relation of the nasopharyngeal tonsil to the orifice of the auditory tube. Understand that enlarged adenoids will obstruct the ostium, thus interfering with the air exchange between nasopharynx and middle ear cavity.

Oral Pharynx or Oropharynx (*Atlas, 578*). The oral pharynx is bounded by the soft palate above and the epiglottis of the larynx below. Push your finger anteriorly into the oral cavity. Palpate the posterior ⅓ of the tongue. Note two folds of mucous membrane which descend from the soft palate (*Atlas, 587*). The anterior fold, the **palatoglossal arch,** descends to the junction of anterior ⅔ and posterior ⅓ of the tongue. The palatoglossal arch forms a dividing line between oral cavity and oral pharynx. The posterior fold, the **palatopharyngeal arch,** descends downward along the lateral wall of the pharynx. Between the two arches lies the **palatine tonsil.** Examine the arches and the tonsil on a cross section through the head (*Atlas, 584*). Identify the right and left palatine arches in the cadaver.

Examine the palatine arches in your fellow students. Notice the two prominent folds in subjects who have undergone tonsillectomy, and observe the empty tonsillar beds. Study the palatine tonsil in several subjects. Note that the tonsils vary in size from person to person.

Laryngeal Pharynx or Laryngopharynx (*Atlas, 578*). This portion of the pharynx extends from the epiglottis to the lower border of the cricoid cartilage. Identify the epiglottis and the inlet (aditus) of the larynx. Palpate the cricoid cartilage through the mucous membrance. Place a probe in the right and left **piriform recesses.** Foreign bodies (bones; food particles) may become trapped here. Define the borders of the piriform recess (*Atlas*, 627): Medially, the larynx; laterally, the thyroid cartilage and the thyrohyoid membrane; posteriorly, the inferior constrictor.

Using the scissor technique, carefully remove the mucosa of the piriform recess. Two nerves, which are submucous, are readily exposed (*Atlas*, 627): **Internal laryngeal nerve** and **recurrent laryngeal nerve.** Observe the nerves. They will be studied more thoroughly during the dissection of the larynx (p. 162).

Bisection of Head

General Remarks and Bony Landmarks

The nasal and oral cavities are not readily accessible in the undivided head. Therefore, the head must be bisected, close to the median plane. For practical purposes, it is best to carry the section just lateral to the nasal septum. Thus, one half of the head will have the nasal septum (*Atlas*, 458); the other half will have its nasal cavity fully opened (*Atlas*, 609).

Usually, the **nasal septum** deviates somewhat to one side. Thus, the nasal cavity is slightly wider on one side, slightly narrower on the side of septal deviation. Refer to one or several skulls, and verify this fact. Logically, the section should be made on the less obstructed side, just lateral to the nasal septum.

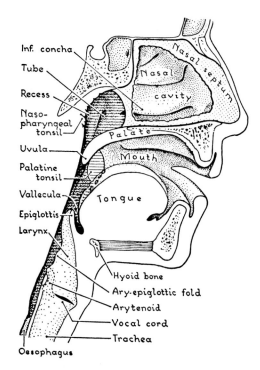

Fig. 8-51. Interior of pharynx (lateral view). (From *Grant's Method of Anatomy*.)

Examine a skull and study the bones through which you must saw:

1. The saw cut must pass through the nasal bone and the remains of the frontal bone (*Atlas*, 460).
2. Subsequently, you must saw just lateral to the crista galli through one of the cribriform plates of the ethmoid bone (*Atlas*, 507). Then, the cut must be carried midsagittally through the body of the sphenoid bone and part of the occipital bone to the anterior margin of the foramen magnum (*Atlas*, 458, 609).
3. You must saw through the hard palate which forms the floor of the nasal cavities and the roof of the oral cavity.

Dissection and Bisection

Cut through the upper lip in the midline. Next, explore each nasal cavity with a probe. Decide on which side of the nasal septum the bisection should be carried out.

On the chosen side, carry out the following procedures:

1. Divide the uvula and the soft palate in the midsagittal plane.
2. Slit open the naris. Cut through the lateral portion of the septal cartilage all the way to the nasal bone (*Atlas*, 468).
3. Insert a small saw into the nasal cavity. Keep the blade close to the septum. Cut upward through the nasal and frontal bones. Subsequently, saw through the cribriform plate, body of sphenoid, dorsum sellae, and basioccipital bone, until you reach the foramen magnum.
4. Saw downward through the floor of the nasal cavity. Divide the hard palate close to the midsagittal plane.

Now, the two upper halves of the head will fall apart from each other. The tongue lies exposed. **Inspect the tongue.** Verify the following statements (*Atlas*, 594):

1. The anterior ⅔ of the tongue lies horizontally in the mouth. This is the **oral part.**
2. The posterior ⅓ of the tongue takes a curved vertical position and forms the anterior wall of the oral pharynx. This is the **pharyngeal part** of the tongue.
3. The boundary between the two parts is marked by the **sulcus terminalis.** This line has the shape of an inverted V (Λ). On each side, it runs from the palatoglossal arch backward to a median pit, the **foramen cecum.**
4. Large and conspicuous **vallate papillae,** 7 to 12 in number, occupy a V-shaped row just in front of the sulcus terminalis. (These papillae contain numerous taste buds.)
5. The anterior ⅔ of the tongue is covered with long **filiform papillae. Fungiform papillae** lie near

the dorsum and margins of the tongue. (These papillae also contain taste buds.)

6. A median fold of mucous membrane, the *median glossoepiglottic fold*, runs from the dorsum of the tongue to the epiglottis. On each side of this fold are the **valleculae.**

7. The surface of the pharyngeal or posterior ⅓ of the tongue is conspicuously different from the oral part. It has no papillae. Its surface is uneven due to the presence of numerous lymphoid follicles. These encapsuled follicles are collectively called the **lingual tonsil.**

8. Realize that the tongue is supplied by 5 (five) different cranial nerves (*Atlas, 593*).

The next objective is to bisect the mandible together with the floor of the mouth and the tongue. Proceed as follows: Turn to the submental triangle between the anterior bellies of the digastrics (*Atlas, 544, 545*). Split the thin median raphe of the **mylohyoids,** and separate the muscles. Identify the underlying paired **geniohyoids.** With probe and scissors, separate these muscles from each other. Clean their pointed mandibular origins. Next, saw through the mandible in the midsagittal plane, exactly between the geniohyoids.

Now, bisect the tongue in the midsagittal plane from the tip to the hyoid bone and to the epiglottis (*Atlas, 595*). Take care not to destroy the epiglottis. Do *not* bisect the hyoid bone and the larynx.

Nasal Cavities

Bony Landmarks

Refer to a skull and, in addition, to a bisected skull. Study the following pertinent features:

The **floor of the nasal cavity** (which is also the roof of the oral cavity) is formed by the **bony palate.** Study its inferior surface (*Atlas, 580*). The anterior ⅔ of the bony palate consists of the **palatine processes of the maxilla.** The posterior ⅓ consists of the **horizontal plates of the palatine bones.** In the midline immediately behind the incisor teeth, find the **incisive foramen.** Medial to the 3rd molar tooth, locate the **greater palatine foramen.** Gently push a thin flexible wire through it into the **greater palatine canal.**

Examine the **vertical part or perpendicular plate of the palatine bone** which forms part of the lateral wall of the nasal cavity (*Atlas, 608, 608.1*). The vertical plate has a **notch** on its superior border. This notch is in contact with the sphenoid bone; thus, the important **sphenopalatine** (pterygopalatine) **foramen** is formed. Identify the foramen in the bisected skull. Next, from the lateral aspect of the skull, look through the **pterygopalatine fossa** (*Atlas, 558*). Detect the **sphenopalatine foramen** in the depth of the fossa. Understand that the foramen is a passage-

way for vessels and nerves from the pterygopalatine fossa to the nasal cavity.

In the bisected skull, examine the body of the **sphenoid bone.** Locate the large **sphenoidal air sinus** (*Atlas, 609*). Usually, the right and left sinuses differ in size. They are partially subdivided by a bony septum. Attempt to find the **posterior opening of the pterygoid canal** (*Atlas, 619.2*). This canal runs postero-anteriorly through the body of the sphenoid. Frequently, the canal causes a ridge on the floor of the sphenoid sinus. Pass a thin flexible wire through the pterygoid canal. Note that the wire connects two foramina: **foramen lacerum** and **sphenopalatine foramen.** These relations are of importance. The greater petrosal nerve, carrying parasympathetic fibers, traverses the foramen lacerum and then the pterygoid canal to reach the sphenopalatine (pterygopalatine) ganglion (*Atlas, 657*).

Preferably in the bisected skull, examine the **lateral wall** of the nasal cavity. Identify the following (*Atlas, 608*):

1. **Frontal process of maxilla.**
2. **Vertical plate of palatine bone.**
3. **Inferior concha** (turbinate)
4. **Middle and superior conchae.** These structures are part of the ethmoid bone. They contain many small air cells. Note the openings of some of these cells.

Just above the inferior concha, find an opening which leads to the large **maxillary sinus** (*Atlas, 608.1, 611.1*). Pass a wire through the **nasolacrimal canal,** and observe that the wire enters the nasal cavity under shelter of and lateral to the inferior concha. Pass a flexible wire from the **frontal air sinus** into the nasal cavity.

Study the bony **roof** of the nasal cavity (*Atlas, 608*). Observe: **Nasal bone;** small part of frontal bone; **cribriform plate** of ethmoid bone; body of **sphenoid.**

Examine the **bony nasal septum** (*Atlas, 605*). Identify the unpaired **vomer.** It articulates with the sphenoid and the bony palate. Identify the unpaired **perpendicular plate of the ethmoid.** Of course, the large septal cartilage is absent in the bony skull. Examine the two **choanae,** the posterior nasal apertures, and review their boundaries (*Atlas, 569*). Review the complex **ethmoid bone** and its relations to the nasal cavity (*Atlas, 614*).

Nasal Septum

Turn to the cadaver. Examine the half of the head which contains the **nasal septum.** Strip the mucoperiosteum completely off and identify the three main components of the septum (*Atlas, 605*): **Perpendicular plate of ethmoid, vomer,** and **septal cartilage.**

Next, carefully remove the bony and cartilaginous parts of the septum. However, *leave intact* the mucoperiosteum lateral to it. Now, the vessels and nerves running along the nasal septum can be examined in the remaining mucoperiosteal membrane.

Arteries. These are difficult to trace, unless they are injected. You are not required to dissect these structures. However, realize that they exist. The arteries form a network which receives its blood supply from various sources (fig. 8-52 or *Atlas, 607*).

Nerves (fig. 8-53 or *Atlas, 606.1*).

1. Close to the cribriform plate is the **olfactory area** which contains olfactory nerve fibers (*Atlas, 651*).
2. *Anterior ethmoidal nerve.* Do not dissect this fine branch of V^1.
3. **Nasopalatine nerve,** a branch of V^2 via the sphenopalatine ganglion (*Atlas, 656 B*). From the palatine side, pierce and mark the incisive canal with a needle. Now, you have a reference point. Using the scissor technique, trace the thin nasopalatine nerve toward the incisive canal.

Remove all remains of the nasal septum, including the mucoperiosteum. Expose the lateral wall of the nasal cavity. The lateral wall of the other side is already exposed.

Lateral Wall of Nasal Cavity

In the cadaver, inspect the **lateral wall** of the nasal cavity (fig. 8-54; *Atlas, 609*). Identify:

1. **Inferior concha.** The space lateral to and inferior to it is the **inferior meatus.** Note that the free edge of the inferior concha is horizontal. About 1.5 cm behind the posterior limit of the inferior concha identify the **pharyngeal orifice of the auditory tube.**
2. **Middle concha.** The space lateral to and inferior to it is the **middle meatus.** Anteriorly, the free edge of the middle concha turns upward.
3. **Superior concha.** This small structure extends from the roof to the front of the sphenoid. Lateral to and inferior to it is the **superior meatus.** The

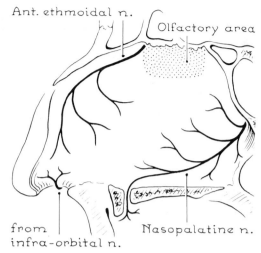

FIG. 8-53. Nerves of nasal septum.

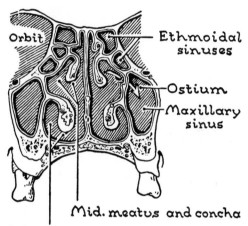

FIG. 8-54. Nasal cavities and adjacent air sinuses (coronal section). (From *Grant's Method of Anatomy.*

space posterosuperior to the superior concha is the **spheno-ethmoidal recess.**

4. **Vestibule,** above the nostril and in front of the inferior meatus. Note the presence of hairs on the mobile part.
5. **Atrium,** above the vestibule and in front of the middle meatus.

With scissors, cut away the **inferior concha** (*Atlas, 610*). Pass a stiff wire from the orbital cavity down through the **nasolacrimal duct** to the **inferior meatus.** Remove the mucoperiosteum from the lateral wall of the inferior meatus. Observe the opening of the bony **nasolacrimal canal** (which contains the nasolacrimal duct).

With scissors, cut away the **middle concha** (*Atlas, 610*). Identify a curved slit, the **hiatus semilunaris.** This hiatus has a sharp lower edge. Its more rounded upper edge is formed by the *ethmoidal bulla,* an elevation of the ethmoidal labrinth.

Identify the opened **frontal air sinus.** Pass a wire downward and backward from the frontal sinus

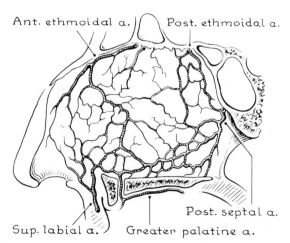

FIG. 8-52. Arteries of nasal septum.

through the **frontonasal duct.** Usually, this duct opens into the upper portion of the **infundibulum.** The infundibulum is a narrow passage anterosuperior to the hiatus semilunaris. In frontal sinus infections, irrigation of the sinus may be necessary. This is done with a specially curved cannula which is passed through the infundibulum and through the frontonasal duct. Study these important relations in the cadaver.

Realize that the **ethmoidal air cells** (or sinus) are located lateral to the middle and superior conchae (fig. 8-54). Stay above the hiatus semilunaris, and break into the *middle ethmoidal cells* of the ethmoidal bulla. Anteriorly, identify the *anterior ethmoidal cells.* Remove the superior concha to display one or more of the *posterior* ethmoidal cells (*Atlas, 611*). Pick away the partitions between the ethmoidal cells until you reach the thin *orbital plate* (lamina papyracea) of the ethmoid bone (fig. 8-54). If you break through this plate, you will enter the orbital cavity.

If time permits, explore the sphenoidal air sinus. Find its orifice or ostium which opens into the spheno-ethmoidal recess. The size of the ostium may vary from 0.5 to 4 mm. Irrigation of an infected sphenoid sinus can be accomplished by inserting a special curved cannula through the ostium. Examine the orifice. Understand that it may not be accessible when the middle concha is too large or the septum is deviated. In that case, a trocar must be pushed directly through the anterior wall of the sphenoid into the sinus. Study these relations.

Explore the **hiatus semilunaris.** In it is the **ostium for the maxillary sinus** (fig. 8-54; *Atlas, 610*). Pass a probe into the maxillary sinus. An infected maxillary sinus may be irrigated through its ostium. However, if difficulties are encountered, an artificial route of drainage is chosen. A curved trocar is pushed through the medial wall of the inferior meatus into the maxillary sinus, close to its floor. With a probe, break through the thin medial wall of the inferior meatus and create an artificial opening.

Now, with the aid of bone forceps, remove the medial wall of the maxillary sinus. Notice that it is a three-sided hollow pyramid. The average adult capacity is approximately 15 ml. Verify that the upper wall separates the sinus from the orbital cavity.

With forceps, remove the mucoperiosteum lining the maxillary sinus. Note a ridge on the orbital and anterior surfaces. This ridge is caused by the **infraorbital canal.** With a probe, break into the canal, open it along its length, and identify its contents: **Infraorbital nerve** and accompanying **vessels.**

Examine the floor of the maxillary sinus. Look for the roots of teeth which may project into the sinus. Sometimes the roots are covered only with mucoperiosteum (*Atlas, 616.3*). Understand that an infection from a decaying tooth may readily spread into the sinus. During extraction of a molar or premolar tooth, the membrane over the projecting root may be torn.

As a result, a fistula between mouth and sinus may occur.

Sphenopalatine Foramen and Pterygopalatine Fossa

Once again, review essential bony landmarks (p. 154). Identify the sphenopalatine foramen and the pterygopalatine fossa. Gently push a thin, flexible wire upward through the greater palatine foramen into the greater palatine canal. Note that the wire emerges in the pterygopalatine fossa close to the sphenopalatine foramen. Review the course of the maxillary nerve V^2 (*Atlas, 655*). Once again, identify the pterygoid canal.

The conchae and the medial wall of the maxillary sinus were removed earlier. The perpendicular plate of the palatine bone and the closely related greater palatine canal are still intact (*Atlas, 608*). Now, strip the mucoperiosteum from the perpendicular plate of the palatine bone. In doing so, you will encounter the *posterior lateral nasal artery.* This artery is a branch of the **sphenopalatine artery** (*Atlas, 607*). After traversing the sphenopalatine foramen, the sphenopalatine artery divides into a *posterior septal branch* (for the septum) and the posterior lateral nasal branch. Most of its small branches have been cut during removal of the conchae. Do not dissect the arterial network of the lateral nasal wall. However, realize that it exists.

The next objective is to expose the **sphenopalatine foramen** and its contents. The greater palatine canal leads to this foramen. Make use of this fact. Insert a needle (about 30 mm or 1¼ in. long) into the greater palatine foramen, just medial to the 3rd molar tooth (*Atlas, 580*). Probe, until you find the opening. Then, push the needle all the way up the greater palatine canal. The tip of the needle will be located in front of the sphenoid bone and just lateral to the sphenopalatine foramen. Leave the needle in place. Now, use a probe, and break down the medial wall of the greater palatine canal. This procedure will expose the contents of the canal: **Greater palatine nerve** (fig. 8-55; *Atlas, 606*) and **greater palatine artery,** a terminal branch of the maxillary artery (*Atlas, 560, 583*).

Follow the greater palatine nerve upward to the sphenopalatine foramen. Here, find the **sphenopalatine (pterygopalatine) ganglion** (fig. 8-55; *Atlas, 606*). If time permits, find the *nerve of the pterygoid canal.* Proceed as follows: Remove the mucoperiosteum from the sphenoid sinus. Find the ridge produced by the pterygoid canal. With a probe, open the canal. Follow the delicate nerve toward the sphenopalatine ganglion. Realize that the nerve of the pterygoid canal (Vidian nerve) consists of preganglionic parasympathetic fibers from the greater petrosal nerve, and postganglionic sympathetic fibers from the deep petrosal nerve (*Atlas, 657*).

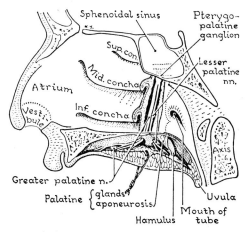

FIG. 8-55. Greater palatine canal and sphenopalatine (pterygopalatine) ganglion. (From *Grant's Method of Anatomy*.)

Next, turn the specimen over and approach it from its lateral aspect. Deep in the **pterygopalatine fossa**, identify the following pertinent structures (*Atlas*, 560):

1. **Maxillary artery,** giving off the **greater palatine artery** and the **sphenopalatine artery.** The sphenopalatine artery is the one passing through the sphenopalatine foramen.
2. **Maxillary nerve V²,** coursing from the foramen rotundum behind to the inferior orbital fissure in front.
3. **Sphenopalatine ganglion.** Attempt to find it. It is attached to the maxillary nerve by two short stout medially running nerve branches (*Atlas*, 655).

If you cannot satisfactorily see the ganglion in relation to nerve V², do not hesitate to remove the floor of the orbital cavity. Follow the infraorbital nerve backward. Compare your field of dissection with the one depicted in *Atlas*, 560.2.

Palate, Tonsil, and Pharyngeal Wall

Hard Palate and Soft Palate

The palate consists of two portions: (1) The **hard palate,** comprising the anterior ⅔; and (2) the mobile **soft palate,** constituting the posterior ⅓ of the palate. Small mucous glands, the **palatine glands,** are abundant over the palate. The pinpoint orifices of their ducts are evident (*Atlas*, 581).

Mark the greater palatine foramen by a needle, as described earlier (p. 156). The **greater palatine nerve and vessels** emerge from this foramen to be distributed to the hard palate (fig. 8-55; *Atlas*, 582, 583). To demonstrate nerve and vessels, proceed as follows: About 5 mm posterior to the marked greater palatine foramen, make a transverse cut through the thickness of the mucoperiosteum of the hard palate. With the

rounded handle of the knife, ease the mucoperiosteum off the bony palate. Free the greater palatine nerve and vessels (*Atlas*, 582). Cut the reflected tissue close to the alveolar processes of the teeth.

Examine the soft palate which had been cut earlier in the midsagittal plane. Observe (fig. 8-56):

1. The thickness of the soft palate is due mainly to glands.
2. The strength of the soft palate depends on its aponeurosis situated in its anterior ⅓.
3. Its mobility is due to muscles situated in its posterior ⅔. These muscles will be studied later (p. 159).

Palatine Tonsil

The right and left **palatine tonsils** lie on each side of the oropharynx. The tonsil is called 'palatine' because its upper ⅓ extends into the soft palate, a matter of clinical importance. Each tonsil is located in the triangular interval between the **palatoglossal arch** and the **palatopharyngeal arch** (fig. 8-57; *Atlas*, 584). In older individuals, the palatine tonsil may be inconspicuous.

Enucleation. If the tonsil is present, remove it. Proceed as follows (fig. 8-57; *Atlas*, 586): Incise the mucous membrane along the palatoglossal arch. Using blunt dissection, free the anterior border and the upper part of the tonsil. This is easily done because the rounded lateral aspect of the tonsil has a fibrous capsule. This capsule is separated from the pharyngeal wall by a layer of loose areolar tissue. Work in the areolar space. Free the posterior part of the tonsil. Finally, detach the lower part where the tonsil is most adherent. Note that the lower pole is continuous with the lymphoid tissue of the tongue, the so-called *lingual tonsil*.

Examine the enucleated palatine tonsil. Section it. Observe the **crypts** that extend from the free surface of the tonsil to almost the level of the capsule (*Atlas*, 585).

Examine the **bed of the palatine tonsil** (*Atlas*,

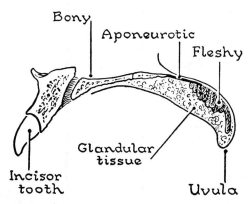

FIG. 8-56. Hard palate and soft palate on sagittal section. (From *Grant's Method of Anatomy*.)

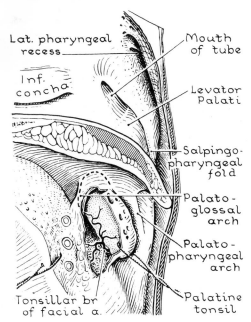

FIG. 8-57. First step in removal of palatine tonsil.

588). The thin fibrous sheet covering the bed of the tonsil is part of the *pharyngobasilar fascia*. Remove it, and expose two muscles: **Palatopharyngeus** and **superior constrictor**. These muscles are part of the muscular coat of the pharynx. The superior constrictor has a delicate, free, arched lower border which does not reach the lower third of the tonsil bed. If engorged, you may see the *paratonsillar vein*. This vein is often responsible for hemorrhage following tonsillectomy.

Push a probe under the free lower border of the superior constrictor. Using the probe as a protective guide, carefully remove a small part of the superior constrictor just anterior to the palatopharyngeus (fig. 8-58; *Atlas*, 589). Now, the styloglossus and the glossopharyngeal nerve are exposed. Identify the **styloglossus**. It is a thick muscular band which passes from the tip of the styloid process to the lateral aspect of the tongue (*compare Atlas*, 549.1). Find the **glossopharyngeal nerve** (IX). It passes through the gap between the superior and the middle constrictors just lateral to the stylopharyngeus. The nerve spreads out to the mucosa of the posterior ⅓ of the tongue. Follow the nerve centrally to the base of the skull (*Atlas*, 573). Review the distribution and functions of nerve IX (*Atlas*, 659).

Pharyngeal Wall

Carefully remove the mucous membrane from both surfaces of the soft palate, from the lateral pharyngeal wall, and from the nasopharynx. When removing the mucosa from the palatoglossal arch, the **palatoglossus** is displayed (*Atlas*, 588). After removal of the mucosa from the palatopharyngeal arch, the **palato-**

pharyngeus is exposed. This muscle is divided into 3 distinct parts (fig. 8-58): *Tubal*, several strands of muscle reaching the cartilage of the auditory tube; *palatine*, to the posterior portion of the soft palate; *tonsilar*, spreading over the bed of the palatine tonsil. These parts of the palatopharyngeus and the **stylopharyngeus** form the longitudinal musculature of the pharynx.

The next objective is to display the **origin of the superior constrictor** from the pterygomandibular raphe (lig.). This raphe connects two bony landmarks: **Hamulus of medial pterygoid plate** (*Atlas*, 580), and an area of the **mandible** just behind the 3rd molar tooth. Observe these bony landmarks in the skull. Then, palpate the hamulus in the cadaver. Now, you can positively identify the fibrous pterygomandibular raphe (*Atlas*, 590). Verify that two muscles meet at the raphe: **Superior constrictor** and **buccinator**. In addition, examine these relations from the lateral aspect of the head (*Atlas*, 574).

Examine the upper free border of the superior constrictor. The gap between this border and the base of the skull is closed by the pharyngobasilar fascia. Passing through this gap are (fig. 8-59; *Atlas*, 588): **Auditory tube, levator palati,** and *ascending pharyngeal artery*.

Auditory Tube (Pharyngotympanic Tube; Eustachian Tube). It connects the nasopharynx with the tympanic cavity (*Atlas*, 633). It is about 36 mm long, and consists of a cartilaginous and a bony portion. Refer to the base of a skull, and look for the opening of

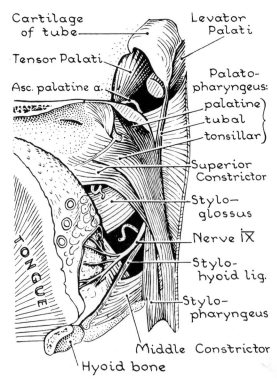

FIG. 8-58. Bed of tonsil. Pharyngeal muscles.

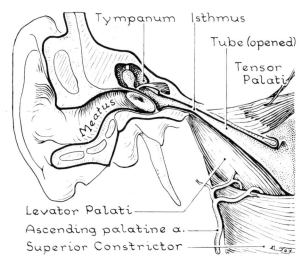

FIG. 8-59. Tube, levator, and artery crossing the upper border of the superior constrictor.

the **osseous portion of the auditory tube** (*Atlas*, *569*). Pass a thin, flexible wire through the canal. Now, look into the external ear canal. You will see the wire in the middle ear cavity (in the cadaver, external ear canal and middle ear cavity are separated by the tympanic membrane).

The anterior ⅔ of the auditory tube is cartilaginous. Observe that the cartilage forms only the upper and medial walls of the tube (*Atlas*, *588*). The lower and lateral walls are membranous. The bony and the **cartilaginous portions** of the auditory tube meet at the *isthmus*. Here, the lumen of the tube is very narrow (fig. 8-59). In the cadaver, pass a thin, flexible wire through the ostium of the auditory tube, and push it into the tube for about 3 cm.

Levator Palati (fig. 8-58; *Atlas*, *588*). At the base of the skull, it arises from the petrous bone and the medial portion of the cartilage of the auditory tube. The levator palati elevates and retracts the soft palate. Identify the muscle which is slightly thicker than a pencil. Pass the handle of a scalpel between the levator and the floor of the auditory tube. Separate the two structures from each other. Cut the levator close to the base of the skull, and reflect it.

Free the **auditory tube** from the medial pterygoid plate. Cut it, and remove its anterior portion. Observe the collapsed, slit-like lumen of the tube. Note the cartilaginous and membranous walls.

Now, the **tensor palati** lies exposed (fig. 8-58; *Atlas*, *590*). The muscle arises from the *scaphoid fossa*. Identify this bony landmark on the skull. Find the fossa at the upper end of the posterior border of the medial pterygoid plate (*Atlas*, *569*). Once again, identify the *hamulus* of the medial pterygoid plate, which serves as a pulley for the tensor palati. In order to render the soft palate 'tense,' the right and left tensors must pull it laterally (the *red arrow* in *Atlas*, *619.2* illustrates how this is accomplished). The thin, ribbon-like muscle ends in a tendon which winds

around the hamulus. In the cadaver, palpate the hamulus. Find the tendon of the tensor palati as it passes medialward to its insertion into the palatine aponeurosis (*Atlas*, *582*).

Continue dissecting the specimen from its medial side (*Atlas*, *590*). Retract the tensor palati superiorly, or remove its superoposterior portion. This procedure will expose the **mandibular nerve** (V³) as it emerges from the **foramen ovale**. Coming from the medial side, carefully pass the tip of a probe through the foramen. Immediately below the foramen and on the medial aspect of V³ lies the small **otic ganglion** (*Atlas*, *598*). The ganglion is difficult to find. Be aware of its functional importance (*Atlas*, *659*).

Mouth and Tongue

Inspection and Palpation

Vestibule of the Mouth (*Atlas*, *465.1*, *591*). It is the U-shaped space bounded externally by the lips and cheeks, and internally by the teeth and gums. The teeth and gums separate the vestibule from the oral cavity proper. With a clean index or middle finger, explore the vestibule of your own mouth. Have a skull on hand for reference. Palpate the following structures:
1. **Mentalis,** passing from the incisive fossa of the mandible to the skin of the chin (*Atlas*, *470*).
2. Lower border of **zygomatic arch.**
3. **Maxilla,** its anterior (facial) and infratemporal surfaces.
4. **Ramus** and **coronoid process of mandible** (*Atlas*, *553.1*). **Tendon of temporalis,** attached to coronoid process.
5. **Masseter,** easily palpated when the teeth are clenched.
6. Behind the last molar teeth, the communication between vestibule and oral cavity proper.
7. **Frenulum** of upper lip; and frenulum of lower lip. The two frenula [L., frenum = bridge] are folds of mucosa attaching the lips to the gums in the median plane.
8. **Orifice of the parotid duct.** A slightly elevated, whitish, constricted opening opposite the 2nd upper molar tooth. Usually, this papilla can be readily palpated with the tip of the tongue. Examine the right and left orifices.

Oral Cavity Proper. Define its **borders:** Laterally and anteriorly the **teeth and gums;** superiorly, the **hard palate** (*Atlas*, *592*); inferiorly, the **tongue;** posteriorly and laterally, the **palatoglossal arch,** marking the border between oral cavity and oropharynx. In the living, inspect or palpate the following structures of the oral cavity proper:
1. **Sublingual region.** This region is located below the mobile portions of the tongue, laterally and in front.

2. **Frenulum linguae,** connecting the tongue to the floor of the mouth. Raise the tip of the tongue to see this median fold.

3. **Deep lingual veins,** easily seen on each side of the frenulum.

4. **Opening of submandibular duct.** Observe it on each side of the root of the frenulum (compare *Atlas, 597*).

5. **Plica sublingualis** (*Atlas, 592, 597*), overlying the upper border of the sublingual salivary gland. Several small sublingual ducts open onto this plica.

6. *Hamulus* of medial pterygoid plate (*Atlas, 580, 590*).

Dissection of Sublingual Region

Briefly refer to a bony mandible. Examine its medial aspect (*Atlas, 553.1*), and identify two important bony landmarks:

1. **Mylohyoid line,** for attachment of mylohyoid muscle.

2. **Sublingual fossa,** for the sublingual gland and associated soft structures above the level of the mylohyoid muscle.

Turn to the bisected head of the cadaver. Briefly examine the muscles of the floor of the mouth and of the tongue, as they can be seen on median section (*Atlas, 595*): **Mylohyoid, geniohyoid,** and the large fan-shaped **genioglossus.**

The next objective is to expose the **sublingual gland.** Before dissecting, it is important that you understand the following (*Atlas, 592*):

1. Dissection of the lateral aspect of the gland is relatively simple, since no important structures intervene between gland and sublingual fossa of mandible.

2. Dissection medial to the gland will require great care. Important structures (nerve, duct, vessels) will be found in the space between gland and genioglossus muscle of the tongue.

3. The sublingual gland rests on the mylohyoid muscle.

With these facts in mind, proceed as follows: Incise the mucous membrane between *plica sublingualis* and *mandible*. Start at the frenulum of the tongue. Carry the incision backwards, but not beyond the 2nd molar tooth. With a probe and handle of a scalpel, displace the **sublingual gland** medially. Identify the sublingual fossa of the mandible. Inferior to it, observe the origin of the mylohyoid.

Next, carefully incise the mucous membrane along the furrow between the *plica sublingualis* and the *tongue*. With a blunt instrument (probe or handle of scalpel), displace the gland laterally and the tongue medially. Identify the following (fig. 8-60; *Atlas, 597*):

1. **Sublingual salivary gland.** It is enveloped in a sheath of areolar tissue which fixes the gland to the floor of the mouth. Tease the tissue between upper border of sublingual gland and plica

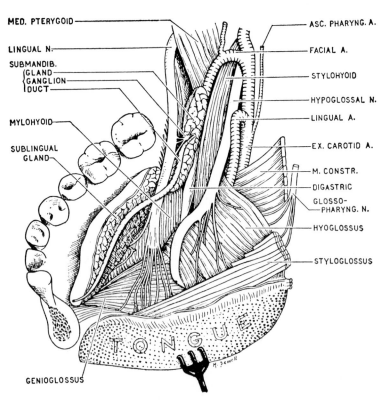

FIG. 8-60. Dissection of right side of floor of mouth. (From *Grant's Method of Anatomy*.)

sublingualis, and identify several very short and fine ducts. There are about 12 ducts which open on the summit of the plica.

2. **Submandibular duct.** It runs diagonally across the medial aspect of the sublingual gland. Follow the duct anteriorly to its papilla just lateral to the frenulum linguae. Then, follow the duct posteriorly to the substance of the **submandibular salivatory gland.**

3. **Lingual nerve.** Pick up the nerve behind the last molar tooth. Once again, verify that the nerve runs between ramus of mandible and medial pterygoid (*Atlas, 559, 597*). Trace the lingual nerve forward. The nerve describes a spiral around the submandibular duct. In successive order, the relations of the nerve to the duct are: Lateral and superior to; inferior to; inferior and medial to; and finally superior and medial to the duct. Observe that the nerve divides into several branches to the tongue. These branches lie immediately beneath the mucosa of the anterior ⅔ of the tongue (fig. 8-60; *Atlas, 549*).

4. *Submandibular ganglion* (fig. 8-60; *Atlas, 547*). Far back, in the vicinity of the 3rd molar tooth, look for the submandibular ganglion. This small ganglion is suspended from the lingual nerve by two or more short branches. Carefully tease the inferior surface of the lingual nerve to reveal the ganglion. Understand the functional importance of the ganglion (*Atlas, 547.1, 657*).

5. **Hypoglossal nerve** (XII). Pick up the nerve as it runs forward between submandibular gland and hyoglossus, well inferior to the lingual nerve (compare *Atlas, 548*). Follow the nerve to the musculature of the tongue.

Dissection of the Tongue

Approach the bisected head from its lateral aspect. With a probe, define the attachment of the **mylohyoid** to the hyoid bone (*Atlas, 547*). Subsequently, detach the muscle from the hyoid bone and reflect it upward. Now, the **hyoglossus** is fully exposed (*Atlas, 548*). Observe the two important nerves which cross the hyoglossus laterally: **Hypoglossal nerve** and, more superiorly, the **lingual nerve.**

With a probe, locate the origin of the **lingual artery** (fig. 8-61; *Atlas, 548, 549.1*). Understand that this artery runs medial to the hyoglossus. To expose the course of the artery, this muscle must be reflected. Proceed as follows: Pass a probe deep to the attachment of the hyoglossus to the hyoid bone. Cut the muscle, and reflect it upward.

Now the course of the **lingual artery** is exposed. Follow its branches to the musculature of the tongue. Search for fine branches to the sublingual gland.

Styloglossus (fig. 8-61; *Atlas, 549*). Trace the muscle from the styloid process to the lateral aspect of the tongue. Note that its fibers interdigitate with those of the hyoglossus.

Genioglossus and Geniohyoid. Once again, examine these two muscles on median section (*Atlas, 595*). Separate the muscles with a probe. The geniohyoid is the one attached to the hyoid bone. Observe the large fan-shaped genioglossus. With a probe, define its apical attachment to the genial tubercle of the mandible.

Next, cut the **genioglossus** close to the mandible. Observe that, as a result of this section, the tongue becomes quite mobile. Raise the tongue well backward into the pharynx. Now, the underlying **geniohyoid** is exposed. Examine the attachments of this muscle to mandible and hyoid bone (*Atlas, 599*).

On only one side of the bisected head, make a cross section through the tongue. Note the **intrinsic musculature of the tongue.** It consists of *vertical, transverse,* and *longitudinal fibers* (*Atlas, 592*). Review the hypoglossal nerve (*Atlas, 662*).

Be aware of the functional significance of the **genioglossus.** This muscle protrudes the tongue. If it is paralyzed, the tongue has a tendency to fall back and to obstruct the vital airways of the oropharynx (risk of suffocation). Total relaxation of the genioglossi can be expected during general anesthesia. Therefore, the tongue of the anesthetized patient must be prevented from relapsing (place patient on side; hold tongue in protruded position by special instrument).

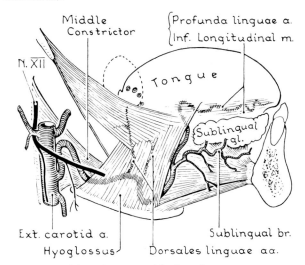

FIG. 8-61. Lingual artery and its branches.

Larynx

General Remarks

The **skeleton of the larynx** (*Atlas, 623–625*) is responsible for maintaining the shape of this organ. It consists of a series of articulating cartilages which are united by membranes. The **cricoid cartilage** [Gk., krikos = ring] is shaped like a signet ring; its large plate or lamina is positioned posteriorly, its arch anteriorly.

The inferior horns or cornua of the **thyroid cartilage** articulate with the cricoid cartilage at special facets. At these facets, the thyroid cartilage can be tilted forward or backward in a visor-like manner.

On the upper border of the lamina of the cricoid are the articular facets for the paired **arytenoid cartilages.** These small pyramidal cartilages are capable of various movements:
1. Tilting forward and backward.
2. Sliding toward or away from another.
3. Rotary motion.

The posterior ends of the **vocal ligaments** are attached at the vocal processes of the arytenoid cartilages (*Atlas, 625*). The anterior ends of the vocal ligaments converge at the angle formed by the laminae of the thyroid cartilage.

The **epiglottic cartilage** lies behind the tongue and hyoid bone. The stalk of this cartilage is attached in the angle between the thyroid laminae, just superior to the vocal ligaments (*Atlas, 625*).

Laryngeal Muscles

The mucosa of the piriform recess was removed earlier, and the **internal laryngeal** and **recurrent laryngeal nerves** were already partially exposed (*Atlas, 627*).

Now, strip the mucosa from the entire pharyngeal aspect of the larynx. This procedure will expose the following intrinsic laryngeal muscles:
1. **Posterior crico-arytenoids** (*Atlas, 627*). A pair of muscles arising from the posterior lamina of the cricoid and inserting into the muscular processes of the arytenoid cartilages.
2. **Arytenoideus.** It unites the two arytenoid cartilages by transverse fibers. Some superficial oblique fibers cross to the opposite side and toward the epiglottis. This part of the muscle is known as the *aryepiglotticus.*

Define the **cricothyroid joint** (*Atlas, 623, 628*). Just posterior to the joint runs the recurrent laryngeal nerve. Cut through the ligamentous bands which hold the joint together. Disarticulate this synovial joint.

The next objective is to reflect a portion of the thyroid lamina in order to expose the remaining laryngeal muscles (*Atlas, 628*). Proceed as follows: Saw or cut the lamina of the thyroid cartilage about 8 mm to the left of the midline. Reflect the thyroid lamina which is attached to the cricoid by the cricothyroid muscle.

Now, the following laryngeal muscles can be identified and studied (*Atlas, 628*):
1. **Cricothyroid,** stretching from the surface of the cricoid to the lower border and inferior horn of the thyroid cartilage.
2. **Lateral crico-arytenoid,** passing from the upper border of the cricoid and the cricothyroid ligament to the muscular process of the arytenoid cartilage.
3. **Thyro-arytenoid,** positioned superior to the lateral cricoarytenoid. It passes from the thyroid cartilage anteriorly to the arytenoid cartilage posteriorly. Its upper and most medial fibers are the *vocalis.*
4. **Vocalis,** applied lateral and inferior to the vocal ligament.
5. *Thyroepiglotticus*, from thyroid cartilage to epiglottis.

Manipulate the arytenoid cartilages. Understand their movements in response to the actions of various laryngeal muscles (fig. 8-62). Only the **posterior cricoarytenoid** is capable of opening the rima glottidis. Thus, this muscle is vital in maintaining the respiratory airway. All other intrinsic laryngeal muscles close the rima glottidis. The cricothyroid muscle tilts the thryoid cartilage forward and thus tenses the vocal cord (higher pitch of voice; *Atlas, 530.2*). Review the nerve supply to the laryngeal muscles (*Atlas, 543.1, 660*).

Interior of Larynx

The **cavity of the larynx** has three compartments (fig. 8-63 or *Atlas, 631.1*):

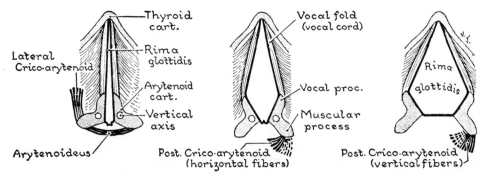

FIG. 8-62. The rima glottidis is controlled by various laryngeal muscles. (From *Grant's Method of Anatomy.*)

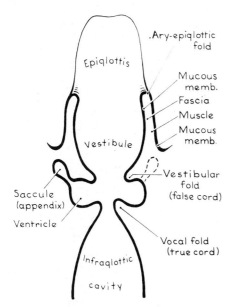

FIG. 8-63. Subdivisions of interior of larynx.

1. **Vestibule,** the upper compartment above the vestibular folds.
2. **Ventricle,** the middle compartment between vestibular and vocal folds.
3. **Infraglottic cavity,** below the vocal folds and continuous with the trachea.

Inspect the interior of the larynx from above. Observe the **vestibular folds** (ventricular folds; false cords) lying superolateral to the vocal cords (true cords).

The next objective is to expose the interior of the larynx. With heavy scissors, split the trachea, lamina of cricoid, and arytenoid muscle in the posterior median plane. In addition, cut the arch of the cricoid cartilage in the anterior median plane. Now, unfold the larynx (*Atlas, 632*).

Identify the **vestibular** and **vocal folds** (*Atlas, 632*). On each side, the depression between the two folds is the ventricle. The ventricle may extend into a recess, the *saccule* (fig. 8-63). With a probe, explore ventricles and recesses.

Remove the mucous membrane from one half of the interior of the larynx (fig. 8-64; *Atlas, 632*). Start at the cricoid cartilage and work upward. Strip the mucosa from the triangular **cricothyroid ligament or conus elasticus.** Observe that this membrane is attached inferiorly to the upper border of the cricoid ring. Superiorly, the free edge of the conus elasticus is thickened as the **vocal ligament.** The vocal ligament forms the basis for the vocal fold.

Next, remove the mucosa from the epiglottis and expose the epiglottic cartilage. Examine its attachment to the thyroid lamina.

Peel the mucosa from the area extending between lateral border of epiglottic cartilage and arytenoid cartilage (fig. 8-64; *Atlas, 632*). The exposed membrane is the **quadrangular membrane.** Its free lower

border is the vestibular ligament which supports the vestibular fold.

Realize that the laryngeal mucosa above the vocal cords is supplied with sensory fibers by the **internal laryngeal nerve** (*Atlas, 660*). Once again, trace this nerve through the thyrohyoid membrane toward the interior of the larynx.

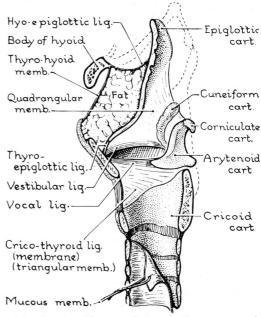

FIG. 8-64. Interior of larynx, after removal mucous membrane.

Middle Ear

General Remarks

The middle ear cavity or **tympanic cavity** is an air space contained within the temporal bone. Refer to schematic diagrams of the middle ear (fig. 8-65; *Atlas, 633–633.2*), and study its boundaries:

1. *Laterally,* the **tympanic membrane.** The small portion of tympanic cavity above the tympanic membrane is the **epitympanic recess.**
2. *Posteriorly,* the mastoid wall. The superior portion of the wall is open. Here, the **aditus** leads to the **antrum** and **air cells** of the **mastoid process.**
3. *Anteriorly,* the **auditory tube** leads to the nasopharynx. Just inferior to the auditory tube and anterior to the tympanic cavity is the **carotid canal** (fig. 8-65 or *Atlas, 640.1*).
4. *Medially,* the structures of the inner ear are contained within the temporal bone.
5. *Inferiorly,* the floor of the tympanic cavity is closely related to the **jugular fossa** in which the superior jugular bulb is located (fig. 8-65 or *Atlas, 640.1*).

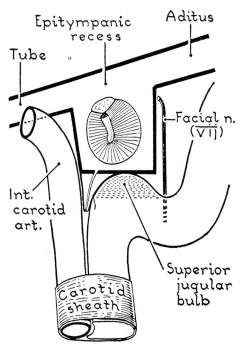

FIG. 8-65. The tympanic cavity and its relations to major vessels and nerve VII. (From *Grant's Method of Anatomy.*)

6. *Superiorly,* the roof or **tegmen tympani** is formed by a plate of the petrous portion of the temporal bone (*Atlas, 633.1*). The tegmen tympani separates the middle ear from the middle cranial fossa.

Each tympanic cavity contains a chain of 3 **auditory ossicles** which connect the tympanic membrane with the inner ear. The middle ear cavity and its associated recesses and air cells are covered with mucous membrane.

The **facial nerve** (VII) traverses the temporal bone. Its course is closely related to the inner and the middle ear. A branch of the facial nerve, the chorda tympani, passes between two of the auditory ossicles.

Bony Landmarks

Refer to a skull and identify the following pertinent bony landmarks:
1. **Mastoid process** (*Atlas, 557*).
2. **External acoustic meatus.**
3. **Suprameatal spine,** just behind the upper part of the external acoustic meatus.
4. **Internal acoustic meatus** (*Atlas, 512*).
5. **Hiatus of facial canal,** for greater petrosal nerve.
6. **Tegmen tympani,** a plate of the petrous part of the temporal bone, located in the middle cranial fossa.
7. **Jugular fossa** and jugular foramen (*Atlas, 569*).
8. Bony portion of **auditory tube.**

9. **Carotid canal.**
10. **Stylomastoid foramen.**

Dissection

Carry this dissection out on one side only. The objectives of this dissection are: (1) to display the mastoid air cells; (2) to expose the structures housed in the tympanic cavity; and (3) to explore the walls of the tympanic cavity.

First Saw Cut. Saw coronally through the temporal bone. Start the saw cut just behind the suprameatal spine (*Atlas, 557*). Carry the cut into the cranial cavity, dividing the bone into two pieces. Now, examine the **mastoid air cells.** Find the **antrum.** From the antrum pass a fine nylon thread through the **aditus** into the tympanic cavity (*Atlas, 633.1*).

Identify certain soft structures which are relevant to this dissection. In the *middle cranial fossa,* remove the trigeminal ganglion and its 3 divisions. Define the **internal carotid artery** and the **middle meningeal artery** (or the foramen spinosum). In the *posterior cranial fossa,* identify the **facial nerve** (VII) and the **vestibulocochlear nerve** (VIII) as they pass through the internal acoustic meatus. Pass a probe into the meatus to gauge its length (approximately 12 mm). Then, remove the roof of the meatus. The bone is very hard. Use fine bone pliers. Protect your eyes against flying chips of bone. Observe the course of the **facial nerve** (*Atlas, 648*). Identify the **geniculate ganglion** and the **greater petrosal nerve.** Review these nervous structures (*Atlas, 657*).

Next, carefully remove the tegmen tympani. With sharp, pointed forceps remove the **incus.** The incus is the strongest and the intermediate of the 3 auditory ossicles. Leave the malleus attached to the tympanic membrane.

Second Saw Cut.* Stabilize the temporal bone as much as possible. Insert a fine saw into the gap created by the removal of the incus. The saw cut is slightly oblique and parallel to the slope of the tympanic membrane. In front, the cut passes between internal carotid artery and middle meningeal artery (foramen spinosum). Carefully split the bone into a medial and lateral piece. With skill, the auditory tube will also be split longitudinally (*Atlas, 641.1*).

---

* This exposure was devised by R. D. Laurenson: *A Rapid Method of Dissecting the Middle Ear.* Anatomical Record, Vol. 151, 1965.

Remove the lateral piece. On it, examine the *lateral wall* of the tympanic cavity (*Atlas, 641*). Note the **tympanic membrane** with the attached handle of the **malleus.** The head of the malleus rises into the epitympanic recess. The **chorda tympani** is covered with mucous membrane. Identify it as it crosses the handle of the malleus medially. On the isolated piece, break down the anterior and inferior walls of the bony external acoustic meatus (*Atlas, 634*). Now, examine the lateral aspect of the tympanic membrane. Note that the membrane faces laterally, downward, and forward.

Anteriorly, the tympanic cavity leads to the **auditory tube**. Posteriorly, it leads to the *aditus ad antrum* (*Atlas, 639, 641*). Verify these facts in the cadaver.

Examine the *medial wall* of the cavity (*Atlas, 637, 641.1*). The features verge on the microscopic. Therefore, a magnifying lens is of great assistance. Observe at least the following features:

1. *Promontory*, a gentle elevation on the medial wall, facing the tympanic membrane.
2. *Stapes*, still in position in the *fenestra vestibuli* (oval window). You may be able to make out the delicate *stapedius tendon*, about 1 mm long, passing from the pyramid to the stapes.
3. *Fenestra cochleae* (round window), at the bottom of a depression postero-inferior to the promontory (*Atlas, 637.1*).
4. *Semicircular canals*. Remove the mucosa from the medial wall of the tympanic cavity. With a probe, break into one of the 3 semicircular canals (*Atlas, 637*).
5. *Tensor tympani* (*Atlas, 641.2*), passing in a mucous fold from the medial wall to the upper part of the handle of the malleus. (Its tendon was divided by the saw cut.)
6. *Facial nerve* in the facial canal (*Atlas, 641.1*). Follow the nerve centrally from the stylomastoid foramen. Use a probe to force the canal open.

If you wish to dissect the inner ear in detail, utilize a decalcified temporal bone, Refer to the following figures: *Atlas, 648, 648.1, and 658.*

I.
FETUS

Estimate the age of the human fetus available for dissection. The age of the fetus is often determined from its crown-rump length (sitting height). Estimation of age may also be based on the *total length* (vertex to heel). Utilize this simple and easily remembered formula to determine the approximate age of the fetus:

Time In Lunar Months (1 lunar month = 4 weeks)	Total Fetal Lengths (vertex to heel)

$$1 \times 1 = 1 \text{ cm}$$
$$2 \times 2 = 4 \text{ cm}$$
$$3 \times 3 = 9 \text{ cm}$$
$$4 \times 4 = 16 \text{ cm}$$
$$5 \times 5 = 25 \text{ cm}$$
$$6 \times 5 = 30 \text{ cm}$$
$$7 \times 5 = 35 \text{ cm}$$
$$8 \times 5 = 40 \text{ cm}$$
$$9 \times 5 = 45 \text{ cm}$$
$$10 \times 5 = 50 \text{ cm}$$

Examples: After 3 lunar months or 12 weeks, the total length of the fetus is approximately 9 cm. A fetus measuring 20 cm in total length is approximately 4½ lunar months or 18 weeks old. After 10 lunar months or 40 weeks, the mature newborn measures 50 cm from vertex to heel.

Display of Thoracic and Abdominal Viscera

Thoracic Incisions (fig. A-1). Make two transverse incisions through the skin (*A* to *B; C* to *D*). Reflect skin and pectorales muscles. With scissors, cut through the soft, pliable ribcage from *D* to *B* and from *C* to *A*. Next, cut across the ribcage and sternum from *A* to *B*. Elevate the anterior chest wall. Cut across it from *C* to *D*, at a level above the diaphragm. Now, the thoracic viscera are exposed.

Abdominal Incisions (fig. A-1). These incisions must be made in such a manner that the umbilical vein and the two umbilical arteries are not destroyed. Starting at point *C*, cut with scissors through the thin diaphragm and enter the abdominal cavity. Cut

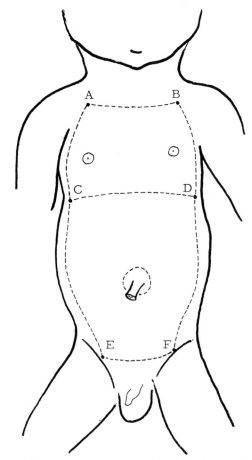

FIG. A-1. Incisions to expose thoracic and abdominal viscera of fetus.

through all layers of the abdominal wall, and carry the incision to the midinguinal point (*E*). Make an equivalent incision on the left side of the fetus (*D* to *F*). Carefully lift up the right triangular flap of abdominal wall (*D* to *C* to *E*), and identify the *umbilical ring* at the inner surface of the abdominal wall. Here, several structures converge:

1. *Falciform ligament.* Along its free margin identify the relatively thick *umbilical vein.*

2. *Right and left umbilical arteries.*
3. *Urachus*, contained in the median umbilical fold between the two umbilical arteries.

Using the scissor technique, dissect these structures (1.–3.) from the abdominal wall, but leave them attached to the umbilical ring. Remove the entire abdominal wall, with the exception of a small circular region around the umbilicus. Now, the abdominal viscera are exposed. The umbilical region and the important structures converging upon it are still intact.

Cardiovascular and Respiratory Systems

Observe that the unexpanded *lungs* do not conceal the *pericardial sac*. The *thymus* is large and covers the upper part of the pericardial sac anteriorly.

Identify the *umbilical vein*. In the living fetus, this vessel carries oxygenated blood. Follow the vein along the free margin of the falciform ligament to the *left portal vein*. Most of the blood by-passes the liver via the *ductus venosus*, which connects the left portal vein with the inferior vena cava. The ductus venosus occupies a fissure behind the liver. To expose this duct, dissect the liver away piece by piece. Demonstrate the continuity of the ductus venosus with the *inferior vena cava*.

To facilitate examination of the heart, remove the lungs, the thymus, and the brachiocephalic veins. Throw a piece of lung tissue into water. Does it float or sink? Of forensic importance: The compact lungs of a still-born child sink. In contrast, aerated lungs float in water.

Incise the *pericardial sac*. Open the *right atrium*. Identify the large *foramen ovale*. Realize that most of the blood from the *inferior vena cava* passes through the foramen ovale into the left atrium. From there, the blood passes through the left ventricle to the ascending aorta and the aortic arch. Follow the course of blood from the *superior vena cava* through the right atrium, the tricuspid orifice, and through the right ventricle into the *pulmonary trunk*. From there, follow its course through the large *ductus arteriosus* into the aorta. Note that the ductus arteriosus reaches the aortic arch just inferior to the origin of the left subclavian artery (fig. A-2).

Observe that the diameter of the pulmonary trunk is equal to that of the aorta. In the fetus, the wall of the right ventricle is as thick as that of the left.

Follow the two *umbilical arteries* from the internal iliac ateries to the umbilical cord. Are there any sensory nerves in the umbilical cord? Is it painful for the newborn to have his or her umbilical cord cut?

In the *thoracic cavity*, find the *two vagi* and the *phrenic nerves*. Identify the *splanchnic nerves*. The *diaphragm* is only a thin translucent membrane.

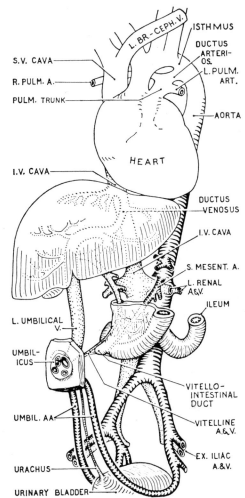

Fɪɢ. A-2. Fetal circulation (After Cullen). (From *Grant's Method of Anatomy.*)

Gastrointestinal System

The *liver* is very large. Note the empty *stomach*. The *cecum*, with the attached appendix, may not yet be fully descended. The cylindrical *rectum* almost fills the lesser pelvis. Identify the various parts of the gastrointestinal tract. The intestines are either empty or contain black meconium (consisting of epithelial cells, mucus, and bile). The *spleen* is conspicuous.

Remove the gastrointestinal tract, the liver, and the spleen. Find the pancreas.

Genito-urinary System

Observe the large *suprarenal glands* covering the upper poles of the *kidneys*. Note the lobulated surface of the kidneys. Follow the sizeable *ureters* to the *urinary bladder*. Identify the *urachus* which extends from the apex of the bladder to the umbilical ring.

If the fetus is a *male*, look for the *testes*. How far have they descended? During the 7th month, the testes are at the level of the inguinal canal. By the end of the 8th month, they are usually within the scrotal sac. Is the *processus vaginalis* patent? Note that the *scrotum* of younger specimens is formed but empty.

If the fetus is a *female*, note *uterus, uterine tubes,* and *ovaries*.

Head and Neck

Cut away the auricle. Remove the scalp. Note the following (*Atlas, 602 A,B,C*):
1. There is no bony external acoustic meatus, but only a *tympanic ring*.
2. The *tympanic membrane* is very close to the surface.
3. There is no mastoid process. This leaves the *facial nerve* relatively unprotected (injury to facial nerve after application of obstetrical forceps).
4. The *primary teeth* have not yet erupted. Cut across the maxilla or the mandible, and look for a *developing tooth*.
5. There are no air sinuses. Therefore, the face is small.
6. Identify the *anterior fonticulus* (fontanella) and the *posterior fonticulus*. These structures are of obstetrical and pediatric importance. Note the thin and pliable bones of the calvaria.
7. Observe the *frontal or metopic suture* which separates the two halves of the frontal bone (fig.

A-3 or *Atlas, 602 A*). Remember: In the adult, this suture is normally absent (*compare Atlas, 460*); but in about 2% of all cases it persists.

Further Examination

Feel free to examine any structure of interest. If the brain is well preserved, note its incomplete development. Examine eyelids, digits, nails, and hair. Make a longitudinal section through a long bone. It starts to ossify during the 2nd fetal month. Observe that the ends of the bone are cartilaginous.

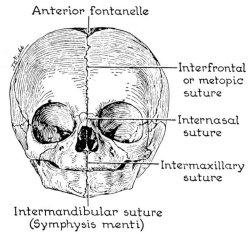

FIG. A-3. The skull at birth (norma frontalis). (From *Grant's Method of Anatomy*.)

II.
LUMBAR APPROACH TO KIDNEY

General Remarks and Orientation

The **lumbar renal approach or retroperitoneal approach** to the kidney is an efficient surgical procedure. Contamination of the peritoneal cavity is avoided. Thus, the lumbar renal approach is indicated in a variety of renal disorders (inflammatory renal disease; renal cystic disease; tumors; calculi).

Level of Kidneys (fig. A-4 or *Atlas, 104.2 D*). In the recumbent position, the kidneys are at the level of vertebrae T_{12} to L_3. Usually, the right kidney is slightly lower (1 cm) than the left one. The kidneys may move up and down, depending on changes in

posture and on respiratory movements. Also, there are individual variations in the precise positions of the kidneys.

Essential Posterior Relations (fig. A-4 or *Atlas, 104.2 D*). These relations must be understood before attempting the retroperitoneal approach. The **upper pole** or end of the right kidney rises to the level of **rib 12**. The upper pole of the left kidney may be positioned as high as rib 11. The upper extremities of the kidneys (with the attached suprarenal glands) are separated from the pleural cavities by the diaphragm. The medial aspect of the posterior surface of the kidney is in contact with the **quadratus lumborum.**

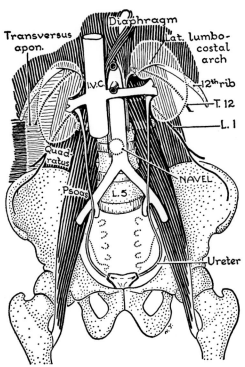

FIG. A-4. Posterior relations of kidneys. (From *Grant's Method of Anatomy*.)

The lateral aspect of the posterior surface is in contact with the **aponeurosis of the transversus abdominis.** The lumbar renal approach is greatly facilitated by the fact that the quadratus lumborum has an *oblique lateral border.* Appreciate this fact. (If the quadratus lumborum were square, and if it were running from the iliac crest to the entire length of rib 12, this thick muscle would greatly impede the lumbar renal approach.)

Two nerves, which must not be cut during surgery, are in close relation to the posterior surface of the kidney (fig. A-4 or *Atlas, 104.2 D*): **Subcostal nerve** (T_{12}), just below rib 12; and **iliohypogastric nerve** (L_1), crossing obliquely the inferior pole of the kidney.

Important topographic knowledge can be gained by studying a transverse section through the abdomen and kidneys (*Atlas, 178*). Again, note that the posterior surface of the kidney is related to the quadratus lumborum and the aponeurosis of the transversus abdominis.

Review the tissues surrounding the kidney (*Atlas, 178*):

1. **Fatty renal capsule** (adipose capsule; perinephric fatty tissue). This fat surrounds the kidney. It is thickest at the margins of the kidney. At the hilus, the renal vessels and the ureter are embedded in the fatty tissue.

2. **Renal fascia** (of Gerota). It encloses both the kidney and its fatty capsule. It will be obvious that the renal fascia must be incised in order to gain access to the kidney. Dorsal to the renal fascia is the **paranephric fat.**

Dissection

Place the cadaver into the prone or the lateral position. If not already done, remove the skin superior to the iliac crest as indicated in *Atlas, 173*. Identify the *thoracolumbar fascia*, the **latissimus dorsi,** and the **external oblique** of the abdominal wall.

Now, incise the latissimus dorsi along the course of rib 12. Reflect the muscle. Palpate rib 12. Identify the thin *serratus posterior inferior.*

Next, incise the **external oblique** just inferior to the tip of rib 12, and turn it laterally (*Atlas, 174*). Make an incision through the **internal oblique** parallel to the free posterior border of the external oblique. Carry the cut all the way to the iliac crest. Reflect the internal oblique medially. Now, the **aponeurosis of the transversus abdominis** is exposed. Note that the aponeurosis is pierced by the **subcostal** and **iliohypogastric nerves.** These nerves must not be cut. Accordingly, the aponeurosis of the transversus must be incised between the two nerves (*Atlas, 175*).

Divide the aponeurosis of the transversus abdominis (*Atlas, 175*). Reflect the aponeurosis medially and expose the **quadratus lumborum.** Extend the incision upward. If necessary, detach the serratus posterior inferior from rib 12. Using blunt dissection, remove any fat you may encounter. This is the *paranephric fat* outside the renal fascia.

Now, the **renal fascia** is exposed. Incise it. Palpate the kidney. Remove the **fatty renal capsule** posterior to the kidney. The structures of the hilus (renal artery, vein, renal pelvis and ureter) lie just anterior to the quadratus lumborum (fig. A-4 or *Atlas, 104.2 D*). Gain access to these structures by retracting the quadratus lumborum medially and gently pulling the kidney laterally. Understand that the right kidney is less freely movable than the left one, since the right renal vein is much shorter than the left renal vein. Identify the **renal pelvis.** Realize that the actual surgical approach must be more delicate than the gross anatomical exposure of the kidney.

As was pointed out earlier (pp. 45–46), on occasion it is advantageous to reach the kidneys and their vessels via the transabdominal route.

III.

JOINTS

Joints of the Lower Extremity

Sacroiliac Joint

The **sacroiliac joint** was briefly discussed earlier (chap. 4, p. 50). On the right side, the hip bone was partially disarticulated to allow better access to the structures contained in the pelvis (chap. 4, p. 55). Use an intact sacroiliac joint for the following dissection (left side of cadaver, or separate specimen).

The synovial sacroiliac joint (articulation) is formed between the auricular surfaces of the **sacrum** and the **ilium** (*Atlas*, 222). Obtain an isolated hip bone (os coxae), and observe the articular **auricular surface** of the ilium. Note the corresponding **auricular surface** in the isolated sacrum. Note that each bone has a **tuberosity** dorsal to its auricular surface. Procure an articulated pelvis and observe:

1. The auricular surfaces are in apposition (*Atlas*, 219, 221, 223).
2. The tuberosities are separated by a deep cleft (fig. A-5 or *Atlas*, 223).

Turn to the cadaver which should be in the prone position (face down). Clean the following ligaments:

1. **Sacrotuberous ligament.** Scrape the gluteus maximus from it. Define the attachments of the ligament, and clean its upward extension to the posterior iliac spines.
2. **Sacrospinous ligament.** Define its attachments (figs. A-6, A-7).
3. **Posterior sacroiliac ligaments** (fig. A-6). Observe long and short fasciculi which pass between sacrum and ilium in various directions.
4. **Interosseous sacroiliac ligament** (figs. A-5; A-7). It is exceedingly strong. It is the essential ligament of the joint. The interosseous sacroiliac ligament binds together the sacral and iliac tuberosities. This fact is best appreciated on cross section (fig. A-5 or *Atlas*, 223). To expose the ligament, you must remove the posterior (dorsal) sacroiliac ligaments.

In front, identify the thin **ventral sacroiliac ligament.** Cut through this ligament which forms the ventral part of the joint capsule. Forcibly separate ilium and sacrum. Examine the cartilage-covered auricular surfaces of the joint.

Understand: Considerable weight is transmitted to the sacrum by the superimposed vertebral column.

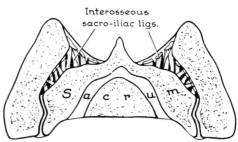

FIG. A-5. Sacroiliac joint on transverse section. Note the interosseous sacroiliac ligaments anchoring the sacrum to the right and the left ilium. (From *Grant's Method of Anatomy*.)

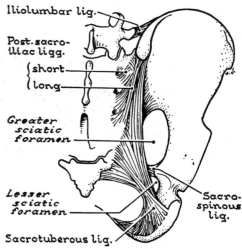

FIG. A-6. Ligaments of the pelvis; posterior view. (From *Grant's Method of Anatomy*.)

This force causes a tendency of the upper end of the sacrum to rotate forward, and of the lower end of the sacrum to rotate backward (fig. A-7). The forward rotation of the sacrum is mainly resisted by the interosseous sacroiliac ligaments and the posterior sacroiliac ligaments. The backward rotation of the sacrum is resisted by the sacrospinous and sacrotuberous ligaments (fig. A-7). On occasion, you will find synostosis (bony fusion) of the joint (*Atlas*, 223.1).

Hip Joint (see chap. 5, pp. 87–88)

Knee Joint (see chap. 5, pp. 86–87)

Ankle Joint (see chap. 5, p. 85)

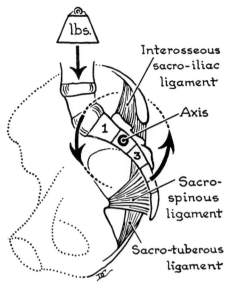

FIG. A-7. Ligaments resisting rotation of the sacrum. (From *Grant's Method of Anatomy*.)

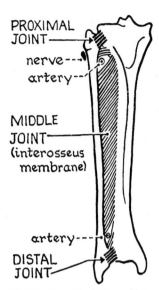

FIG. A-8. The tibiofibular articulations. Note unity of direction of ligamentous fibers. (From *Grant's Method of Anatomy*.)

Tibiofibular Joints

Tibiofibular Joints (fig. A-8). The fibula is moored to the tibia at its upper end, along its shaft, and at its lower end, at proximal, middle, and distal joints.

Examine an isolated fibula and a tibia. Note (*Atlas*, 315): A small, flat, round facet on the head of the fibula; a similar facet on the posterolateral aspect of the lateral condyle of the tibia.

In the cadaver, remove the popliteus tendon and the popliteus bursa posterior to the **proximal tibifibular joint**. Note that the joint capsule is strengthened by strong anterior and weak posterior fibers. Open the capsule, and observe the small synovial cavity of this gliding joint.

The *middle* and *distal tibiofibular joints* are *syndesmoses*. The **interosseous membrane (middle joint)** extends down the respective sides of tibia and fibula, producing a sharp line on each bone. Strip the muscles from the front and the back of the interosseous membrane. Note the oval aperture between proximal tibiofibular joint and upper free margin of interosseous membrane: The *anterior tibial artery* passes through this opening (fig. A-8). Observe the gap between distal tibiofibular joint and the lower free margin of interosseous membrane: The *perforating branch of the peroneal artery* passes through this opening (fig. A-8; *Atlas*, 244).

Clean the anterior and posterior ligaments of the **distal tibiofibular joint** (fig. A-8; *Atlas*, 332, 338, 340). These are the strong **anterior inferior and posterior inferior tibiofibular ligaments**. Grasp tibia and fibula well above the ankle, alternately squeezing the bones together and relaxing them. Note the yielding of the distal tibiofibular joint.

Joints of the Foot

Joints of Inversion and Eversion (see chap. 5, pp. 85–86)

Joints Distal to the Transverse Tarsal Joint

Intertarsal, Tarsometatarsal, and Intermetatarsal Joints. Review the bones of the foot (*Atlas*, 311–314, 343). Frequently refer to *Atlas 332 and 343*. Observe the **dorsal cuneonavicular ligament**. Cut through the ligaments, and open the **cuneonavicular joint** from the dorsum of the foot. Carry the incision to the **cubonavicular joint**. Explore the extent of the joint: Anteriorly, it is continuous with the **intercuneiform and cuneocuboid joints**.

Note the bursa deep to the insertion of the tibialis anterior. This bursa communicates with the **first cuneometatarsal joint** (*Atlas*, 332, 343). Open this joint from the dorsum of the foot. Leave the plantar ligaments (*Atlas*, 342) intact to act as hinges. Coming from above, open the joints between the tarsal and metatarsal bones. Note and open the **intermetatarsal joints** (between metatarsal bones).

Metatarsophalangeal and Interphalangeal Joints (*Atlas*, 343). These are hinges, like the corresponding joints in the hand (compare Appendix, Joints of the Upper Extremity, p. 173). Identify the **plantar ligaments** (plates) of the metatarsophalangeal joints. Observe the two sesamoid bones beneath the head of the first metatarsal (*Atlas*, 331). Examine an **interphalangeal joint**. Observe that it possesses a plantar ligament and collateral ligaments.

Joints of the Upper Extremity

Sternoclavicular Joint

In the articulated skeleton, observe the relations

between **sternum** and **clavicle** (*Atlas, 391*). Identify the **clavicular notch** of the manubrium sterni (*Atlas, 393*). This notch and the adjacent parts of the first costal cartilage articulate with the enlarged sternal (medial) end of the clavicle.

Turn to the cadaver. Anterior to the **sternoclavicular joint** is the tendon of the sternomastoid. Remove it. Dorsal to the joint are the broad, fleshy, strap-like sternohyoid and sternothyroid muscles (*Atlas, 533*).

Note the superolateral direction of the dense, parallel fibers of the anterior part of the **joint capsule**. This is the anterior sternoclavicular ligament (*Atlas, 533*). The costoclavicular ligament runs obliquely from the first costal cartilage to the inferior surface of the clavicle near its medial end (*Atlas, 19; not labelled*). Clean the ligaments.

Cut through the anterior sternoclavicular ligament. In doing so, keep the blade of the scalpel close to the manubrium. Reflect the ligament. Now, the **articular disc** is exposed (*Atlas, 534*). Note that it divides the articular cavity into two parts. Observe that the articular disc is attached in such a manner as to resist medial displacement of the clavicle: Inferiorly, it is attached to the first costal cartilage; superiorly, it is attached to the clavicle (fig. A-9).

On yourself, palpate the **movements** at the sternoclavicular joint. Move the scapula, and with it the clavicle. Observe that the sternoclavicular joint allows a limited amount of movement in nearly every direction.

Acromioclavicular Joint

Review the essential bony landmarks relevant to the acromioclavicular articulation and its associated ligaments (*Atlas, 1*): **Acromion** and **coracoid process** of scapula; **lateral end of clavicle.**

Remove the deltoid and the trapezius from the acromion and the lateral end of the clavicle. Thus, expose the **acromioclavicular joint** (*Atlas, 35*). The joint is subcutaneous; below it lies the subacromial bursa.

Identify the strong and important **coracoclavicular ligament** (fig. A-9; *Atlas, 36; 36.1*). Clean the

two parts of the ligament (conoid lig. and trapezoid lig.).

Open the synovial acromioclavicular joint from above. Look for a small articular disc hanging into the joint cavity. Remove the joint capsule completely; i.e. separate acromion from lateral end of clavicle.

Now, with the acromioclavicular joint disarticulated, the important functions of the coracoclavicular ligament can be studied. Observe (fig. A-9; *Atlas, 36.1*):

1. The ligament prevents the scapula from being driven medially.
2. As long as the ligament remains intact, the acromion cannot be driven under the clavicle.

On yourself, palpate the subcutaneous acromioclavicular joint. Observe: The joint enables the scapula to move vertically on the chest wall (as when shrugging the shoulders). It is essential to free elevation of the upper limb.

Shoulder Joint (see chap. 7, p. 112)

Elbow Joint (see chap. 7, p. 112)

Radio-ulnar Joints

The two bones of the forearm are united at the proximal, intermediate or middle, and distal radio-ulnar joints. The necessary rotary movements during supination and pronation take place in the proximal and distal radio-ulnar joints (fig. A-10).

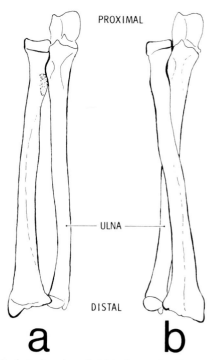

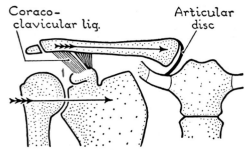

FIG. A-9. Structures having unity of function: Articular disc and coracoclavicular ligament. (From *Grant's Method of Anatomy.*)

FIG. A-10. Anterior view of right ulna and radius; *a*, in supination; *b*, in pronation. Note proximal and distal radio-ulnar joints.

The **proximal radioulnar joint** (articulation) was considered with the elbow joint (see chap. 7, pp. 111–112).

Intermediate (Middle) Radio-ulnar Joint (*Atlas*, 52). The shafts of the radius and ulna are united by the **interosseous membrane.** Remove or reflect all muscles from the anterior and posterior forearm, and expose the interosseous membrane. Note the direction of its fibers. The general direction of the fibers of the membrane is such that an upward thrust to the radius is transmitted to the ulna. Understand: During an upward thrust (fall on the hand), the forces are transmitted from hand via wrist joint to radius, from radius via interosseous membrane to ulna, from ulna (and radius) to humerus.

Note that blood vessels are closely applied to the interosseous membrane, and that small vessels pierce the membrane (*Atlas*, 52).

Distal Radio-ulnar Joint (fig. A-10). Cut through the anular ligament and release the head of the radius. Cut the interosseous membrane. Pass the blade of the scalpel through a sac-like recess, the **sacciform recess** (*Atlas*, 90). Now, enter the distal radio-ulnar joint. Do not injure the triangular **articular disc** (*Atlas*, 90, 91, 94).

Swing the radius laterally and view the **articular disc.** Observe:

1. It is fibrocartilaginous. Its apex and its anterior and posterior margins are ligamentous.
2. The apex is attached to the styloid process of the ulna.
3. The base of the triangular disc is attached to the ulnar notch of the radius.
4. The ligamentous borders of the disc spread far laterally on the radius.
5. Commonly, the cartilaginous part of the disc is perforated (the disc is subjected to constant pressure and friction).

Wrist Joint (see chap. 7, pp. 111–112)

Small Joints of the Hand

Review the bones of the hand (*Atlas*, 62, 86). The osseofibrous **carpal tunnel** has already been opened (chap. 7, p. 107). Remove all contents from the carpal tunnel. Trace the tendon of the flexor carpi radialis through its special tunnel to the 2nd metacarpal (*Atlas*, 72). Observe that the tubercle of the scaphoid acts as a pulley for the tendon. Note that the lunate bulges conspicuously into the carpal tunnel (*Atlas*, 91).

Clean the **intercarpal, carpometacarpal,** and **intermetacarpal ligaments.** Open all joints from the palmar aspect. First, open the **midcarpal joint (transverse carpal joint)** by entering the scalpel between tubercle of scaphoid and tubercle of trapezium (*Atlas*, 93). Observe the sinuous surfaces of the opposed bones. Note that synovial folds project into the joint.

Next, open the **carpometacarpal joints** (*Atlas*, 95). Observe that the carpometacarpal joint of the thumb (digit 1) has a loose capsule with parallel fibers. Manipulate the metacarpal bones. Observe the hinge movements at the bases of the 4th and 5th carpometacarpal joints. The flexion possible at these two joints allows the grip of the hand to be more secure (*Atlas*, 95.2).

Joints of the Digits

In the clefts between the fingers, the lumbrical muscles and the digital nerves and vessels pass anterior to the **deep transverse metacarpal ligaments.** The interossei pass dorsal to the ligaments (*Atlas*, 69–72). Define the upper and lower borders of the quadrate ligaments (*Atlas*, 72). On each side, the deep transverse metacarpal ligaments are continuous with the palmar ligaments which form the proximal limit of the posterior wall of the fibrous digital flexor sheath (*Atlas*, 72).

Metacarpophalangeal Joints (*Atlas*, 96). Cut one or more of the deep transverse metacarpal ligaments. Remove the interossei and the dorsal extensor expansion. Clean a pair of collateral ligaments. They are triangular and important. A *cord-like part* passes to the base of the adjacent phalanx; a *fan-like part* passes to the side of the palmar ligament. Verify: The strong, cord-like parts of the collateral ligaments are eccentrically attached to the flat metacarpal heads. The ligaments are slack during extension and taut during flexion. Therefore, the fingers cannot be spread (abducted) unless the hand is opened.

Interphalangeal Joints (*Atlas*, 96). Note the collateral ligaments of the interphalangeal joints. These are hinge joints. Explore the synovial cavity of the joints. Note the articular surfaces which are covered with smooth cartilage.

IV.

DISSECTION OF EYEBALL OF BULL

General Remarks

The dissection of the *eyeball of the bull* is a convenient way to acquire a general knowledge of the gross anatomical features of the human eye.

The **eyeball or bulbus oculi** has **three concentric coats** (figs. A-11, A-12; *Atlas, 523.1*):

1. **External or fibrous coat:** *sclera* and *cornea*.
2. **Middle or vascular coat:** *choroid, ciliary body* and *iris*.
3. **Internal or retinal coat:**
   a. *Outer layer* of pigmented cells
   b. *Inner layer.* The cells of this layer are nervous (visual) posterior to the ora serrata.

The **four refractive media** are:

1. *Cornea*
2. *Aqueous humor*
3. *Lens*
4. *Vitreous body*

Dissection

Clean the exterior of the eyeball or bulb by removing the adherent fat, muscles, and vessels. Leave the stump of the optic nerve intact. In front, sever the conjunctiva at the corneoscleral junction (margin), and remove it.

Divide the bulb into posterior and anterior halves by cutting with a sharp scalpel (new blade!) around the equator. During the process, you will successively cut the sclera, choroid, retina, and the vitreous body.

Examination of Posterior Half; Inner Aspect. The **retina** is dull and gray like an exposed photographic film, and exceedingly friable. It is held in position, applied to the choroid, by the vitreous body.

Gently scoop out the jelly-like **vitreous body** with the handle of a scalpel. Now, the **retina** is no longer firmly applied to the choroid. As a result, it falls into folds, except at the optic disc. The **optic disc** is the site where the fibers of the optic nerve pierce the sclera, choroid, and outer retinal layer to spread out into the inner (optic) layer of the retina. The disc is a blind spot.

The **choroid** is the thin and pigmented vascular middle coat (fig. A-12). Generally, it is easily detached intact from the sclera. At several spots, however, the choroid is bound to be sclera of the posterior half of the bulb:

1. Where it is pierced by the optic nerve;
2. Where the vorticose veins leave it near the equator to pierce the sclera.

There are certain differences between the human eye and the bull's eye: The pupil of the bull's eye is not round. There is no macula in the eye of the bull. In the bull, but not in man, a wide

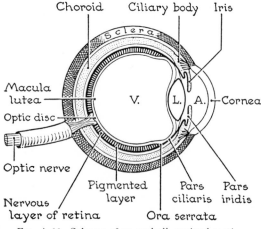

FIG. A-11. Scheme of an eyeball, sagittal section. (From *Grant's Method of Anatomy*.)

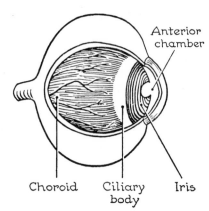

FIG. A-12. Eyeball of a bull, middle coat exposed. (From *Grant's Method of Anatomy*.)

triangular area of the choroid above the level of the optic disc has a greenish-blue metallic sheen. This is due to the presence of a fibrous sheet, the tapetum, between the layers of the choroid.

Examination of Anterior Half; Inner Aspect

(*Atlas, 523.2 D*). Observe the anterior part of the vitreous body. Gently remove it. The dull gray optic part of the retina ends well in front of the equator in a slightly scalloped margin, the **ora serrata.**

Anterior to the ora serrata lies the ciliary zone. Here, about 70 black finger-like ridges, the **ciliary processes,** converge on the equator of the **lens.** Note that the lens is suspended by numerous **zonular fibers** (*Atlas, 523.1, 523.2 D*).

Dissection from the Front (fig. A-13). The sclera is white and tough. It is continuous with the transparent **cornea.** Through the cornea observe the dark **iris** which surrounds the **pupil.** Behind the pupil is the lens.

With a sharp scalpel, incise the cornea vertically. With scissors, cut horizontally along the corneoscleral junction. Leave the right quarter of the cornea intact. You have now opened the **anterior chamber** which, in the living, is filled with aqueous humor. Place a probe into the angle between iris and cornea, the **iridocorneal angle** (fig. A-14; *Atlas, 523.1*). Pass the point of a probe through the pupil and into the space between lens and posterior surface of iris. The probe is now in the **posterior chamber.**

Remove a section of the **iris** (fig. A-15). Examine the thus exposed **posterior chamber** which is triangular on cross section. It is bounded anteriorly by the iris, posteriorly by the lens and zonular fibers, and laterally by the ends of the ciliary processes (*Atlas, 523.1*).

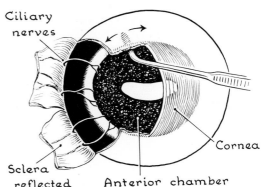

Fig. A-14. Bull's eye, dissection from the front, II.

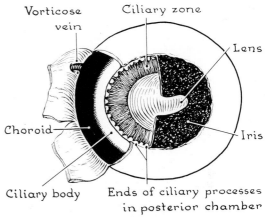

Fig. A-15. Bull's eye, dissection from the front, III.

Cut horizontally through the front of the capsule of the lens. The lens will pop out; if not, it can be easily expressed. Note that the anterior surface of the lens is less curved than the posterior surface.

Place the point of a probe in the iridocorneal angle (fig. A-14). Break through the firm attachment of the ciliary muscle to the anterior limit of the sclera. Detach the ciliary muscle widely. Press the probe against the sclera in order not to damage the delicate choroidal coat. With strong scissors, cut a sector of sclera and reflect it posteriorly. Observe the following (fig. A-14):

1. A white circular band, about 4 mm in width. This is the outer surface of the **ciliary body.** The ciliary body contains the ciliary muscle and the ciliary processes.

2. Numerous white streaks. These are the **ciliary nerves.** They run toward the ciliary body and iris. Understand the function of these nerves (*Atlas, 653*).

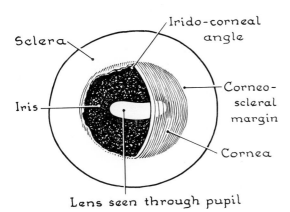

Fig. A-13. Bull's eye, dissection from the front, I.